MOLECULAR VOLUMES IN CHEMISTRY AND BIOLOGY:
Applications including Partitioning and Toxicity

MOLECULAR VOLUMES IN CHEMISTRY AND BIOLOGY: Applications including Partitioning and Toxicity

JOHN C. McGOWAN, M.A., D.I.C., Ph.D., D.Sc.
formerly Research Chemist
Imperial Chemical Industries plc, Welwyn Garden City

and

ALAN MELLORS, B.Sc., Ph.D.
Professor, Guelph-Waterloo Centre for Graduate Work in Chemistry
Department of Chemistry and Biochemistry
University of Guelph, Canada

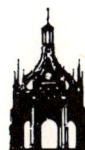

ELLIS HORWOOD LIMITED
Publishers · Chichester

Halsted Press: a division of
JOHN WILEY & SONS
New York · Chichester · Brisbane · Toronto

First published in 1986 by
ELLIS HORWOOD LIMITED
Market Cross House, Cooper Street,
Chichester, West Sussex, PO19 1EB, England
The publisher's colophon is reproduced from James Gillison's drawing of the ancient Market Cross, Chichester.

Distributors:

Australia and New Zealand:
JACARANDA WILEY LIMITED
GPO Box 859, Brisbane, Queensland 4001, Australia

Canada:
JOHN WILEY & SONS CANADA LIMITED
22 Worcester Road, Rexdale, Ontario, Canada

Europe and Africa:
JOHN WILEY & SONS LIMITED
Baffins Lane, Chichester, West Sussex, England

North and South America and the rest of the world:
Halsted Press: a division of
JOHN WILEY & SONS
605 Third Avenue, New York, NY 10158, USA

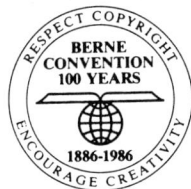

© 1986 J. McGowan and A. Mellors/Ellis Horwood Limited

British Library Cataloguing in Publication Data
McGowan, John, *1914–*
Molecular Volumes in Chemistry and Biology:
applications including partitioning and toxicity. —
(Ellis Horwood series in inorganic chemistry)
1. Biological chemistry   2. Molecules — Toxicology
I. Title   II. Mellors, Alan
574.19′283   QP514.2

Library of Congress Card No. 86–10520

ISBN 0–7458–0081–5 (Ellis Horwood Limited)
ISBN 0–470–20353–6 (Halsted Press)

Printed in Great Britain by Butler & Tanner, Frome, Somerset.

Table of Contents

Authors' Preface   9

List of Symbols   13

1   Introduction   17

2   Molecular Volumes (Systems of One Component)
    (a)   Compressibility and Pressure   24
    (b)   Properties of Liquids and Characteristic Volumes   25
    (c)   Factors for Calculation of Characteristic Volumes   27
    (d)   Examples of Determination of Characteristic Volumes
        from Properties   29
    (e)   Volumes and Chemical Reactivities of Strained Molecules   30
    (f)   van der Waals Volumes   34

3   Molecular Volumes in Mixtures
    (a)   Partial Molar Volumes of Non-electrolytes   36
    (b)   Partial Molar Volumes of Electrolytes   40
    (c)   Characteristic Volumes of Compounds Including Salts
        in Solution   42

4   Solutions of Unassociated Compounds in Unassociated
    Solvents without Interaction
    (a)   Regular Solutions   53
    (b)   Solubilities, Free Volumes and Isothermal Compressibilities   55
    (c)   Volume Changes when Unassociated Liquids are Mixed   58
    (d)   Molecular Volumes and Solubilities of Unassociated
          Compounds   62
    (e)   The Distribution Law   68
    (f)   Concentration Units   70
    (g)   Solubilities of Gases, Vapours and Solids   73
    (h)   Estimation of Characteristic Temperature and Solubilities
          by Computer   79
    (i)   Characteristic Volumes and Mutual Solubilities of
          Unassociated Liquids   82

5   Specific Interactions and Associated Liquids
    (a)   The Process of Solution   85
    (b)   Interactions between Solvent and Solutes   88
    (c)   Solvents other than Water   95
    (d)   Corrections for Differences in Compressibility   100
    (e)   Mixed Solvents and Chromatography   101
    (f)   Solubilities in Solutions of Salts   104
    (g)   Solubilities of Salts   108
    (h)   Salts and Unassociated Liquids   113

6   Physical Toxicity
    (a)   Physical Toxicity and Living Cells   120
    (b)   Physical Toxicity and Enzymes   123
    (c)   Estimation of Physical Toxicities   123
    (d)   Physical Toxicity in Systems Containing Aqueous and
          Non-aqueous Phases   129
    (e)   Physical Toxicities with Salt Solutions   134
    (f)   Further Aspects of Physical Toxicity   138
    (g)   Hydration and Sweetness of Certain Carbohydrate
          Derivatives   138
    (h)   Properties of the Biophase   141
    (i)   The 'Cut-off'   143
    (j)   1-Octanol/Water Partitions   145
    (k)   Variations in Properties of the Biophase   149

7   The Site of Action of Physically Toxic Substances
    (a)   Are Proteins the Targets of Anaesthetics?   151
    (b)   Inhibition of Enzymes by Physically Toxic Substances   152

   (c)   Other Proteins as targets of anaesthetics and Physcially
        Toxic Substances   162
   (d)   Partitioning of Proteins   163

8   Physical Toxicities of Vapours
   (a)   Toxicities of Vapours   168
   (b)   Physical Toxicities of Vapours and Boiling Points   171
   (c)   Physical Toxicity and Human Exposure   172
   (d)   Physical Toxicity and Industrial Hygiene   173

9   Chemical and Physical Toxicity
   (a)   Chemical Reactivity and Toxicity   178
   (b)   Actions of Physically Toxic Compounds   182
   (c)   Specific Interactions and Chemical Toxicity   184
   (d)   Conclusion   185

**Appendix I.   Instructions and examples for computer programs
                dealing with molecular volumes in chemistry and
                biology**   187

**Appendix II.   Computer programs, written in BASIC, for the
                estimation of characteristic temperature, density,
                isothermal compressibility, surface tension, viscosity
                and solubility of liquids, and for the estimation of
                concentrations required for physical toxicity**   198

Appendix III.   Data for estimation of solubilities   212

References   219

Formula index   239
Subject index   249
Author index   252

Authors' Preface

The importance of molecular volumes has not been appreciated in recent years. There are only two well-known books on molecular volumes and they were both published over 50 years ago. The book by W. Blitz, *Raumchemie der festen Stoffe* (Leopold Voss, Leipzig, 1934) deals with molecular volumes at the absolute zero. These molecular volumes, 'characteristic volumes', were obtained by extrapolation from values at the boiling point of nitrogen and at other low temperatures. They can be calculated from atomic and structural factors. As the temperature is raised above the absolute zero, substances expand so that the molecular volumes at, say room temperature, are not proportional to the characteristic volumes. However, molecular volumes measured at what are known as 'corresponding states' are proportional to characteristic volumes. At their critical points, compounds are in corresponding states and critical volumes are about 3.8 times the characteristic volumes. Compounds at their boiling points are approximately in corresponding states. Kopp and his coworkers measured many molecular volumes, at boiling points, and showed that these were made up of atomic and structural factors.

As well as molecular volumes, other properties of compounds vary with temperature and combinations of properties can be independent of temperature and proportional to characteristic volumes. S. Sugden used a function of molecular volume and surface tension which did not vary with temperature and called this the 'parachor'. In his book, *The Parachor and Valency* (Routledge, London, 1929), Sugden gave a list of factors which could be used to calculate parachors. Other lists of such factors have been suggested since then and perhaps the best known of these is the set given by O.R. Quayle (*Chemical Reviews* 1953, **53**, 439–589). The factors in these sets do not clearly follow the order of the sizes of atoms. This deficiency is corrected here, and in this book the characteristic volumes are related to the known sizes of atoms. Other properties besides surface tension can be used to obtain characteristic volumes at temperatures above the absolute zero. The isothermal compressibility, for example, may be used and because it is a property of the bulk of the liquid, it is to be preferred to the surface tension.

The characteristic volume can be found (except for compounds with molecules having strained structures) by the addition of atomic factors and the subtraction of the same factor for each covalent bond regardless of whether this is a single, double or triple bond. Characteristic volumes can be used to estimate properties of unassociated liquids and this of value to chemists, physicists and engineers, especially those in industry. Some properties, or combination of properties of unassociated liquids and this is of value to chemists, physicists and constant for all the liquids, are functions of the characteristic volumes. When the property varies with temperature, a characteristic temperature is required for the estimation of properties of a compound, and can be found from a single experimental value of a property, such as the density, of the liquid. In this book, discussion is confined to relationships between molecular volumes and properties. The wider aspects of molecular and macroscopic approaches to the study of liquids are given in another book in this series: viz. *Liquids and their Properties* by H.N.T. Temperley and D.H. Trevena (Ellis Horwood, Chichester, 1978).

Molecular volumes are very important for the study of the distribution of a compound between liquid phases. Solubilities have been related to the work required to bring the isothermal compressibilities of the components to that of the solution. For a dilute solution (the compressibility of the solution is taken as equal to that of the solvent)

$$RT \log_e y = P_x V_x X$$

where

R is the gas constant

T is the temperature

y is the volume fraction of the solute

P_x is a constant with the units of a pressure

V_x is the characteristic volume of the solute

X is a function of V/V_x and V'/V_x' where

V $= M/(\rho_L - \rho_g)$ with M the mass per mol of solute and ρ_L and ρ_g the densities of the liquid and of the vapour in equilibrium with it respectively

V' and V_x' are the values for the solvent corresponding to V and V_x for the solute. It is suggested that solubilities might be more satisfactorily correlated with values of V_x/V than with cohesive energy densities.

The partitioning of compounds between unassociated and associated liquids is largely determined by two factors. The first of these is the breaking up of the association, which is proportional to V_x for the compound being partitioned. The second is interactions between molecules of the compounds involved. It has been found that the partition coefficient (C_S/C_W) between water and an organic liquid phase is given approximately by $-\log(C_S/C_W) = kV_x - E$. Here C_S and C_W are the concentrations (mol per unit volume of solution) of the compound in the organic and aqueous phases respectively. The term E, which may be zero, takes into account the interactions and k is a constant at a given temperature. The equation with appropriate changes with k and E can be used for partitioning into associated liquids other than water, such as ethanol, methanol and solutions containing salts if appropriate values are taken for k and E. Further, in the partitioning, one phase can be the pure organic liquid and so the equation can be used to estimate solubilities in associated liquids. When the partitioning is between two phases which both contain more than negligible amounts of water (for methanol or ethanol), the E term depends on the ratio of the total hydroxyl concentrations in the two phases and equals $n \log \Sigma[\text{ROH}]_1/\Sigma[\text{ROH}]_2$. For the partitioning of compounds containing a single interacting group (alcohol, ester, ether or ketone) n is 1, but for electrolytes n is higher (usually at least 6). It is possible to relate the solubilities of electrolytes in mixtures of water, methanol and ethanol.

Biological activities of many compounds depend upon their partitioning into some non-aqueous biophase. The equation given above for partitioning can be used to estimate the toxic concentrations (C_t) of these compounds in water required to give a certain biological effect (e.g. narcosis, death, c-mitosis) which corresponds to a concentration (C_B) in the biophase. The equation

$$-\log_{10}(C_B/C_t) = kV_x - E$$

with similar values for k and E can also be applied to the inhibition of a number of enzymes by 'physically toxic' compounds. The values which have to be taken for the interaction terms E are low and this suggests that the biophase contains much water. Large molecules are insufficiently soluble in the biophase to give biological activity. The existence of this 'cut-off' suggests that the biophase is an associated (liquid) phase. The biophase may be a protein and it is possible that physically toxic compounds convert a phase containing protein and much water into one containing much protein and comparatively little water. Effects arising from what is called 'hydrophobicity' are those attributable to characteristic volume. In higher organisms, such as mammals, which contain appreciable amounts of fat or other non-aqueous phase, most of the physically toxic compounds which have low solubility in water may be in the non-aqueous phase. The partitioning will then in effect be between this phase and the biophase, and the toxic doses given to the system will be almost constant for a given biological effect. Features which distinguish chemically toxic compounds from physically toxic compounds and the estimation of the toxic concentrations of vapours are discussed.

The study of molecular volumes has many practical applications. A value may be suggested for a liquid property which is either unknown or not known under the required conditions. Estimates of solubilities and partition coefficients may be required for separations such as those involving chromatography and purifications, for example in the isolation of products from reactions involving enzymes. Of course, it is often important to know the toxic concentrations of solutions and vapours. Molecular volume is an important consideration in the design of anaesthetics and in human toxicology including solvent abuse ('glue-sniffing') and the setting of safe limits for human exposure to chemical vapours. It may be an advantage to know whether biological activity is of the physical class and useful to choose compounds to maximise or minimise this activity.

In Appendix II, microcomputer programs are given for estimation of properties of unassociated liquids, for solubilities in these liquids and for the correlation and estimation of biological activities. These programs were written for the Amstrad CP464 microcomputer and printed on an Epson RX-80F/T printer. The programs are straightforward and it should be easy to adapt them for other computer systems.

We should like to thank Edward G. Janzen, Chairman of the Department of Chemistry and Biochemistry, University of Guelph and the Faculty of the Guelph-Waterloo Centre for Graduate Work in Chemistry for their assistance and encouragement in the preparation of this book. We are grateful to Dr John Burgess, Department of Chemistry, University of Leicester, for his helpful suggestions; to Mrs Florence Rayner for expert typing; to Mr Ellis Horwood and his staff for their help in publishing this work; and to the Natural Science and Engineering Research Council of Canada for financial support.

John C. McGowan
Alan Mellors

List of Symbols

a	van der Waals constant
a'	Fraction of dissociated molecules
$\underline{a}$	Constant in Collander equation
A	Area of surface
A_L	Cross-sectional area of solvent phase (in chromatography)
A_s	Cross-sectional area of aqueous phase (in chromatography)
AH_{50}	Concentration required to reduce osmotic haemolysis by 50%
b	van der Waals constant
$\underline{b}$	Constant in Collander equation
B	Ratio V/V_X
C	Concentration
C_B	Concentration in biophase for a given biological effect
C_i	Ideal solubility expressed as concentration
C_j	Concentration of ion j
C_L	Concentration of liquid in its own liquid phase
C_P	Specific heat at constant pressure
C_s	Concentration of solute in solution
C_{SB}	Solubility of compound in biophase
C_t	Concentration in water to give a certain biological effect
C_t'	Dose (mol kg^{-1}) of drug required by system (e.g. animal)
C_w	Concentration in aqueous phase in two-phase system
C^* and C'	Constants in equations of the Tait type

dn/dt	Diffusion rate
D	Symbol for density $(\rho_l - \rho_g)$ used in computer program
E	Symbol for viscosity (η) used in computer program
E	Interaction term
E_c	Internal energy
E_{QX}	Extraction constant
E_s	Shorter's steric factors
E_s^c	Taft's steric factors
f	Factor for estimation of physical toxicity
g	Ratio mol solvent to mol solute
I	Ionality or ional concentration of a salt in solution

$$\left(= \sum_j c_j z_j \right)$$

I_A	Ionisation potential of the molecule A
J	Partition coefficient
k	Constant (mol per unit volume) in partition equation
k_2	Dimerisation constant
$k_{1+}, k_{2+}, k_{1-}, k_{2-}$	Rate constants for reactions catalysed by enzymes
k_B	Partition constant involving the biophase
k_{Bc}	Constant for interaction with the biophase
k_E	Constant for Masson plots
k_f'	Forward permeability constant
k_H, k_H', k_H''	Constants in Hansch equation
k_M	Solvent association constant
k_0	Equilibrium constant for complex involving a salt
k_R	Rothmund constant
k_R'	Modified Rothmund constant
$\underline{k}_s$	Setschenow constant
k_Z	Constant for solvation equilibrium
K_i	Concentration equired to produce half-maximal inhibition
K_m	Michaelis–Menten constant
K_p	Association constant
L	Ostwald coefficient – the ratio of volume of gas absorbed to volume of absorbing liquid
L^* and L'	Constants in equations of the Tait type
M	Mass of one mol
M_0	Mass of one mol of solvent
M_s	Mass of one mol of solute
n	Number of molecules of solvent interacting with each molecule of solute in process of solution
n'	Number of solvent molecules coordinately bound to each molecule of salt
N	Number of ions in a salt molecule
p	Vapour pressure

p_s	Vapour pressure of gas over a solution
p_t	Toxic vapour pressure
P	Pressure
P_e	Effective pressure exerted by a salt in solution
P_x	Characteristic pressure ($= 4.455 \times 10^9$ N m^{-2})
r	Correlation coefficient for linear regression
r_A	Molecular radius
R	Gas constant ($= 8.314$ J mol^{-1} K^{-1})
R_F	Retardation factor (in chromatography)
R_m	$\log_{10}(1/R_F - 1)$
S_m	Solubility in salt solution
S_0	Solubility in water
S_p	Solubility under pressure
T	Temperature
T_B	Boiling point
T_c	Critical temperature
T_m	Melting point
T_x	Characteristic temperature
v	Rate of a reaction catalysed by an enzyme in the presence of an inhibitor
v_0	Rate of uninhibited reaction catalysed by an enzyme
V	Molecular volume ($= M/(\rho_l - \rho_g)$) of liquid (or M/ρ_g of a gas)
V_0	Molecular volume V at low pressure
V_g	Molecular volume of vapour
V_{max}	Maximum velocity for a reaction catalysed by an enzyme
V_p	Parachor
V_p^A	Parachor of species A
V_p^M	Parachor of mixture
$\bar{V}_s$	Partial molar volume
$\bar{V}_s^{\circ}$	Partial molar volume at infinite dilution
V_w	van der Waals volume
V_x	Characteristic volume
x	Mol fraction
x_f	Weight of non-aqueous phase
x_w	Weight of aqueous phase
y	Volume fraction
z	Numerical value of charge on ion regardless of sign
α	Coefficient of thermal expansion
α'	Ionisation potential
γ	Surface tension
γ_0	Surface tension of solvent
γ_s	Surface tension of solution
γ_x	Characteristic surface tension ($= 6.46 \times 10^{-2}$ N m^{-1})
δ	Solubility parameter
ΔC_p	Difference between C_p for liquid and solid

ΔE_c	Internal energy change
ΔH	Molar heat of evaporation, i.e. latent heat
ΔH_f	Molar heat of fusion
ΔH^v	Molar internal latent heat $= \Delta H - RT$
ΔS	Entropy change
η	Viscosity
η_x	Characteristic viscosity $((\log_{10}\eta_x(\text{in N s m}^{-2}) = -3.88)$.
θ_L	Temperature-reducing parameter
κ	Isothermal compressibility at low pressure
κ_0	Isothermal compressibility of solvent
κ_p	Isothermal compressibility under pressure
κ_s	Isothermal compressibility of solution
π	Logarithm of ratio of the partition coefficient of a substituted x^s and unsubstituted compound x^H between 1-octanol and water at 300 K
ρ	Rate constant in Hammett equation
ρ_f	Density of non-aqueous phase
ρ_g	Density of saturated vapour
ρ_l	Density of liquid or pure solvent
ρ_s	Density of solution or whole system
ρ_w	Density of aqueous phase
σ	Substituent constant in Hammett equation
Σ	Sum of

1

Introduction

It has often been found, in the past, that the toxicities of many compounds depended upon the physical rather than the chemical properties. Toxicities have been related to boiling points [1–5], vapour pressures [6], solubilities in water [7–10], partition coefficients between water and an organic liquid [11–17] and chemical potential [18–22]. These various properties are all related and it has been found [23] that properties of an unassociated liquid depend upon two constants — a characteristic volume V_x and a characteristic temperature T_x. Compounds chosen for biological tests often have values of T_x which are close to each other so that the concentrations of the compounds for a definite biological effect will depend mainly on their characteristic volumes. This means that these concentrations can be related to properties of the compounds which are functions of V_x. It has been suggested [21, 24] that these relationships arise because the toxic symptoms can be caused by any compound regardless of its composition, if it obtains a definite molar concentration in a certain biophase within the living organism. This biophase appears to be very similar for all organisms [24]. It is possible that the toxic symptoms arise when compounds attain a certain volume fraction in this biophase [25, 26].

Narcotics are often physically toxic. Ferguson [27] has pointed out that: 'Narcotics act as whole molecules. The actual process of narcosis does not involve as a first step any chemical reaction, any breaking of covalent bonds. Many narcotics leave the body unchanged. No traces of break-down products are detected.'

One relationship is that between toxic concentration and solubility in water. According to Bradbury, McCarthy and Suckling [8], Snow [9] in 1858 concluded from observations of anaesthesia produced by several compounds: 'We find that the quantity of each substance in the blood in corresponding degrees of narcotism, bears a certain proportion to what the blood would dissolve – a proportion that is almost exactly the same for all of them'. Richet [7] suggested that the concentrations of compounds required to show a given biological effect were inversely proportional to the solubilities of the compound in water. Führner [10] measured the concentrations, of 40 compounds, required to have the same effect on the heart of frogs as 7% (v/v) ethanol. He found that the ratio of the toxic concentration (in aqueous solution) to the concentration of the saturated solution was not constant but fell within narrow limits and for 29 of the compounds he listed, this ratio lay between 0.3 and 0.5. He noted that the concentrations he required to give the effect on the frogs' hearts were on average 5.4 times those which Overton [11] found were necessary for the narcosis of tadpoles. In Table 1, the results reported by Führner are given.

Table 1. Narcotic concentrations for action on frog's heart and solubilities in water (Führner [10]).

Compound	Narcotic concentration ($mol\ m^{-3}$)	Solubility	Ratio
1-Butanol	109	919	0.12
1-Propanol, 2-methyl-	135	1351	0.10
1-Butanol, 3-methyl-	39	230	0.17
2-Butanol, 2-methyl-	184	1420	0.13
1-Heptanol	3	8	0.38
1,3,5-Trioxane, 2,4,6-trimethyl- (paraldehyde)	150	909	0.17
Ethane, 1,1'-oxybis- (ether)	292	875	0.17
Acetic acid, ethyl ester	130	732	0.18
Acetic acid, 1-propyl ester	35	203	0.17
Acetic acid, 2-propyl ester	62	267	0.23
Acetic acid, 2-methyl-1-propyl ester	15	46	0.33
2,4, (1H,3H,5H)-Pyrimidinetrione, 5,5-diethyl (veronal)	27	27	1.00
Benzene	11	18	0.61
2-Propanol, 1,1,1-trichloro-2-methyl- (chloreton)	9	28	0.32
1,1-Ethanediol, 2,2,2-trichloro- (chloral hydrate)	30	4040	0.01

Table 1 (cont'd)

Compound	Narcotic concentration (mol m^{-3})	Solubility	Ratio
Methane, dichloro-	16	209	0.08
Methane, trichloro- (chloroform)	7	63	0.11
Methane, tetrachloro- (carbon tetrachloride)	3	4	0.75
Methane, dibromo-	14	65	0.22
Methane, tribromo-	1	5	0.20
Methane, iodo-	64	100	0.64
Ethane, chloro-	46	88	0.52
Ethane, 1,2-dichloro-	31	75	0.41
Ethane, 1,1-dichloro-	10	60	0.17
Ethane, 1,1,2,2-tetrachloro-	2	11	0.18
Ethane, bromo-	33	93	0.35
Ethane, iodo-	12	25	0.48
Propane, 1-chloro-	17	51	0.33
Propane, 1-bromo-	8	22	0.36
Propane, 2-bromo-	10	26	0.38
Propane, 1-iodo-	5	5	1.00

More recently, an example of the relationship between solubility and toxicity for quite a different kind of biological activity was given by Hutchinson, Hellebust, Tam, Mackay, Mascarenhas and Shiu [28]. They measured the concentrations of hydrocarbons and halogenated hydrocarbons (38 compounds in all) required to reduce the photosynthesis of two algae, *Chlamydomonas angulosa* and *Chlorella vulgaris*, by 50%. They compared the toxic concentrations (C_t) with the solubilities in water (C_s), some of which they measured [29] and others they took from the literature. The results are given in Table 2 and lead to the relationship for *C. angulosa*

$$\log_{10} C_t = 0.826 \log_{10} C_s - 0.101$$

and for *C. vulgaris*

$$\log_{10} C_t = 0.804 \log_{10} C_s - 0.069$$

These experiments will be discussed further in Chapter 6 (section (i)) in connection with what is known as the 'cut-off' of physical toxicity; the significance of the characteristic volume V_x will then be clarified.

Table 2. Concentrations (C_t) required to halve the photosynthetic activities of algae [28].

Compound	$V_x(\text{m}^3\ \text{mol}^{-1}) \times 10^5$	Solubility $C_s(\text{mol m}^{-3})$	*Chlamydomonas angulosa*		*Chlorella vulgaris*	
			$C_t(\text{mol m}^{-3})$	C_t/C_s	$C_t(\text{mol m}^{-3})$	C_t/C_s
Dichloromethane	4.944	228.5	17.40	0.076	27.00	0.012
Trichloromethane	6.168	66.6	3.20	0.048	3.40	0.051
Cyclopentane	7.046	2.22	1.72	0.77	1.66	0.75
Benzene	7.164	22.79	5.90	0.26	4.00	0.18
l,1,1-Trichloroethane	7.577	5.39	2.10	0.39	1.15	0.21
Chlorobenzene	8.388	4.19	0.50	0.12	0.88	0.21
Cyclohexane	8.455	0.65	0.46	0.70	0.38	0.58
Methylcyclopentane	8.455	0.50	0.46	0.91	0.32	0.63
Toluene	8.573	5.59	1.45	0.26	2.25	0.40
1,2,3-Trichloropropane	8.986	12.88	0.76	0.059	1.15	0.089
Hexane	9.541	0.11	9.4×10^{-2}	0.85	>Sat	–
3-Methylpentane	9.541	0.15	>Sat	–	0.145	0.99
Methylcyclohexane	9.864	0.14	0.107	0.75	0.107	0.75
Ethylbenzene	9.982	1.43	0.48	0.34	0.59	0.41
1,4-Dimethylbenzene	9.982	1.74	0.43	0.25	0.99	0.57
1,1,2,2,2-Pentachloroethane	10.025	2.37	0.12	0.05	0.15	0.06
1,2,3-Trichlorobenzene (s)	10.834	9.1×10^{-2}	1.9×10^{-2}	0.21	3.4×10^{-2}	0.37
Naphthalene (s)	10.854	2.47×10^{-1}	7.5×10^{-2}	0.30	0.15	0.61
Cyclo-octane	11.272	7.0×10^{-2}	2.65×10^{-2}	0.38	2.4×10^{-2}	0.35
1-Ethyl-4-methylbenzene	11.392	0.78	0.45	0.58	0.40	0.51

Table 2 (continued)

Compound	V_x(m³ mol⁻¹) × 10⁵	Solubility C_s(mol m⁻³)	Chlamydomonas angulosa		Chlorella vulgaris	
			C_t(mol m⁻³)	C_t/C_s	C_t(mol m⁻³)	C_t/C_s
1-Ethyl-2-methylbenzene	11.392	0.77	0.16	0.20	0.34	0.44
Propylbenzene	11.392	0.46	0.15	0.33	0.14	0.29
(2-Propyl) benzene	11.392	0.42	7.3 × 10⁻²	0.17	0.18	0.42
1,2,3,5-Tetrachlorobenzene (s)	12.060	1.65 × 10⁻²	7.3 × 10⁻³	0.44	1.16 × 10⁻²	0.70
1-Methylnaphthalene	12.263	0.20	1.2 × 10⁻²	0.06	3.6 × 10⁻²	0.18
2-Methylnaphthalene (s)	12.263	0.18	3.15 × 10⁻²	0.18	6.3 × 10⁻²	0.35
Octane	12.360	5.7 × 10⁻³	>Sat	—	>Sat	—
Butylbenzene	12.801	9.4 × 10⁻²	2.6 × 10⁻²	0.28	2.3 × 10⁻²	0.24
2-Methylpropylbenzene	12.801	7.5 × 10⁻²	2.3 × 10⁻²	0.31	2.6 × 10⁻²	0.35
1,2,4,5-Tetramethylbenzene (s)	12.801	7.2 × 10⁻²	>Sat	—	>Sat	—
Decalin	13.005	4.48 × 10⁻²	1.4 × 10⁻²	0.32	7.3 × 10⁻³	0.16
Biphenyl (s)	13.242	4.5 × 10⁻²	8.3 × 10⁻³	0.18	2.5 × 10⁻²	0.56
Phenanthrene (3)	14.543	7.2 × 10⁻³	5.3 × 10⁻³	0.74	6.8 × 10⁻³	0.94
Anthracene (s)	14.543	2.3 × 10⁻⁴	>Sat	—	>Sat	—
Decane	15.178	3.65 × 10⁻⁴	>Sat	—	>Sat	—
Pyrene (s)	15.846	6.7 × 10⁻⁴	>Sat	—	>Sat	—
Dodecane	17.996	2.22 × 10⁻⁵	>Sat	—	>Sat	—
Tetradecane	20.354	1.15 × 10⁻⁵	>Sat	—	>Sat	—

(s) Indicates the compound is a solid.

Ferguson [21, 22, 30–32] showed that, although the concentration of many compounds required to give a biological effect might vary widely, the ratio of the toxic concentration in some phase (usually aqueous solution or vapour) to the concentration required to saturate that phase fell in narrow limits. The biological activity thus appears in many cases to depend on partitioning and for this reason (and others besides), it is important to discover the factors upon which partitioning depends.

Smith [33] studied the partitioning of a number of organic acids and bases between water and xylene and between water and chloroform. He concluded that in any series of compounds having the same 'intrinsic intensity of secondary valence', there was a linear relationship between the logarithm of the partition coefficient between water and a given organic liquid and the molecular volume of the compound. By secondary valence Smith meant the force that binds molecules together or, in other words, the cohesion. Smith [34] extended his studies to partitions between ether and water and later [35] to partitions between the two phases formed when glycerol and acetone are mixed. He found [36] support for his views from these studies and results taken from the literature. Some of Smith's results are given in Table 3.

A method was devised [26, 37, 38] for the estimation of partition coefficients of compounds between a phase consisting of an unassociated liquid and water in the absence of specific interactions. It was assumed that, as a first approximation, the unassociated liquids could all be taken as having the same solvent properties. Further, water is an associated liquid and the assumption was made that the free energy required to transfer a compound from the unassociated liquid to water was proportional to the extent of breakdown of the association in water, i.e. to the molecular volume of the compound. In the simplest cases

$$\log_{10} \frac{[\text{concentration in organic phase}]}{[\text{concentration in water}]} = kV_x \tag{1}$$

Relationship (1) resembles that proposed by Smith, but here k is a constant and V_x is the characteristic molecular volume and not the molecular volume, at the temperature of the experiment, of the compound being partitioned. Applications and extensions of this treatment will be discussed. In the next two chapters, different measures of molecular volumes will be described and relationships between them discussed. A description will then be given of the use of work of compressibility to account for the differences, often relatively small, between unassociated organic compounds as solvents. The treatment proposed is compared with that based on the idea of regular solutions. In the next chapter the simple equation given above is extended to compounds giving specific interactions with solvent. Estimates are made for partition coefficients and solubilities including those of salts in certain systems. The final chapters are devoted to the actions of aqueous solutions and vapours of physically toxic compounds on living cells and the nature of the biophase, and include some relevant studies on the inhibitions of enzymes.

Table 3. Molecular volumes of amines and their partition coefficients between water and organic solvents

Amine	Molecular volume (m^3 mol^{-1})	Partition coefficients between water and			Ratio of the coefficients for chloroform and xylene
		Xylene [33]	Chloroform [33]	Ether [34]	
Ethanamine (ethylamine)	6.46×10^{-5}	0.077	0.396	0.172	5.15
Methanamine, N-methyl- (dimethylamine)	6.63×10^{-5}	0.12	0.588	0.231	4.90
Methanamine, N,N-dimethyl- (trimethylamine)	8.80×10^{-5}	0.47	2.38	0.660	5.06
Piperidine	1.088×10^{-4}	0.44	2.15	0.655	4.90
Ethanamine, N-ethyl-	1.093×10^{-4}	0.44	2.2	0.652	5.00
Pentanamine	1.275×10^{-4}	1.46	7.3	–	5.00
Ethanamine, N,N-diethyl-	1.526×10^{-4}	3.17	16.0	–	5.07

2

Molecular Volumes (Systems of One Component)

(a) COMPRESSIBILITY AND PRESSURE

The molecular volume of a compound is the volume occupied by one mole so that it equals the mass of one mole (often called the molecular weight) divided by the density. For a perfect gas, the molecular volume V is given by the gas law (2)

$$PV = RT \tag{2}$$

where P is the pressure, T is the temperature and R is the gas constant equal to $8.314 \, J \, mol^{-1} \, K^{-1}$. From this equation, the isothermal compressibility

$$\kappa = -\frac{1}{V}\left(\frac{\delta V}{\delta P}\right)_T = \frac{1}{P}$$

and equation (2) can be written as (3)

$$V = RT\kappa \tag{3}$$

Equations (2) and (3) have to be modified for imperfect gases. The van der Waals equation and modifications of it are often used for these gases. Attempts have been made [39–41] to treat liquids in the same way but in the authors' opinion these attempts have not been very successful. Whilst the isothermal compressibilities of permanent gases at room temperature and atmospheric pressure are around $10^{-5} \, N \, m^{-2}$, those of unassociated liquids [42], such as benzene and carbon tetrachloride, are about $10^{-9} \, N \, m^{-2}$. The very strong forces between molecules in liquids that resist compression and expansion can be considered as giving rise to 'internal pressures' and are responsible for the surface tensions.

(b) PROPERTIES OF LIQUIDS AND CHARACTERISTIC VOLUMES

It has been found [23] that many properties of unassociated liquids can be estimated with the aid of two constants characteristic of each liquid. One constant is the characteristic volume V_X mentioned above and the other is a characteristic temperature T_X. Since the effect of external pressure on properties of liquids is only appreciable at high pressures and the results to be considered here are measured at low pressures (around atmospheric), the effect of pressure has been neglected. Equations allowing for the effects of pressure have been given [23]. The equations (4), (5) and (6) have been used for the estimation of the density ρ_l, isothermal compressibility κ and surface tension γ respectively at temperature T.

$$V_X(\rho_l - \rho_g)/M = (1 - T/T_X)^{0.3} \tag{4}$$

$$\frac{1}{\kappa} = P_X(1 - T/T_X)^{1.8} \tag{5}$$

$$\gamma = \gamma_X(1 - T/T_X)^{1.2} \tag{6}$$

The constants $P_X = 4.455 \times 10^9$ N m^{-2} and $\gamma_X = 6.46 \times 10^{-2}$ N m^{-1} seem to be the same for all unassociated liquids. The surface tension for water at 298.2 K is 7.197×10^{-2} N m^{-1} and for this associated liquid equation (6) cannot be used. The high value for γ indicates that there are special forces of attraction acting between the molecules besides those normally present in unassociated liquids. Equation (4) refers not to the molecular volume M/ρ_l but to the mass of one mole (M) divided by the difference between the density of the liquid ρ_l and that of the vapour in equilibrium with it ρ_g. The density of the vapour can often be neglected. At the absolute zero ($T = 0$) the molecules will be at rest, ρ_g will be zero and $V_X = M/\rho$. This provides a method for the determination of V_X. Biltz and co-workers [43, 44] measured densities at the boiling point of nitrogen and at other low temperatures and extrapolated their results to the absolute zero. They give many values of V_X measured in this way and found the densities of solids and liquids (i.e. glasses) differ little at the absolute zero.

Values of V_X and T_X can be found from the variation of $\rho_l - \rho_g$ with temperature and the use of equation (4). If the term involving temperature is eliminated between equations (4) and (5), equation (7) is obtained

$$V_X = \frac{M}{(\rho_l - \rho_g) \kappa^{1/6} P_X^{1/6}} \tag{7}$$

This equation can be used to obtain V_X from densities and isothermal compressibilities [45]. The parachor V_P is given by equation (8) and is a molecular volume which is independent of temperature.

$$V_P = \frac{M_\gamma^{1/4}}{\rho_1 - \rho_g} = \gamma_x^{1/4} \, V_X \tag{8}$$

Equations (7) and (8) show that plots of log V against log κ and against log γ will give straight lines with slopes 6 and -4 respectively. Reed [46] has found that plots of log κ against log V (neglecting ρ_g) give straight lines of slope close to 6. In earlier papers [5, 26, 37, 38, 47–49] the parachor V_P was used in place of V_X, which is now favoured [23, 50]. The use of the parachor does suggest that surface tension is involved in the estimation of the solubilities. The parachor does not have the units of volume (its units are $m^{1/2}$ l^3 $t^{-1/2}$) and conversion between different units is rather complicated. The parachor is usually given in CGS units and to convert parachors in CGS units to V_X values is SI units, division by 2.835×10^6 is required. The viscosity η of an unassociated liquid with molecules which are not too large is related [23, 51] to the characteristic volume by the relationship (9)

$$V_x^6 = \frac{69 R T M^5 \log_{10}(\eta/\eta_x)}{P_x (\rho_1 - \rho_g)^5} \tag{9}$$

The symbols have already been used above with the exception of η_x and $\log_{10}(\eta_x$ in N s m^{-2}) is -3.88. The relationship (9) can be used to obtain values of V_X.

Certain volumes are approximately proportional to V_X and the following relationships have been suggested [52]:

critical volume = 3.8 V_X
molecular volume at the boiling point = 1.4 V_X
van der Waals b term = 1.9 V_X

For approximately 50 years from about 1840 onwards, Kopp [53] studied molecular volumes at the boiling points and found them to be approximately additive. About the same time, Schroeder [54, 55] showed that the molecular volume (cm^3 mol^{-1}) for saturated compounds of carbon, hydrogen, oxygen and nitrogen was equal to roughly the number of atoms multiplied by seven. One had to be added to the number of atoms for each ethylenic linkage (C$=$C) and each carbonyl (C$=$O) before the multiplication by seven. This relationship has recently been examined by Reid, Prausnitz and Sherwood [56], who found the value was surprisingly good and gave molecular volumes at the boiling point within about 3 to 4% of the observed values, except for highly associated liquids. The Schroeder method may be used to estimate values of V_X if 5×10^{-6} m^3 mol^{-1} is used as the atomic factor for each carbon, nitrogen, oxygen and hydrogen atom in saturated compounds and 5×10^{-6} m^3 mol^{-1} added to the total of these factors for every ethylenic and carbonyl double bond in the molecule of the compound.

From equations (4), (5) and (6), it will be seen that for any unassociated liquids, when the T/T_X values are equal, the isothermal compressibilities and surface tensions will be equal and $M/(\rho_1 - \rho_g)$ will be proportional to V_x; the molecular volumes can then be estimated by means of atomic and structural factors. Extensive use has been made of factors for the calculation of parachors V_p (see equation (8)) which can be described as molecular volumes compared when liquids have equal surface tensions.

(c) FACTORS FOR CALCULATION OF CHARACTERISTIC VOLUMES

Sugden, who introduced the idea of the parachor, gave one set of factors [57–59]. Exner [60] lists these together with sets of Quayle [61] and Vogel [62] and a set of his own. Another set has been given by Mumford and Phillips [63]. Any of these sets of factors may be used to calculate the parachors V_p and hence V_x (in SI units) = V_p (in CGS units) $\div$ 2.835 $\times$ 10^6. Vogel and coworkers [62] allotted parachor values to bonds. Exner [64] states that no physical meaning can be attributed to bond molecular volumes and Benson and Buss [65] point out that compared with atomic factors, the bond system represents a higher degree of approximation and needs a greater number of constants.

It would be expected that atomic parachors would be a measure of the volumes of the atoms, but the atomic factors given in the sets listed above bear little relationship to the sizes of the atoms determined by X-ray and other methods or to the electronic structures. Copley [66] suggested that the parachors of atoms with equal numbers and kinds of complete electron shells varied linearly with the atomic numbers. Thus, the change from tetravalent carbon to trivalent nitrogen would produce the same change in parachors as the change from trivalent nitrogen to divalent oxygen. This idea was extended by McGowan [52, 67], who gave a set of atomic parachors in which for a given electronic configuration around a central nucleus, an increase of one unit in the positive change on the nucleus lowers the atomic parachor by the same amount. He also found that molecular parachors can be calculated by the addition of these atomic parachors and, except in strained structures, the substraction of the same factor (6.56×10^{-6} m^3 mol^{-1}) for every bond regardless of whether it is a single, double or triple bond. The differences in the characteristic volumes for atoms with successive atomic numbers and the same electronic configuration is 1.96×10^{-6} m^3 mol^{-1} from hydrogen to potassium; 1.605×10^{-6} m^3 mol^{-1} from potassium to caesium; and about 1.25×10^{-6} m^3 mol^{-1} from caesium onwards. In Table 4, values of atomic V_x are listed. In the atomic parachors listed originally [52], values were given for all the elements in the periodic table and the parachors of compounds containing transitional metals were discussed. The parachors (and characteristic volumes) of such compounds depend upon the electronic configuration of the transition metal atom and this often does not correspond with that of an inert gas of group zero and may not even be the same in different compounds of the metal. It is not proposed to discuss this subject here.

Table 4. Atomic constants for characteristic volumes V_X (m³ mol⁻¹).

Outside shell with electrons	Period	Group I	II	III	IV	V	VI	VII	Zero group
K	I	He 8.71×10^{-6}							He 6.755×10^{-6}
L	II	Li 2.224×10^{-5}	Be 2.028×10^{-5}	B 1.832×10^{-5}	C 1.635×10^{-5}	N 1.439×10^{-5}	O 1.243×10^{-5}	F 1.047×10^{-5}	Ne 8.51×10^{-6}
K		4.80×10^{-6}	2.84×10^{-6}						
M	III	Na 3.270×10^{-5}	Mg 3.074×10^{-5}	Al 2.878×10^{-5}	Si 2.683×10^{-5}	P 2.487×10^{-5}	S 2.291×10^{-5}	Cl 2.095×10^{-5}	A 1.899×10^{-5}
L		6.55×10^{-6}	4.59×10^{-6}	2.63×10^{-6}					
N	IV	K 1.704×10^{-5}	Ca 1.543×10^{-5}		Ge 3.102×10^{-5}	As 2.942×10^{-5}	Se 2.781×10^{-5}	Br 2.621×10^{-5}	Kr 2.460×10^{-5}
M									
O	V	Rb 2.300×10^{-5}	Sr 2.139×10^{-5}		Sn 3.935×10^{-5}	Sb 3.774×10^{-5}	Te 3.614×10^{-5}	I 3.453×10^{-5}	Xe 3.293×10^{-5}
N									
P	VI	Cs 3.132×10^{-5}	B 3.007×10^{-5}		Pb 4.344×10^{-5}	Bi 4.219×10^{-5}			
O									

A bond between two atoms —6.56×10^{-6}

(d) EXAMPLES OF DETERMINATION OF CHARACTERISTIC VOLUMES FROM PROPERTIES

In Figure 1, the use of equation (4) for the determination of V_x from the variation of densities with temperature is illustrated. When $[(\rho_1 - \rho_g)/M]^{10/3}$ is plotted against temperature, the points fall near straight lines which cut the horizontal axis at T_x and have a slope of $1/(T_x \times V_x^{10/3})$. The densities of liquid and saturated vapour for carbon tetrachloride are those of Young [68].

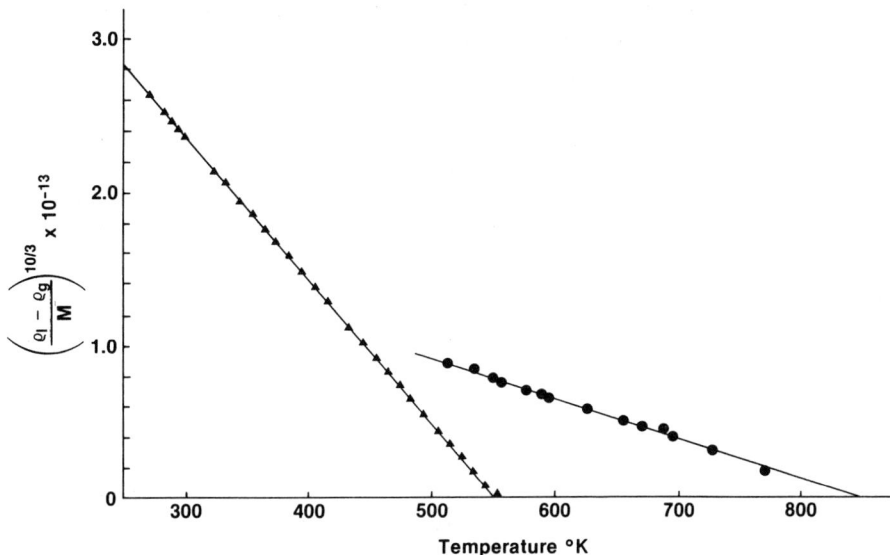

Fig. 1. Variation of $\dfrac{\rho_1 - \rho_g}{M}$ with temperature. ▲ Carbon tetrachloride [68] ● Molybdenum pentachloride [69].

From the line, V_x comes to 7.70×10^{-5} m^3 mol^{-1} and T_x to 552 K. For the other example, the densities of liquid and saturated vapour for molybdenum pentachloride given by Nisel'son and Sokolova [69] have been used and T_x equals 852 K with V_x apparently 9.94×10^{-5} m^3 mol^{-1}. Ewens and Lister [70] studied the electron diffraction of the vapour of molybdenum pentachloride and found this was monomeric. However, when the crystal structure was studied later by Sands and Zalkin [71], they found that in the solid state molybdenum pentachloride existed as a dimer Mo_2Cl_{10} with the chlorine atoms forming two octahedra which share a common edge. When V_x is obtained as above from the variation of density with temperature, it is not possible to distinguish between monomer and dimer because the relationship uses the ratio of V_x and M, which will be the same for both provided the number of bonds is the same. The relationship (9) can be written

$$V_x = \frac{69RT\log_{10}(\eta/\eta_x)}{P_x(1 - T/T_x)^{1.5}} \tag{10}$$

and this gives V_x from the viscosity and T_x independently of M. Nisel'son and Sokolova [69] measured some viscosities of liquid molybdenum pentachloride and in Table 5 their values have been used to find V_x with the value of $T_x = 852$ K found from the density plot. Although there is a drift among these figures, they clearly point to a dimeric structure for molybdenum pentachloride in the liquid state. The atomic factor (V_x) for molybdenum, calculated from Mo_2Cl_{10} (12 bonds), is $(1.988 \times 10^{-4} - 1.308 \times 10^{-4})/2 = 1.7 \times 10^{-5}$ m^3 mol^{-1}. There does seem to be a tendency for the molecules of the heavier transition elements to contain more than one atom of the transition element. It has, for example, been found [72, 73] that the $ReCl_4^-$ ion, in $CsReCl_4$, is, in fact, a trimer $Re_3Cl_{12}^{3-}$.

Table 5. Estimation of V_x from viscosities [69] of molybdenum pentachloride and $T_x (= 852$ K).

T (K)	Viscosity (N s m^{-2})	$V_x = \dfrac{69RT\log_{10}(\eta/\eta_x)}{P_x(1 - T/T_x)^{1.5}}$
483.7	8.56×10^{-4}	1.78×10^{-4} m^3 mol^{-1}
494.2	7.90×10^{-4}	1.82×10^{-4} m^3 mol^{-1}
503.7	7.32×10^{-4}	1.85×10^{-4} m^3 mol^{-1}
513.7	6.87×10^{-4}	1.90×10^{-4} m^3 mol^{-1}
525.7	6.21×10^{-4}	1.92×10^{-4} m^3 mol^{-1}
537.2	5.99×10^{-4}	2.02×10^{-4} m^3 mol^{-1}
549.2	5.64×10^{-4}	2.11×10^{-4} m^3 mol^{-1}
562.7	5.25×10^{-4}	2.19×10^{-4} m^3 mol^{-1}
584.7	4.79×10^{-4}	2.40×10^{-4} m^3 mol^{-1}

(e) VOLUMES AND CHEMICAL REACTIVITIES OF STRAINED MOLECULES

The method given above for the calculation of characteristic molecular volumes gives satisfactory results for liquids with molecules having normal valency angles and bond lengths but the agreement between observed and calculated characteristic volumes is not so good for compounds with 'strained' or 'sterically overcrowded' molecules. Such molecules can often be recognised by their chemical reactivity.

The characteristic volume of carbon tetrachloride calculated from the factors given in Table 4 is 7.39×10^{-5} m^3 mol^{-1}, which is considerably smaller than the value of 7.76×10^{-5} m^3 mol^{-1} found from densities and surface tensions (i.e. the parachor) and 7.7×10^{-5} m^3 mol^{-1} from the variation of density with temperature (Fig. 1). This suggests that four chlorine atoms are too large to fit without strain around the rather small carbon atom. The reactions of carbon tetrachloride support the view that it is a strained molecule: the carbon–chlorine bonds can be broken fairly readily in all of the three possible ways. Carbon tetrachloride, like most other carbon compounds of chlorine, reacts with active anions like methoxide and the chlorine is split off as a negative chloride ion

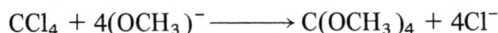

$$CCl_4 + 4(OCH_3)^- \longrightarrow C(OCH_3)_4 + 4Cl^-$$

In addition, there are reactions of carbon tetrachloride in which the carbon to chlorine bond is split homolytically. For example, carbon tetrachloride is a transfer agent in the free-radical polymerisation of ethylene under high pressure

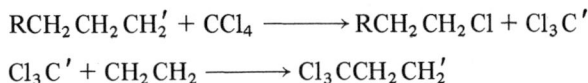

$$RCH_2CH_2CH_2' + CCl_4 \longrightarrow RCH_2CH_2Cl + Cl_3C'$$

$$Cl_3C' + CH_2CH_2 \longrightarrow Cl_3CCH_2CH_2'$$

Also, the damage caused to the liver by carbon tetrachloride is believed [74, 75] to involve trichloromethyl radicals which can be trapped and identified by reaction with α-phenyl-N-t-butylnitron [76]. Atherton and Todd [77] used the reaction of dialkyl phosphites and certain halogen compounds such as carbon tetrachloride for the phosphorylation of amines. They suggested that the reaction involved the splitting off of positive halogen

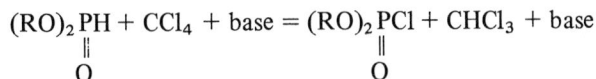

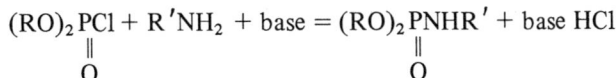

$$\underset{\underset{O}{\|}}{(RO)_2PH} + CCl_4 + base = \underset{\underset{O}{\|}}{(RO)_2PCl} + CHCl_3 + base$$

$$\underset{\underset{O}{\|}}{(RO)_2PCl} + R'NH_2 + base = \underset{\underset{O}{\|}}{(RO)_2PNHR'} + base\ HCl$$

In general, they found that the reactivity for the halogen containing compounds was decreased by the introduction of fluorine and increased by substitution with the larger atoms, bromine or iodine for chlorine. Carbon tetrabromide, tribromomethane and iodoform were active but chloroform did not give the reaction [78]. Carbon tetraiodide, which, as would be expected, gave the phosphorylation reaction, and a number of organic compounds of iodine have been found to be fungistatic. All the compounds which, at low concentrations, inhibited the germination of *Botrytis allii* spores, showed positive iodine in the phosphorylation reaction [78]. Some of Muirhead's results are given in Table 6. Here the characteristic volume would seem to be a measure of strain and hence of chemical and biological activity. Too reactive a compound may be destroyed in side reactions and so there may well be some characteristic volume which might give maximum activity. Quaternary carbon atoms are under strain. An interesting example of the breaking of a carbon—carbon bond at a quaternary carbon atom is the formation of vitamin Ds by the action of light on ergosterol and related compounds: the B ring opens and the methyl group between the A and B rings becomes a methylene.

Attempts to provide factors for the correction of strain and steric effects have been reviewed by Quayle [61]. The strain in any particular series of compounds will be unique and such factor will, at the best, be only approximately correct.

Table 6. Inhibition of germination of *Botrytis allii* spores by Halogen compounds [78].

Compound	V_X $(m^3\ mol^{-1})$	Phosphorylation reaction	Least concentration inhibiting germination of *B. allii* spores $(kg\ m^{-3})$
Cl₂C=CCl₂ (tetrachloroethylene)	8.35×10^{-5}	Negative	> 0.25
(H)(I)C=C(I)(H)	8.61×10^{-5}	Negative	> 0.25
CHI_3	10.23×10^{-5}	Positive	> 0.1
Br₂C=CBr₂	10.45×10^{-5}	Not known	> 0.1
(I)(Br)C=C(I)(Br)	12.12×10^{-5}	Positive	0.05
CI_4	12.81×10^{-5}	Positive	0.025
(I)(I)C=C(I)(Br)	12.98×10^{-5}	Not known	$0.025-0.05$
(I)(I)C=C(I)(I)	13.78×10^{-5}	Positive	0.0125

The factor required to correct the calculated value of the characteristic volume for carbon tetrachloride is $3 \times 10^{-6}\ m^3\ mol^{-1}$. This factor will not be of use for other compounds since carbon tetrachloride is the only compound with tetravalent carbon attached to four chlorines. Larger factors would be expected to be required if the chlorine atoms were replaced by bromine or iodine atoms and smaller ones if the chlorine were replaced by fluorine or hydrogen.

Attempts have been made to give measures of steric effects which depend on shape as well as on size. Shorter [79] takes the methyl group as a standard and lists E_s factors which are derived from the ratio of the rate of a reaction for this group compared with that for some other group X in an *ortho*-substituted benzene

$$\log\frac{k_{CH_3}}{k_X} = C\,E_s$$

where C is a constant for any given reaction. In Fig. 2, values of E_s are plotted against the atomic characteristic volumes of halogens (from Table 4). Here only single atoms are involved and so the shape factor will be minimised. It will be seen that the points fall close to a straight line. Shorter attributes steric effects to the intense repulsive forces which operate when two non-bonded atoms approach each other very closely.

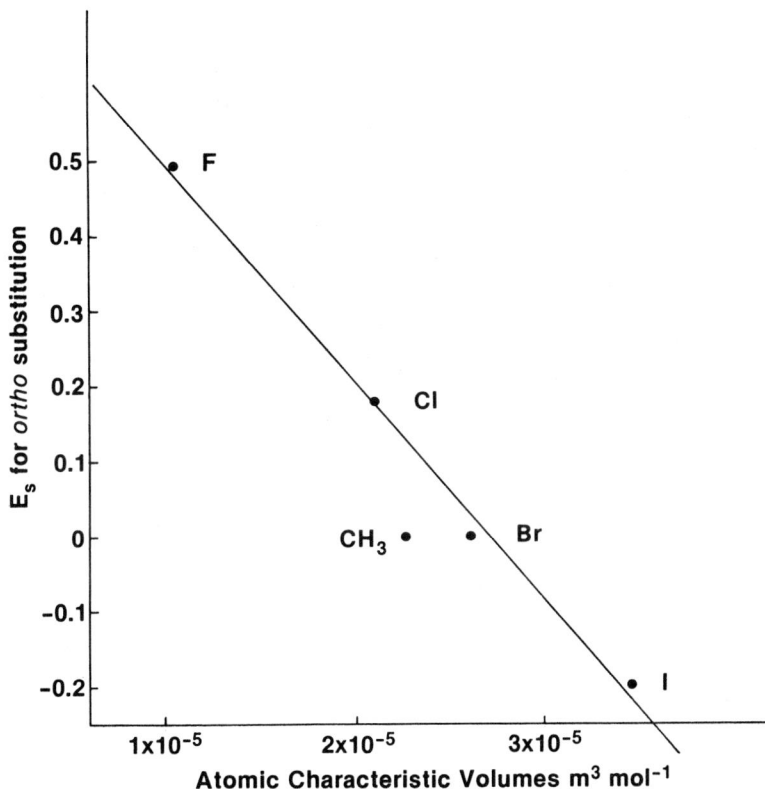

Fig. 2. Steric factors and characteristic volumes.

Taft [80] uses, as a measure of steric effects, the changes brought about by substituents upon the acid-catalysis compared with the base-catalysed hydrolysis of esters. He gives examples of reactions in which the rates are largely controlled by steric effects. Hancock, Meyers and Yeger [81] give E_s^c values, which are Taft's values corrected for hyperconjugation. In correlations for biological activity, steric factors have proved of value [16]. Hansch [82], for example, has been able to correlate the inhibition constants for a set of p-nitrophenyl phosphorus esters on cholinesterase activity of human serum with E_s^c as follows

$$\log K_i = 2.58\, E_s^c + 7.94, \quad n = 13, \quad r = 0.927$$

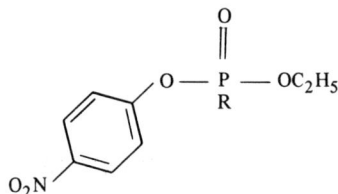

$$
\begin{array}{c}
\quad\quad\quad\quad\quad\quad O \\
\quad\quad\quad\quad\quad\quad \parallel \\
O\!-\!P\!-\!OC_2H_5 \\
\quad\quad\quad\quad\;\; R
\end{array}
$$

(p-nitrophenyl phosphorus ester structure: O_2N–C$_6$H$_4$–O–P(=O)(R)–OC$_2$H$_5$)

R = normal or branched alkyl

(f) VAN DER WAALS VOLUMES

Mention should be made here of van der Waals volumes V_w used by Bondi and Simkin [83]. These were calculated [84] from bond distances and van der Waals radii. Bondi lists a number of values of V_w and some of these are compared in Table 7 with the characteristic volumes derived from the atomic volumes given in Table 4. It has already been pointed out [85] that V_w is roughly equal to 0.7 V_x. Bondi and Simkin [83] also used a temperature-reducing parameter θ_L, which is approximately equal [85] to T_x.

The calculation of characteristic volumes based on the factors given in Table 4 has the advantage of having the minimum number of constants, namely one for each atom with its normal electronic configuration and a single value for a covalent bond. Moreover, the atomic constants given are related to the known sizes of the atoms.

Table 7. van der Waals volumes [84] and characterstic volumes.

Structure	V_W (m^3 mol^{-1})	V_X (m^3 mol^{-1})	V_W/V_X
Methane	1.71×10^{-5}	2.495×10^{-5}	0.69
Ethane	2.73×10^{-5}	3.904×10^{-5}	0.70
Ethene	2.39×10^{-5}	3.474×10^{-5}	0.69
Ethyne	2.31×10^{-5}	3.044×10^{-5}	0.76
$-CH_2-$	1.023×10^{-5}	1.409×10^{-5}	0.73
$-S-$	1.08×10^{-5}	1.635×10^{-5}	0.66
$-\underset{\overset{\parallel}{O}}{C}-$	1.17×10^{-5}	1.566×10^{-5}	0.75
Benzene	4.836×10^{-5}	7.164×10^{-5}	0.68
Naphthalene	7.397×10^{-5}	1.0854×10^{-4}	0.68

3

Molecular Volumes in Mixtures

(a) PARTIAL MOLAR VOLUMES OF NON-ELECTROLYTES

Water has been one component in many studies of molecular volumes in mixtures. Traube [86–92] measured many partial molar volumes of compounds in aqueous solution. The partial molar volume $\bar{V}_s$ is defined by (11)

$$\bar{V}_s = \frac{M_s + gM_0}{\rho_s} - \frac{gM_0}{\rho_1} \tag{11}$$

where M_s and M_0 are the 'molecular weights' (mass of one mole) of the solute and solvent respectively, g is the ratio of the number of moles of solvent present to the number of moles of solute in solution and ρ_s and ρ_L are the densities of the solution and pure solvent respectively. Traube found that partial molar volumes of compounds in water could be estimated by the use of factors [88, 89, 92]. Some of the factors given by Traube [88, 89] are listed in Table 8. At first sight, there would appear to be little resemblance between these factors and the characteristic volumes V_x from the values given in Table 4. However, on closer examination, there is clearly a relationship between the two sets of values. Molecules can be considered to be made up of two terminal atoms or groups with a number of linkage units between. For the linkage unit $-CH_2$, Traube's factors for carbon and two hydrogens $(9.9 + 2 \times 3.1) \times 10^{-6} = 1.61 \times 10^{-5}$ m^3 mol^{-1} would give $\bar{V}_s$. The $-C=CH$ linkage unit consists of two carbon atoms, two hydrogen atoms and a double bond and so its factor is $(2 \times 9.9 + 2 \times 3.1 - 1.7) \times 10^{-6} = 2.43 \times 10^{-5}$ m^3 mol^{-1}. In Table 9, $\bar{V}_s$ values calculated from Traube's factor given in Table 8 are compared with the V_x values calculated as already described from the factors in Table 4. The values are fairly close.

Table 8. Factors [88, 89] for the estimation of partial molar volumes $\bar{V}_s$ (m^3 mol^{-1}) in aqueous solution at about 291 K.

Hydrogen	3.1×10^{-6}
Carbon	9.9×10^{-6}
Nitrogen (III)	1.5×10^{-6}
Oxygen in $-$OH	2.3×10^{-6}
Oxygen in $>$CO and C$-$O$-$C	5.5×10^{-6}
Oxygen in OH of $-$COOH	4×10^{-7}
Sulphur	1.55×10^{-6}
Double bond	-1.7×10^{-6}

Partial molar volume $\bar{V}_s$ = sum of factors plus 1.24×10^{-5}. If the compound is ionised, 1.35×10^{-5} has to be subtracted.

Table 9. Partial molar volumes $\bar{V}_s$ from Traube factors and characteristic volumes V_x of linking groups (m^3 mol^{-1}).

Group	$\bar{V}_s$ (from factors)	V_x
$-$CH$_2$	1.61×10^{-5}	1.409×10^{-5}
$-$CH$=$CH	2.43×10^{-5}	2.388×10^{-5}
$-$O	5.5×10^{-6}	5.87×10^{-6}
$-$CO	1.54×10^{-5}	1.566×10^{-5}
$-$S	1.55×10^{-5}	1.635×10^{-5}

The ratio of the factors for the $-$CH$_2$ group, $\bar{V}_s/V_x = 1.14$ and this is based on many experimental values. In Table 10, experimental values of $\bar{V}_s$ for organic compounds studied by Traube [88, 89] are compared with $1.14\,V_x$. The figures for carboxylic acids and for bases have been left off in order to shorten the table and because corrections might be necessary for ionization. The compounds which contain more than one hydroxyl group have been separated. For these compounds and for acetamide, urea and thiourea, $\bar{V}_s$ is considerably smaller than $1.14\,V_x$. Apart from these, $\bar{V}_s$ values are mostly slightly larger than $1.14\,V_x$. Traube considered that molecules dissolved in water gave an expansion of 1.24×10^{-5} m^3 mol^{-1}. This he called a 'co-volume' and added it to the total sum of his factors. From the figures in Table 10, it appears that this co-volume correction is unnecessary and can be taken into account by a change in the factors for the terminal groups.

Traube [90] suggested that the reason why the polyhydroxy and certain other compounds have low $\bar{V}_s$ values compared with what might be expected, was that the 'attractive pressure' (or the reciprocal of the compressibility) of

Table 10. Partial molar volumes [88, 90] (at about 291 K) and characteristic volumes of organic compounds.

Compound	$\bar{V}_s$ (m^3 mol^{-1})	1.14 V_x (m^3 mol^{-1})
Methyl acetate (6.12 $\times$ 10^{-2})	7.17 $\times$ 10^{-5}	6.91 $\times$ 10^{-5}
Ethyl acetate (5.07 $\times$ 10^{-2})	8.81 $\times$ 10^{-5}	
Methyl propionate	8.78 $\times$ 10^{-5}	8.51 $\times$ 10^{-5}
n-Propyl formate	8.86 $\times$ 10^{-5}	
n-Propyl acetate	1.050 $\times$ 10^{-4}	1.1012 $\times$ 10^{-4}
Ethyl propionate	1.040 $\times$ 10^{-4}	
Allyl acetate	9.80 $\times$ 10^{-5}	9.63 $\times$ 10^{-5}
Ethyl acetoacetate	1.175 $\times$ 10^{-4}	1.158 $\times$ 10^{-4}
Methanol (7.05 $\times$ 10^{-2})	3.70 $\times$ 10^{-5}	3.51 $\times$ 10^{-5}
Ethanol (6.73 $\times$ 10^{-2})	5.28 $\times$ 10^{-5}	5.12 $\times$ 10^{-5}
n-Propanol (5.89 $\times$ 10^{-2})	6.89 $\times$ 10^{-5}	6.73 $\times$ 10^{-5}
i-Propanol	6.87 $\times$ 10^{-5}	
i-Butanol (4.49 $\times$ 10^{-2})	8.48 $\times$ 10^{-5}	8.33 $\times$ 10^{-5}
i-Pentanol (3.05 $\times$ 10^{-2})	1.016 $\times$ 10^{-4}	9.94 $\times$ 10^{-5}
Dimethylethylcarbinol (4.35 $\times$ 10^{-2})	9.95 $\times$ 10^{-5}	
Allyl alcohol	6.33 $\times$ 10^{-5}	6.23 $\times$ 10^{-5}
Phenol (5.31 $\times$ 10^{-2})	8.43 $\times$ 10^{-5}	8.84 $\times$ 10^{-5}
o-Cresol	9.97 $\times$ 10^{-5}	
m-Cresol	1.011 $\times$ 10^{-4}	1.044 $\times$ 10^{-4}
p-Cresol	1.010 $\times$ 10^{-4}	
Acetone (6.48 $\times$ 10^{-2})	6.66 $\times$ 10^{-5}	6.24 $\times$ 10^{-5}
Acetamide (7.20 $\times$ 10^{-2})	5.48 $\times$ 10^{-5}	5.77 $\times$ 10^{-5}
Urea (7.30 $\times$ 10^{-2})	4.31 $\times$ 10^{-5}	5.30 $\times$ 10^{-5}
Thiourea (7.30 $\times$ 10^{-2})	5.36 $\times$ 10^{-5}	6.45 $\times$ 10^{-5}
Ethyl mercaptan	6.67 $\times$ 10^{-5}	6.45 $\times$ 10^{-5}
Acetonitrile (6.9 $\times$ 10^{-2})	4.62 $\times$ 10^{-5}	4.61 $\times$ 10^{-5}
Compounds containing more than one hydroxyl group		
1,2-Ethanediol (7.24 $\times$ 10^{-2})	5.42 $\times$ 10^{-5}	5.79 $\times$ 10^{-5}
Glycerol (7.29 $\times$ 10^{-2})	6.89 $\times$ 10^{-5}	8.07 $\times$ 10^{-5}
Erythritol	8.67 $\times$ 10^{-5}	1.034 $\times$ 10^{-4}
Mannitol (7.33 $\times$ 10^{-2})	1.167 $\times$ 10^{-4}	1.489 $\times$ 10^{-4}
Quercitol	1.053 $\times$ 10^{-4}	1.298 $\times$ 10^{-4}
Xylose	9.56 $\times$ 10^{-5}	1.213 $\times$ 10^{-4}
Glucose (7.33 $\times$ 10^{-2})	1.114 $\times$ 10^{-4}	1.440 $\times$ 10^{-4}
Fructose	1.102 $\times$ 10^{-4}	
Sucrose (7.35 $\times$ 10^{-2})	2.087 $\times$ 10^{-4}	2.827 $\times$ 10^{-4}
Catechol	8.54 $\times$ 10^{-5}	
Resorcinol	8.84 $\times$ 10^{-5}	9.51 $\times$ 10^{-5}
Hydroquinone	8.71 $\times$ 10^{-5}	

Table 10 (continued)

Compound	$\bar{V}_s$(m³ mol⁻¹)	1.14 V_x(m³ mol⁻¹)
Pyrogallol	8.56 × 10⁻⁵ ⎫	
Phloroglucinol	8.94 × 10⁻⁵ ⎭	1.018 × 10⁻⁴

The figures in brackets after the names of compounds are surface tensions [90, 92] (N m⁻¹) for 250 mol m⁻³ aqueous solutions at 288 K. The value for water itself is 7.30 × 10⁻².

their solutions in water was high compared with that of other compounds. The isothermal compressibilities of most organic compounds are considerably higher than that of water, which is 4.6×10^{-10} m² N⁻¹ at 298 K: examples are [42] methanol 11.5×10^{-10}, ethyl acetate 11.8×10^{-10} and acetone 12.4×10^{-10} m² N⁻¹. The isothermal compressibilities of some compounds with more than one hydroxyl group are, however, about equal to that of water or even lower: that of 1,2-ethanediol [42] is 3.7×10^{-10} and of glycerol [94, 95] 2.2×10^{-10} m² N⁻¹. Not only will a compound of low compressibility have a low molecular volume itself but, if the solution has a lower compressibility than that of the solvent, the molecular volume of the solvent will also be lowered. This will lower the apparent partial molar volume of the solute since partial molar volumes are worked out from equation (11) on the assumption that the molar volume of the solvent is unchanged. Traube [90, 92] measured the surface tensions of aqueous solutions and he considered that these gave a measure of the 'attractive pressures'. His values for solutions with 250 mol m⁻³ at 288 K are shown in brackets after the names of the compounds in Table 10. When these surface tensions are greater or near 7.3×10^{-2} N m⁻¹, the value of water itself, $\bar{V}_s$ is less than 1.14 V_x. When the surface tension of the solution is well below 7.3×10^{-2} N m⁻¹, $\bar{V}_s$ is greater than 1.14 V_x. The presence of groups giving interaction with water does not appear to have any appreciable effect on partial molar volumes of compounds in aqueous solutions.

Traube [91] has summarised his work and suggested that many physical and biological properties can be correlated with 'attractive pressures'. For example, he has related the concentrations for narcotic action on frog's heart measured by Fühner [10] (see Table 1) and the effects of additions of non-electrolytes on the solubilities of salts in water (see Chapter 5) to 'attractive pressures'. It would seem, however, that although 'attractive pressures' (i.e. reciprocal of compressibility of the solution) may have some influence on such properties, they depend mainly on the characteristic volumes.

It has been found [93, 96] that the partial molar volumes of proteins in aqueous solution can be calculated quite accurately from the factors given in Table 11. These factors are those given by Traube with slight modifications.

Table 11. Factors [93, 96] for the calculation of partial molar volumes of proteins in aqueous solutions at about 293 K.

Group	Factor (m^3 mol^{-1})	V_X(m^3 mol^{-1})
—CH_2—	1.63×10^{-5}	1.409×10^{-5}
—CONH—	2.0×10^{-5}	2.564×10^{-5}
—NH_2	7.7×10^{-6}	1.204×10^{-5}
—COOH	1.89×10^{-5}	2.359×10^{-5}

(b) PARTIAL MOLAR VOLUMES OF ELECTROLYTES

Traube measured the partial molar volumes of many electrolytes. Some of his results [97] are given in Table 12. He noted a number of relationships amongst the $\bar{V}_s$ values of electrolytes. Some ions had about the same partial molar volume: for example, Pb^{2+} (-1.55×10^{-5}), Ca^{2+} (-1.785×10^{-5}) and Sr^{2+} (-1.816×10^{-5}): also NH_4^+ (1.786×10^{-5}) and Rb^+ (1.407×10^{-5}); and ClO_4^- (4.412×10^{-5}) and MnO_4^- (4.25×10^{-5}). All the ions Ag^+ (-0.21×10^{-7}), Na^+ (-1.21×10^{-6}), H^+ (standard zero), Li^+ (-8.8×10^{-7}), Cu^+, Au^+ and Hg^+ were roughly the same size and there was the same difference in the partial molar volumes between the pair K_2SeO_3 and K_2SO_3 as between the pair K_2SeO_4 and K_2SO_4. Other ions had about the same volume, including Fe^{2+} (-2.47×10^{-5}), Mn^{2+} (-1.77×10^{-5}), Ni^{2+} (-2.3×10^{-5}) and Cu^{2+} (-2.776×10^{-5}); and the pair Zn^{2+} (-2.16×10^{-5}) and Mg^{2+} (-2.117×10^{-5}). The atoms palladium, iridium and platinum had equal volumes and so had molybdenum and tungsten. However, $\bar{V}_s$ varies with the concentration of the solution and it is usual to estimate its value $\bar{V}_s^\circ$ at infinite dilution. In order to do this, plots of $\bar{V}_s$ against the square root of the concentration produced back to zero have been used, as suggested by Masson [98]. It should be pointed out that $\bar{V}_s^\circ$ still depends on temperature. Redlich and Rosenfeld [99, 100] applied the Debye–Hückel theory to the variation of partial molar volumes $\bar{V}_s$ of electrolytes with concentration c and gave the relationship (12)

$$\bar{V}_s = \bar{V}_s^\circ + k(\Sigma_i n_i z_i^2)^{3/2} \sqrt{c} \dots \dots \tag{12}$$

where n_i is the number of ions of species i and z_i is the valency (i.e. charge) of that ionic species. Redlich [101] gives limiting slopes of 5.91×10^{-14}, 3.07×10^{-13}, 4.725×10^{-13}, 8.68×10^{-13} and 1.87×10^{-12} $m^{9/2}$ $mol^{-3/2}$ for the slopes of plots of $\bar{V}_s$ against $\sqrt{c}$ with 1:1, 2:1, 2:2, 3:1 and 4:1 electrolytes respectively at 298 K in water. It should be noted that the relationship (12) only applies to very dilute solutions and the slopes found are not the same as those given by Masson plots for fairly concentrated solutions. The equation (12) is for electrolytes and according to Redlich [101], the partial molar volumes of non-electrolytes vary linearly with the concentration. A number of reviews on

Table 12. Partial Molar volumes and characteristic volumes of some electrolytes.

Electrolyte	Calculated characteristic Volume V_X (m^3 mol^{-1})	Partial molar volume (m^3 mol^{-1})		$1.08 V_X$ -1.35×10^{-5}
		$\bar{V}_s$ at 291 K [97]	$\bar{V}_s^\circ$ at 298 K [108]	
NaCl	2.751×10^{-5}	1.63×10^{-5}	1.66×10^{-5}	1.62×10^{-5}
NaNO$_3$	3.857×10^{-5}	2.64×10^{-5}	2.78×10^{-5}	2.82×10^{-5}
NaClO$_3$	4.513×10^{-5}	3.43×10^{-5}	3.55×10^{-5}	3.52×10^{-5}
KCl	3.799×10^{-5}	2.55×10^{-5}	2.69×10^{-5}	2.75×10^{-5}
KBr	4.325×10^{-5}	3.35×10^{-5}	3.37×10^{-5}	3.32×10^{-5}
KI	5.157×10^{-5}	4.44×10^{-5}	4.52×10^{-5}	4.21×10^{-5}
KNO$_3$	4.905×10^{-5}	3.59×10^{-5}	3.80×10^{-5}	3.94×10^{-5}
RbCl	4.395×10^{-5}	3.17×10^{-5}	3.29×10^{-5}	3.40×10^{-5}
Na$_2$SO$_4$	5.952×10^{-5}	1.04×10^{-5}	1.16×10^{-5}	5.08×10^{-5}
K$_2$SO$_4$	8.048×10^{-5}	2.95×10^{-5}	3.20×10^{-5}	7.34×10^{-5}

the partial molar volumes of electrolytes have appeared [101–109]. Partial molar volumes are additive and Millero [108] gives a large number of values for $\bar{V}_s^\circ$ for single ions based on the assumption that $\bar{V}_s^\circ$ for H$^+$ is zero: values from Millero are given in brackets after the ions listed above. His values are only in fair agreement with Traube's conclusions. In Table 12, Millero's values of $\bar{V}_s^\circ$ for the salts are compared with Traube's experimental values of $\bar{V}_s$. It will be seen that $\bar{V}_s^\circ$ at 298 K is higher than $\bar{V}_s$ at 291 K: the effect of the rise in temperature raises $\bar{V}_s$ more than the decrease in concentration lowers it.

For water itself, the molecular volume at 298 K is 1.08 times the characteristic volume and this seems to be about the ratio of $\bar{V}_s^\circ$ and V_X of salts. Traube [97] subtracted 1.35×10^{-5} m^3 m^{-1} for the effect of charges on $\bar{V}_s^\circ$ of all electrolytes, and for a number of the compounds studied by Traube, there is good agreement between $1.08 V_X - 1.35 \times 10^{-5}$ and $\bar{V}_s^\circ$ m^3 mol^{-1} (see Table 12). However, in most of the examples given in Table 13, the difference between $1.08 V_X$ and $\bar{V}_s^\circ$ is not about 1.35×10^{-5} m^3 mol^{-1}. For example, for the salts of the small cation Li$^+$, $1.08 V_X - \bar{V}_s^\circ$ is about 1.1×10^{-5} m^3 mol^{-1}, whilst the figure for the small anions F$^-$ and OH$^-$ is over 2×10^{-5} m^3 mol^{-1}. For salts consisting of a divalent ion and two univalent ions, $1.08 V_X - 1.35 \bar{V}_s^\circ$ is between 4×10^{-5} and 5.5×10^{-5} m^3 mol^{-1}. Millero [108] gives Sr^{2+} a lower $\bar{V}_s^\circ$ than Ca^{2+}. Another curious observation [105] is that $\bar{V}_s^\circ$ for IO$_3^-$ is lower than that for BrO$_3^-$, which in turn is lower than that for ClO$_3^-$. There seems to be no clear explanation for these observations at present. Traube's value of 1.35×10^{-5} m^3 mol^{-1} for the decrease in volume for two (single) electrical charges is about the decrease which would be expected for the formation of two covalent bonds, but this does not seem to be significant. Couture and Laidler [103] have

Table 13. Characteristic volumes and partial molar volumes [108] (m^3 mol^{-1}) of electrolytes at infinite dilution in water at 298 K.

Electrolyte	Characteristic volume V_X (m^3 mol^{-1})	$\bar{V}_s^\circ$	$1.08\,V_X - \bar{V}_s^\circ$
LiCl	2.575×10^{-5}	1.695×10^{-5}	1.086×10^{-5}
LiNO$_3$	3.681×10^{-5}	2.855×10^{-5}	1.120×10^{-5}
NaF	1.704×10^{-5}	-2.37×10^{-6}	2.077×10^{-5}
KF	2.751×10^{-5}	7.86×10^{-6}	2.185×10^{-5}
NaOH	2.113×10^{-5}	-5.25×10^{-6}	2.807×10^{-5}
KOH	3.162×10^{-5}	4.98×10^{-6}	2.917×10^{-5}
NaBrO$_3$	5.037×10^{-5}	3.409×10^{-5}	2.031×10^{-5}
NaIO$_3$	5.869×10^{-5}	2.409×10^{-5}	3.930×10^{-5}
NH$_4$Cl	4.394×10^{-5}	3.569×10^{-5}	1.177×10^{-5}
[N(CH$_3$)$_4$]Cl	1.003×10^{-4}	1.074×10^{-4}	9.2×10^{-7}
[N(C$_2$H$_5$)$_4$]Cl	1.567×10^{-4}	1.670×10^{-4}	2.3×10^{-6}
CaCl$_2$	5.733×10^{-5}	1.582×10^{-5}	4.610×10^{-5}
SrCl$_2$	6.329×10^{-5}	1.489×10^{-5}	5.346×10^{-5}
BaCl$_2$	7.197×10^{-5}	2.319×10^{-5}	5.454×10^{-5}
Na$_2$SeO$_4$	6.439×10^{-5}	1.858×10^{-5}	5.096×10^{-5}
Na$_2$S$_2$O$_3$	6.997×10^{-5}	3.158×10^{-5}	4.399×10^{-5}
Na$_2$(oxalate)	4.962×10^{-5}	1.358×10^{-5}	4.001×10^{-5}

attempted to relate partial molar volumes at infinite dilution to the crystal radii of the ions which electrolytes contain.

(c) CHARACTERISTIC VOLUMES OF COMPOUNDS INCLUDING SALTS IN SOLUTION

It is possible to obtain V_X values from measurements of densities of fairly concentrated solutions [45] if corrections are made. These corrections require either the isothermal compressibilities or the surface tensions of the solutions. Hammick and Andrew [110] found that the parachor V_p^M of a mixture of a substance of parachor V_p^X present at mole fraction x and another of parachor V_p^s

$$V_p^m = V_p^s(1-x) + V_p^X x \qquad (13)$$

The use of this relationship enables the parachors of solids and substances not readily available in the liquid state to be found. If the surface tensions of the two components differ by more than $6 \times 10^{-3}\,N\,m^{-1}$, the value for V_X is not constant but the values found give a straight line when plotted against x. Bowden and Butler [111] used the Hammick and Andrew relationship and their results with mixtures containing methyl carbonate are given in Table 14. The value of V_x for methyl carbonate C_3H_6O (11 bonds) given by the addition of the factors from Table 4 is 6.64×10^{-5} m^3 mol^{-1}.

Table 14. Characteristic volumes of methyl carbonate from mixtures at 298.2 K.

x	$\rho_s(kg\ m^{-3})$	$\gamma\ (N\ m^{-1})$	$V_x(m^3\ mol^{-1})$
Methyl carbonate and benzene [111]			
0	872.87	0.02821	—
0.17170	902.58	0.02811	6.92×10^{-5}
0.34401	932.81	0.02810	6.91×10^{-5}
0.51315	963.82	0.02807	6.93×10^{-5}
0.67640	995.03	0.02821	6.91×10^{-5}
0.83748	1027.11	0.02834	6.93×10^{-5}
1.00000	1060.27	0.02846	6.92×10^{-5}
			Mean 6.92×10^{-5}
Methyl carbonate and chloroform			
0	1479.7	0.02621	—
0.14270	1416.1	0.02645	6.88×10^{-5}
0.28121	1355.2	0.02650	6.91×10^{-5}
0.47254	1293.9	0.02677	6.90×10^{-5}
0.56361	1234.1	0.02688	6.94×10^{-5}
0.71110	1174.1	0.02713	6.91×10^{-5}
0.85503	1116.6	0.02994	6.94×10^{-5}
1.00000	1060.3	0.02846	6.92×10^{-5}
			Mean 6.91×10^{-5}
Methyl carbonate and nitrobenzene			
0	1198.1	0.04308	—
0.16259	1180.4	0.03992	6.57×10^{-5}
0.31931	1162.0	0.03727	6.64×10^{-5}
0.47837	1141.9	0.03419	6.73×10^{-5}
0.61267	1123.1	0.03306	6.77×10^{-5}
0.75557	1101.7	0.03145	6.84×10^{-5}
0.87341	1082.6	0.03012	6.89×10^{-5}
1.00000	1060.3	0.02846	6.92×10^{-5}
			Mean 6.77×10^{-5}

Bhagwat, Shukla and Gupta [112] found that the expression of Hammick and Andrew [110], mentioned above for the additivity of parachors, could be applied to moderately concentrated aqueous solutions of simple salts. This is perhaps rather surprising since water is strongly associated. The parachor is found from equation (14), which resembles (11) but includes γ_s and γ_0, the surface tensions of the salt solution and pure water respectively.

$$V_X = \frac{(M_s + gM_0)\,\gamma_s^{1/4}}{\rho_s \gamma_X^{1/4}} - \frac{gM_0\,\gamma_0^{1/4}}{\rho_0 \gamma_X^{1/4}} \tag{14}$$

Figures for potassium chloride are used in Table 15 to test equation (14) and the V_X figures found are around the value of 3.80×10^{-5} m^3 mol^{-1}, which is given by the addition of the factors in Table 4. If one reference is given in the table, both density and surface tension come from this. Two references are given if the surface tension alone is given in the first; the second shows that the densities were taken from *International Critical Tables* [113]. It is perhaps surprising that (14) should give V_X because g and ρ_s refer to the bulk of the solution and the surface tension γ_s is a property of the surface, which would not be expected to have the same concentration or density (but might have the same value for $\gamma^{1/4}/\rho$) as the bulk phase. This objection can be overcome by the use of equation (15) in which isothermal compressibilities at low (e.g. atmospheric) pressure (κ) are used instead of surface tensions.

$$V_X = \frac{(M_s + gM_0)}{\rho_s P_X^{1/6} \kappa_s^{1/6}} - \frac{gM_0}{\rho_1 P_X^{1/6} \kappa_0^{1/6}} \tag{15}$$

Here P_X is the same constant (4.455×10^9 N m^{-2}) as used previously. With both (14) and (15), V_X is found from the difference between two much larger numbers. The last term in (14) and (15) involves the properties of the pure solvent and varies somewhat with temperature. It should be evaluated from experimental values preferably made by those who made the measurements for the solutions. The use of the last term of (14) (and of 15) can be avoided if

$$\frac{(M_s + M_0 g)\gamma_s^{1/4}}{\rho_s\,\gamma_X^{1/4}} \quad \text{or} \quad \frac{M_s + M_0 g}{\rho_s P_X^{1/6}\,\kappa_s^{1/6}}$$

is plotted against g. At each temperature, a straight line will be obtained and each line will intercept the axis $g = 0$ at V_X for the salt. Values [118, 120–122] for potassium bromide are shown in Fig. 3 to illustrate the use of equations (14) and (15). The points fall on lines, all of which are drawn through $V_X = 4.32 \times 10^{-5}$ m^3 mol^{-1} (the sum of the factors for potassium and bromine in Table 4) for $g = 0$.

If water is coordinately bound to the ion, allowance should be made for this. The following ions do not appear to carry coordinately bound water [52]: Li$^+$, Na$^+$, K$^+$, Rb$^+$, NH$_4^+$, Ag$^+$, F$^-$, Cl$^-$, Br$^-$, I$^-$, NO$_3^-$, NO$_2^-$, and SCN$^-$. However, the ionisation constant of the magnesium ion suggested [123–124] that it has six water molecules covalently bound to it giving the ion [Mg.6H$_2$O]$^{2+}$, which would be an octahedral complex of the outer orbital type. In equations (14) and (15), $M_s + M_0 g$ is not altered by solvation because what is taken from the second term is added to the first. If n' is the number of molecules of water

Table 15. Characteristic volume V_x of potassium chloride from surface tension of aqueous solutions.

g	Density ρ_s (kg m^{-3})	Surface tension γ_s (N m^{-1})	V_x	T (K)	References
55.508	1048.1	7.368×10^{-2}	2.97×10^{-5}	298.16	[114, 113]
53.813	1044	7.455×10^{-2}	3.66×10^{-5}	298.16	[115]
53.748	1042.87	7.346×10^{-2}	3.54×10^{-5}	298.16	[116]
37.87	1062.3	7.483×10^{-2}	3.54×10^{-5}	293.16	[117, 113]
37.87	1054.8	7.182×10^{-2}	3.60×10^{-5}	311.16	[117, 113]
28.575	1081.9	7.496×10^{-2}	3.43×10^{-5}	292.3	[118]
27.615	1082.0	7.534×10^{-2}	3.71×10^{-5}	298.16	[114, 113]
26.085	1089.0	7.775×10^{-2}	3.87×10^{-5}	291.16	[119, 113]
26.085	1088	7.613×10^{-2}	3.68×10^{-5}	293.16	[115]
26.037	1086.75	7.506×10^{-2}	3.63×10^{-5}	298.16	[116, 113]
24.58	1093.3	7.599×10^{-2}	3.61×10^{-5}	293.16	[117, 113]
24.58	1085.2	7.297×10^{-2}	3.67×10^{-5}	311.16	[117, 113]
18.193	1120.3	7.673×10^{-2}	3.74×10^{-5}	298.16	[114, 113]
16.782	1129.25	7.676×10^{-2}	3.70×10^{-5}	298.16	[116]
16.751	1129	7.77×10^{-2}	3.79×10^{-5}	293.16	[115]
15.51	1141.6	7.764×10^{-2}	3.63×10^{-5}	291.5	[118]
13.824	1155.0	7.814×10^{-2}	3.74×10^{-5}	298.16	[114, 113]
13.126	1182	7.917×10^{-2}	3.30×10^{-5}	293.16	[115]
12.15	1173.8	8.112×10^{-2}	3.87×10^{-5}	291.16	[119, 113]

coordinated in each molecule of the salt, then since there is one bond (factor 6.56×10^{-6}) per water molecule

V_x for actual salt with coordinated water

$$= V_x \text{ for unhydrated salt} + n'V_x \text{ for water} - 6.56 \times 10^{-6} \, n'$$

$$= \frac{(M_s + M_0 \, g) \gamma_s^{1/4}}{\rho_s \gamma^{1/4}} - gV_x \text{ for water} + n'V_x \text{ for water}$$

and so

$$\frac{(M + M_0 \, g) \gamma_s^{1/4}}{\rho_s \gamma^{1/4}} - \frac{gM_0 \gamma_0^{1/4}}{\rho_0 \gamma_x^{1/4}}$$

$$= V_x \text{ for unhydrated salt} - 6.56 \times 10^{-6} \, n'$$

$$= \text{apparent } V_x \text{ for the salt obtained from equation (13) or (14).}$$

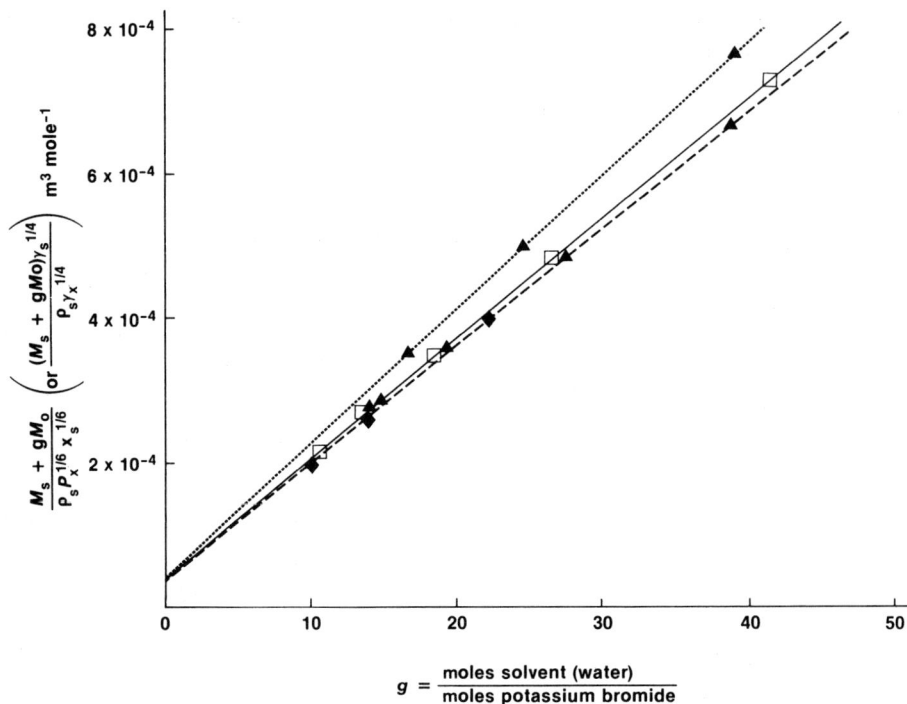

Fig. 3. Variation of $\dfrac{(M_s + gM_0)}{\rho_s P_x^{1/6} \kappa_s^{1/6}}$ or $\dfrac{(M_s + gM_0)\gamma_s^{1/4}}{\rho_s \gamma_x^{1/4}}$ with g, for potassium bromide solutions in water. ▲ from γ_s and ρ_s (Stocker [118] at 291 K); other points from κ_s and ρ_s: □ Gibson [120] at 298.2 K; ▲ Thomas and Perman [121] at 303.2 K; ♦ Scott, Obenhaus and Wilson [122] at 308.2 K.

In Fig. 4,

$$\frac{(M_s + gM_0)\gamma_s^{1/4}}{\rho_s \gamma_x^{1/4}}$$

is plotted against g for magnesium chloride just as it would be if the salt were not solvated. The points [113, 117, 118] fall near a straight line but this line does not cut the vertical axis at $V_x =$ (from the factors for $Mg^{2+} + 2Cl^-$) 4.65×10^{-5} m^3 mol^{-1}. For magnesium in an outer orbital complex (i.e. with an electronic structure like argon), $V_x = 3.074 \times 10^{-5}$ m^3 mol^{-1}, and, if the number of coordinately bound water molecules (n') is 6, the apparent characteristic volume for magnesium chloride will be $3.074 \times 10^{-5} + 4.190 \times 10^{-5}$ (for two Cl^-) $-6 \times 6.56 \times 10^{-6}$ (for six bonds) $= 3.328 \times 10^{-5}$ m^3 mol^{-1}. The line in Fig. 4 has been drawn through this point. The apparent V_x for the magnesium ion is $(3.328 - 4.190) \times 10^{-5}$ m^3 mol$^{-1} = -8.62 \times 10^{-6}$. In Fig. 5, lines through points for calcium chloride will cut the vertical axis at $V_x = 5.734 \times 10^{-5}$ m^3 mol^{-1}, which is the value the factors give for this salt with all the

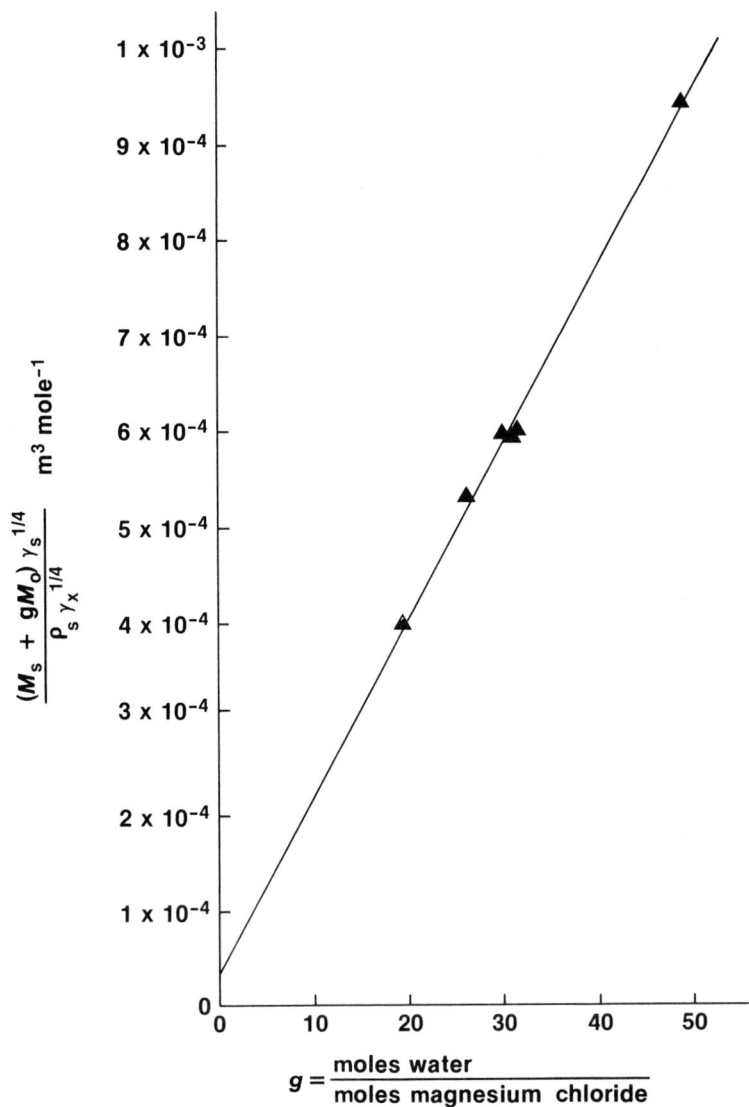

Fig. 4. Variation of $\dfrac{(M_s + gM_0)\gamma_s^{1/4}}{\rho_s\gamma_x^{1/4}}$ with g, for magnesium chloride solutions in water
[113–115].

ions unsolvated. This example is of interest because some of the experimental
points [125–127] are obtained from very concentrated solutions.

The characteristic volume for an ion can be found from measurements on
salts containing the ion and others for which characteristic volumes (real or
apparent) are known. In Fig. 6, this procedure has been used to derive the
characteristic volume for the sulphate ion. From each of the molecular volumes

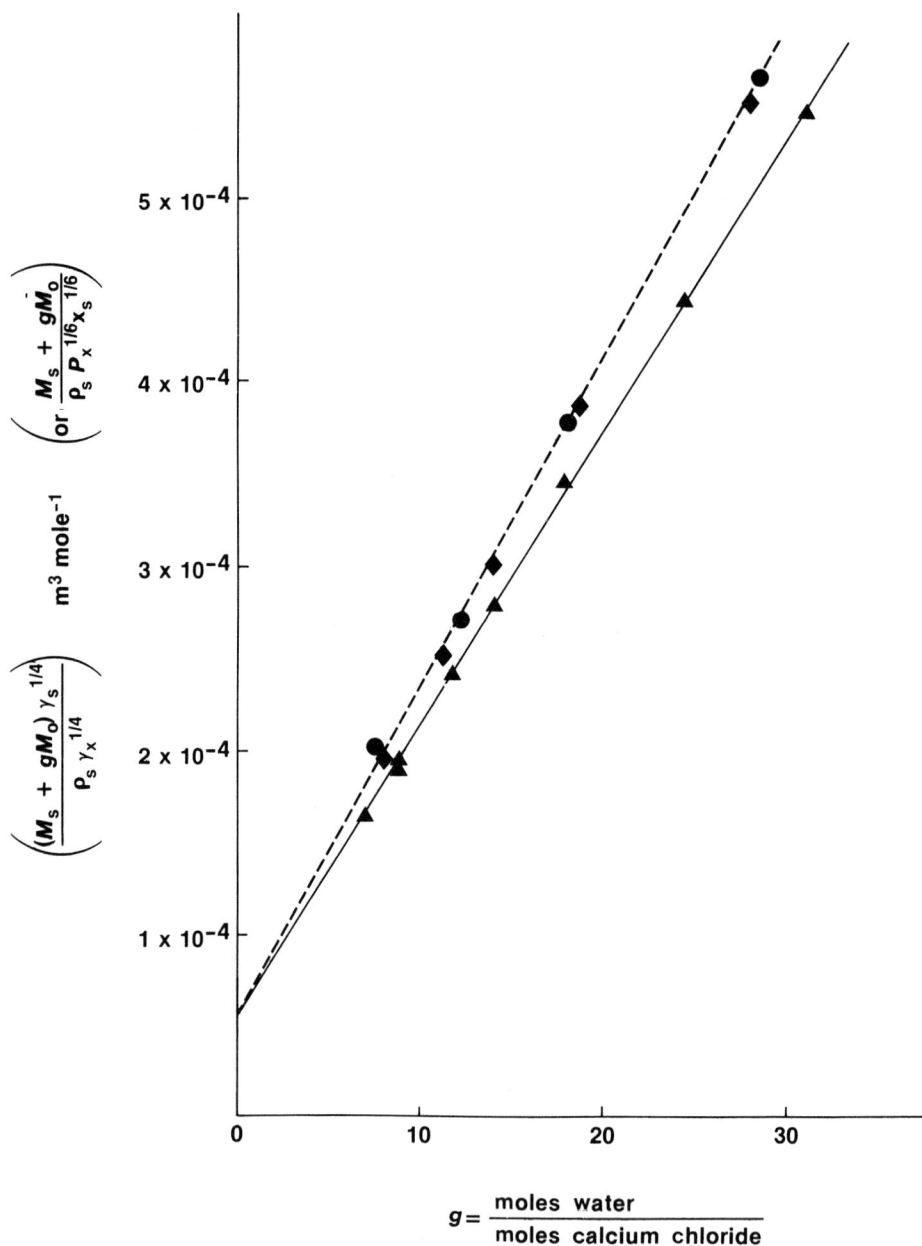

Fig. 5. Variation of $\dfrac{(M_s + gM_0)\gamma_s^{1/4}}{\rho_s\gamma_x^{1/4}}$ or $\dfrac{M_s + gM_0}{\rho_s P_x^{1/6}\gamma_s^{1/6}}$ with g, for solutions of calcium chloride in water. ▲ from κ_s and ρ_s values of Perman and Urry [125] at 303.16 K; ● from γ_s and ρ_s values of Cupples [126] at 298.16 K; ♦ from γ_s and ρ_s values of Hawkins and Gilbert [127] at 298.16 K.

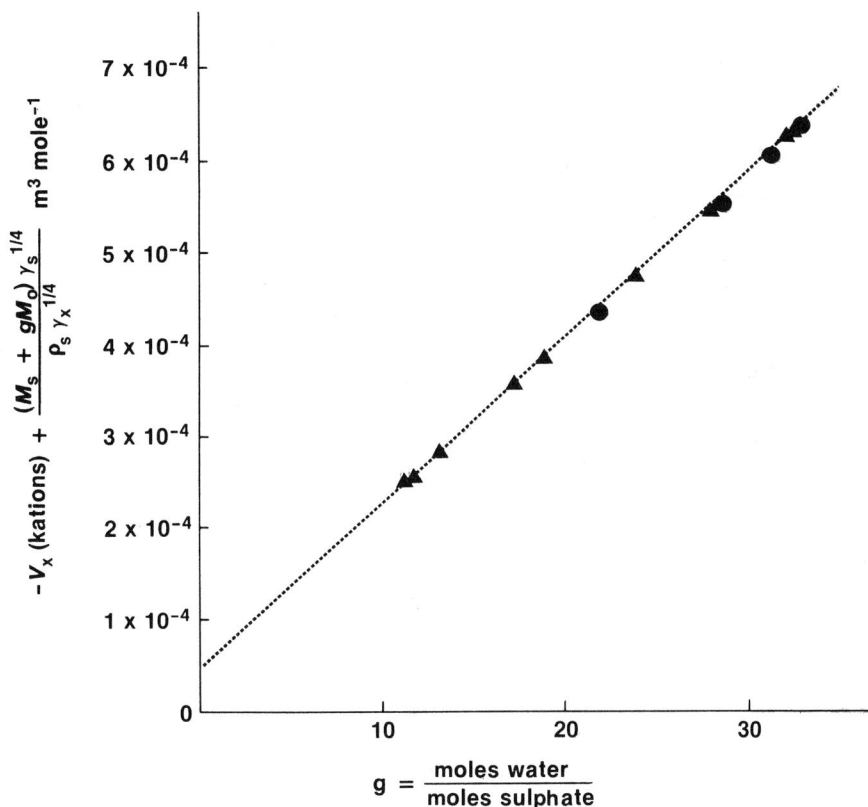

Fig. 6. Variation of $-V_x$ (cations) $+ \dfrac{(M_s + gM_0)\gamma_s^{1/4}}{\rho_s\gamma_x^{1/4}}$ with g, for aqueous sulphate solutions [113, 117, 118, 128, 129]. ▲ Ammonium sulphate; ● magnesium sulphate.

(with surface tension correction) for ammonium sulphate [118, 128] 4.85×10^{-5} m^3 mol^{-1} (for two NH$_4^+$ ions) has been subtracted and, since the apparent characteristic volume for the magnesium ion in water is negative (see above), 8.62×10^{-6} has been added to the values [112, 117, 129] for magnesium sulphate. The points fall close to a straight line which cuts the vertical axis at 4.65×10^{-5} m^3 mol^{-1}, the value from the factors for unsolvated sulphate SO$_4^{2-}$ (four bonds).

Unless figures are available for concentrated solutions ($g = 15$ or less) the extrapolation to $g = 0$ is too long to be made with accuracy. In Fig. 7, an attempt has been made to use the surface tension measurements, on aqueous solutions, of Pappenheimer, Lepie and Wyman [130] and of Belton [131], together with densities measured by Daniel and Cohn [132], to find characteristic volumes of three amino acids. The characteristic volumes calculated from the factors for glycine C$_2$H$_5$NO$_2$ (nine bonds), α-alanine C$_3$H$_7$NO$_2$ (12 bonds) and α-aminobutyric acid C$_4$H$_9$NO$_2$ (15 bonds) are

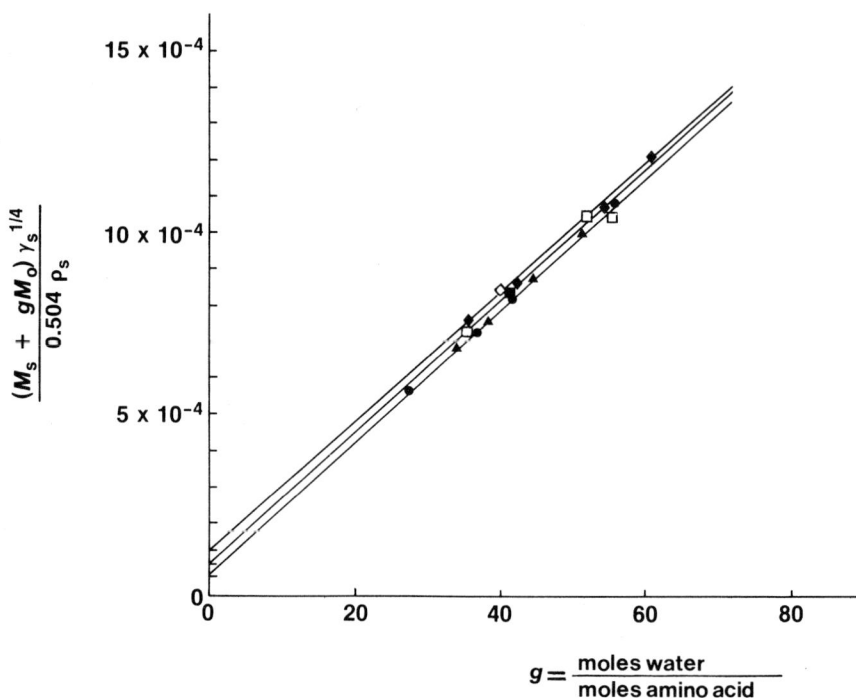

Fig. 7. Variation of $\dfrac{(M_s + gM_0)\gamma_s^{1/4}}{0.504\,\rho_s}$ with g, for aqueous solutions of almino acids. ▲ Glycine; ■ alanine; ◆ α-aminobutric acid [130]; ● glycine; □ alanine; ◇ α-aminobutric acid [131].

5.646×10^{-5}, 7.055×10^{-5} and 8.464×10^{-5} respectively and marks at these points are shown on the vertical axis. Satisfactory lines can be drawn through the experimental points to cut the axis at these values but clearly the characteristic volumes could not be determined with any accuracy from the points.

In the examples given above, the equations (14) and (15) have been used to find the characteristic volumes of compounds with molecules having electric charges. These equations do of course apply to non-electrolytes. In Table 16, values for the characteristic volumes, V_x, have been worked out with formula (14) from surface tensions [133] and densities [134] for some sugars. In Table 17, characteristic volumes of sucrose have been calculated from formula (15) and the isothermal compressibilities and densities of aqueous solutions reported by Perman and Urry [125]. From the factors given in Table 4, sucrose and maltose $C_{12}H_{22}O_{11}$ (46 bonds and two rings) have characteristic volumes equal to 2.2279×10^{-6} m^3 mol^{-1} for the isomeric cellobioise. Glucose and fructose have 24 bonds in the ring structure (pyranoside or furanoside) and from the factors their characteristic volume is 1.1976×10^{-4} m^3 mol^{-1}. In the open-chain structure, there is a carbonyl group. On account of the double bond, there is one bond less than in the ring structure so that the characteristic volume is 1.2632×10^{-4} m^3 mol^{-1}. The figures in Table 17 favour the ring structures for glucose and fructose in aqueous solution.

Table 16. Characteristic volumes of sugars from surface tensions [133].

Carbohydrate	Conc (mol m^{-3})	V_X (m^3 mol^{-1})	V_X calc.
Sucrose	301	2.22×10^{-4}	
	632	2.26×10^{-4}	
	951	2.23×10^{-4}	
			2.2279×10^{-4}
Maltose	214	1.98×10^{-4}	
	444	2.06×10^{-4}	
	694	2.14×10^{-4}	
Glucose	608	1.15×10^{-4}	
	1189	1.15×10^{-4}	
	1830	1.24×10^{-4}	
			1.1976×10^{-4}
Fructose	558	1.19×10^{-4}	
	1240	1.20×10^{-4}	
	1864	1.20×10^{-4}	

Table 17. Characteristic volume of sucrose from isothermal compressibilities at different temperatures.

T (K)	Conc sucrose (mol m^{-3})	V_X (m^3 mol^{-1})
303.2	1667	2.32
	1962	2.32
	2330	2.33
313.2	1657	2.31
	2014	2.32
	2320	2.34
323.2	1653	2.30
	2004	2.32
	2306	2.34
333.2	1642	2.31
	1993	2.30
	2295	2.30
343.2	1635	2.31
	1980	2.32
	2283	2.33
353.2	1627	2.30
	1972	2.31
	2270	2.32

4

Solutions of Unassociated Compounds in Unassociated Solvents without Interaction

(a) REGULAR SOLUTIONS

Solubility of unassociated compounds in unassociated liquids has often been interpreted on the basis of the theory of 'regular solutions' [135–137]. A regular solution is one in which there is no change in entropy when one component is transferred from the solution to an ideal solution. For such solutions it is only necessary to evaluate the heat of mixing in order to calculate free energies and the solubility relations. If there is no compound formation there will be absorption of heat during solution but compound formation will give evolution of heat. Many non-ideal solutions have been treated as regular solutions.

The following outline of the treatment of regular solutions is based on that given by Hildebrand and Scott [136]. The van der Waals [138] equation (16) which relates pressure P, molecular volume V and temperature T for fluids has two constants, a and b.

$$P + \frac{a}{V^2} = RT/(V - b) \tag{16}$$

The term a/V^2 has been used as a rough measure of the internal pressure of a liquid: for liquids it is usually much larger than the pressure P. If the liquid were expanded isothermally until it attained the volume of the saturated vapour V_v, the energy absorbed would be the same as the ordinary vaporisation heat ΔH, hence

$$\Delta H = \int_V^{V_v} \frac{a}{V^2}\, \partial V = a\left[\frac{1}{V} - \frac{1}{V_g}\right] \tag{17}$$

The equation (17) was first derived by Bakker [139, 140]. Partington [141, 142] listed latent heats calculated from equation (17) and found that they were too small (often about two-thirds the experimental values). The $1/V_g$ term can usually be neglected and then the equation gives $\Delta H/v = a/V^2$. The latent heat per unit volume was suggested as a measure of internal pressure by Dupré [143] and by Stefan [144]. The latent heat should have been replaced by what is sometimes called the 'internal latent heat' $\Delta H^v = \Delta H - RT$. The latent heat ΔH includes the work done by the vapour when it expands against the pressure and this work is close to RT when the behaviour of the vapour approximates to that of an ideal gas.

The values of the constants a and b for mixtures of two components with constants a_1 and a_2 and b_1 and b_2 are found [138] from

$$\sqrt{a} = x_1\sqrt{a_1} + x_2\sqrt{a_2} \tag{18}$$

$$b = x_1 b_1 + x_2 b_2 \tag{19}$$

where x_1 and x_2 are the mole fractions of the components.

The heat of mixing ΔH^M (it is assumed that any volume change can be neglected for a regular solution) is given by

$$\Delta H^M = x_1 \int_{V_1}^{\infty} \frac{a_1}{V^2}\, \partial V + x_2 \int_{V_2}^{\infty} \frac{a_2}{V^2}\, \partial V - \int_{V_{mix}}^{\infty} \frac{a_{mix}}{V^2}\, \partial V$$

$$= x_1 \frac{a_1}{V_1} + x_2 \frac{a_2}{V_2} - \frac{a_{mix}}{V_{mix}}$$

If the liquid is unexpanded $V = b$, thus

$$\Delta H^M = x_1 \frac{a_1}{b_1} + x_2 \frac{a_2}{b_2} - \frac{a}{b} \tag{20}$$

and if (20) is combined with (18) and (19)

$$\Delta H^M = \frac{x_1 x_2 b_1 b_2}{x b_1 + x_2 b_2}\left[\frac{a_1^{1/2}}{b_1} - \frac{a_2^{1/2}}{b_2}\right]^2 \tag{21}$$

Now follows what appears to be a curious and inspired step in which the molecular volumes V_1 and V_2 are substituted [145] for b_1 and b_2 so that (21) becomes (22)

$$\Delta H^M = \frac{x_1 x_2 V_1 V_2}{x_1 V_1 + x_2 V_2}\left[\frac{a_1^{1/2}}{V_1} - \frac{a_2^{1/2}}{V_2}\right]^2 \tag{22}$$

Another derivation of this equation was given by Scatchard [146] who modified it to (23)

$$\Delta H^M = [x_1 V_1 + x_2 V_2] y_1 y_2 [\delta_1 - \delta_2]^2 \tag{23}$$

where y_1 and y_2 are the volume fractions and where

$$\delta^2 = \frac{\text{internal latent heat}}{V}$$

for a liquid. The internal latent heat is the latent heat less RT, which is a measure of the work done by the vapour on expansion. The differentiation of (23) yields equations for γ_1 and γ_2, the activity coefficients.

$$RT \log_e \gamma_1 = V_1 y_2^2 [\delta_1 - \delta_2]^2 \tag{24}$$

and

$$RT \log_e \gamma_2 = V_2 y_1^2 [\delta_1 - \delta_2]^2 \tag{25}$$

Values of δ, which is called the solubility parameter, do provide a useful guide for discussion of the properties of solvents and their choice for various purposes. There is, however, an alternative method for treatment of solubilities, which will now be given.

(b) SOLUBILITIES, FREE VOLUMES AND ISOTHERMAL COMPRESSIBILITIES

The isothermal compressibility κ is defined as

$$-\frac{1}{V} \left(\frac{\partial V}{\partial P} \right)_T$$

and its reciprocal is called the bulk modulus. Murnagham [147] suggested the following relationship (26) between the isothermal compressibility κ_p of pressure P for constant temperature

$$\frac{1}{\kappa_p} = \frac{1}{\kappa} + CP \tag{26}$$

κ is the isothermal compressibility at zero pressure which for a liquid does not differ appreciably from the compressibility at one atmosphere: C is about 9 and independent of temperature. Murnagham also gave the itegrated form (27) of (26)

$$CP = \frac{1}{\kappa} (V_0/V)^c + \frac{1}{\kappa} \tag{27}$$

Others [148–157] have put forward equations (26) and (27) and at least some have discovered them independently. Examples showing the application of equation (27) are given in Fig. 8. Moelwyn-Hughes [148] has written equation (26) in the form

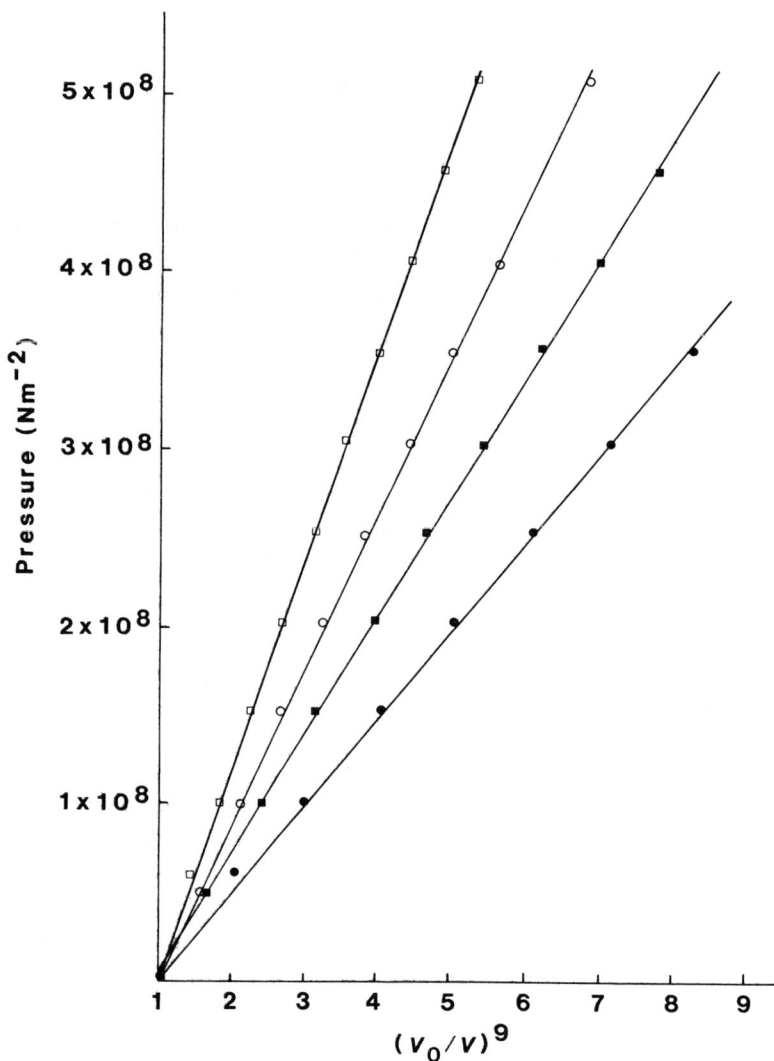

Fig. 8. Relationship between pressure and volume. □ Phosphorus trichloride [158] at 293 K; ○ bromoethane [158] at 293 K; ■ hexane [159] at 298 K; ● hexane [159] at 333 K.

$$C = \frac{1}{\kappa_p^2} \frac{\partial \kappa_p}{\partial P} = \frac{V}{\kappa_p} \cdot \frac{\partial \kappa_p}{\partial V} = \frac{d(\log \kappa_p)}{d(\log V)} \tag{28}$$

Blagoi and Sorkin [160] have plotted $\log \kappa_p$ against $\log \rho_l$ for xenon and krypton. They obtained straight lines with slopes 8.7 and 8.6 respectively. The effects of pressure on compressibilities and densities are discussed further in Chapter 5, section (f). It is of interest that equation (26) can be applied to a perfect gas with $C = 1$ and $1/\kappa = 0$ (see equations (2) and (3)). If κ is eliminated between the equations (7) and (27) and the result combined with equation (4), the following equation [23, 161] can be obtained, which relates the pressure P, density and temperature T of an unassociated liquid compound, where as before M is the molecular weight, V_x

$$\frac{9(P-p)}{P_x} \left(1 - \frac{T}{T_x}\right)^{0.9} = \left(\frac{V_x(\rho_1 - \rho_g)}{M}\right)^9 - \left(1 - \frac{T}{T_x}\right)^{2.7} \tag{29}$$

is the characteristic volume calculated as already described, ρ_1 is the density of the liquid and ρ_g the density of the vapour with vapour pressure p. For all liquids P_x appears to equal 4.455×10^9 N m^{-2} and T_x is a temperature characteristic of each liquid. Now if p can be neglected compared with P, ρ_g can be neglected compared with ρ_1, and V_0, the volume at zero pressure, can be taken as the volume at one atmosphere, the work of compression per unit volume for V_0 to pressure P and volume V is

$$\frac{1}{V_0} \int_{V_0}^{V} P dV$$

and equals [162]

$$P_x(V_x/V_0)^6 \left[\frac{1}{8} - \frac{1}{72}(V_0/V)^8 - \frac{1}{9}(V/V_0)\right] \tag{30}$$

When a liquid has the same compressibility as the original liquid, it follows from equations (4) and (5) that

$$V = \frac{V_0' V_x}{V_x'} \tag{31}$$

Therefore it might be expected that [163]

$$RT\log_e(C_s/C_L) = P_x V_x \left[\frac{1}{8} \left(\frac{V_x}{V}\right)^5 - \frac{1}{72} \left(\frac{V_x'}{V'}\right)^8 \left(\frac{V}{V_x}\right)^3\right.$$
$$\left. - \frac{1}{9} \left(\frac{V_x}{V}\right)^6 \left(\frac{V'}{V_x'}\right)\right] \tag{32}$$

Here V_x and V_0 refer to the solute and V_x' and V_0' to the solvent. The volume fraction y of the solute in the saturated solution equals C_s/C_L.

This work with the value of V from (26) was equated to $RT\log_e y$ where y is the volume fraction of the solute in the saturated solution and if required a term (see equation (64)) was added to allow for the decrease in solubility if the solute is a solid. The final equation was (33)

$$RT \log_e y + \Delta H_f (1 - T/T_m) = P_x V_x \left[\frac{1}{8} (V_x/V)^5 - \frac{1}{72} \left(\frac{V_x'}{V'} \right)^8 \left(\frac{V}{V_x} \right)^3 \right.$$

$$\left. - \frac{1}{9} \left(\frac{V_x}{V} \right)^6 \left(\frac{V'}{V_x'} \right) \right] \qquad (33)$$

Here V_x and V_0 refer to the solute and V_x' and V_0' to the solvent: ΔH_f is the latent heat of fusion and T_m is the melting point of the solid. The volume fraction y of the solute in the saturated solution equals C_s/C_L.

(c) VOLUME CHANGES WHEN UNASSOCIATED LIQUIDS ARE MIXED

Equation (32) given above for the solubility of one unassociated liquid in another does not take into account all the factors involved in the mixing of unassociated liquids. It is based on the assumption that the solute has to be brought to the compressibility of the solvent. This will be approximately true only for dilute solutions and the solubility should in fact be related to the work required to bring the solute and the solvent to the compressibility of the solution. From the composition and the equation (56) given below, M and V_x for a mixture can be found and if the density of the mixture is known, the compressibility can be calculated with the aid of equations (4) and (5). In order to obtain this density, the volume change, when the liquids are mixed, as required. It might be expected that volume changes for mixing would be obtained from the value of the density which corresponded to the minimum work for mixing. This work can be obtained in the following manner.

When two liquids have the same isothermal compressibility κ, it follows from equations (4) and (5) that

$$P_x^{1/6} \kappa^{1/6} = \text{a constant B} = \frac{V}{V_x} = \frac{V'}{V_x'} \qquad (34)$$

where $V(= M/(\rho_L - \rho_g))$ and V_x apply to one liquid and V' and V_x' are the corresponding values for the other liquid. When equation (34) holds, the two liquids have the same free volumes, i.e. their molecules occupy the same fractions of the molecular volumes. The work per mol required to bring one component (mol fraction x_1) and the other to the same compressibility κ is from equation (30).

$$W = x_1 P_x V_x \left(\frac{V_x}{V_0} \right)^5 \left[\frac{1}{8} - \frac{1}{72} \left(\frac{V_0}{P_x^{1/6} \kappa^{1/6} V_x} \right)^8 - \frac{P_x^{1/6} \kappa^{1/6} V_x}{9 V_0} \right]$$

$$+ (1 - x_1) P_x V_x' \left(\frac{V_x'}{V_0'} \right)^5 \left[\frac{1}{8} - \frac{1}{72} \left(\frac{V_0'}{P_x^{1/6} \kappa^{1/6} V_x'} \right)^8 \right.$$

$$\left. - \frac{P_x^{1/6} \kappa^{1/6} V_x'}{9 V_0'} \right] \qquad (35)$$

where V_0 and V_x are the volume per mol and the characteristic volume of one component (e.g. solute) and V_0' and V_x' are the corresponding values for the other component (e.g. solvent). From (35)

$$\frac{dW}{dx_1} = x_1 P_x V_x \left(\frac{V_x}{V_0}\right)^5 \left[\frac{V_0^8}{54 P_x^{4/3} V_x^8 \kappa^{7/3}} - \frac{P^{1/6} V_x}{54 V_0 \kappa^{5/6}}\right]$$

$$+ (1-x_1) P_x V_x' \left(\frac{V_x'}{V_0'}\right)^5 \left[\frac{V_0'^8}{54 P_x^{4/3} V_x'^8 \kappa^{7/3}} - \frac{P^{1/6} V_x'}{54 V_0' \kappa^{5/6}}\right]$$

(36)

This derivative will be zero for values of x giving (maximum or) minimum work, i.e. when

$$\frac{1}{\kappa^{3/2}} \left(\frac{x_1 V_0^3}{P_x^{4/3} V_x^2} + \frac{(1-x_1) V_0'^3}{P_x^{4/3} V_x'^2}\right) = \frac{x_1 P_x^{1/2} V_x^7}{V_0^6}$$

$$+ \frac{(1-x_1) P_x^{1/6} V_x'^7}{V_0'^6}$$

(37)

so that

$$P_x \kappa = \left(\frac{\dfrac{x_1 V_0^3}{V_x^2} + \dfrac{(1-x_1) V_0'^3}{V_x'^2}}{\dfrac{x_1 V_x^7}{V_0^6} + \dfrac{(1-x_1) V_x'^7}{V_0'^6}}\right)^{2/3} = B^6$$

(38)

Aicart, Tardajos and Diaz Pena [164] measured the isothermal compressibilities of mixtures of cyclohexane with a number of n-paraffins. Some of their experimental values are compared with values calculated from equation (38) in Table 18. The molecular volumes for the pure components were derived from the experimental compressibilities and the relationship (34). Compared with cyclohexane, hexane is more compressible, tetradecane less so and decane about the same. The agreement between the experimental and the estimated values is quite good for the mixtures of these rather similar compounds.

The volumes per mol of solution for two components in a mixture can be calculated from (39) and (40). These follow from equation (34), which also applies to the solution.

$$x_1 V = x_1 B V_x$$

(39)

$$(1-x_1) V' = (1-x_1) B V_x'$$

(40)

These volumes may be compared with the volumes before the mixing $x_1 V_0$ and $(1-x_1) V_0'$. The sum of the volumes for the components is the volume per mol of the solution. In Table 19, values of the volumes before mixing of

Table 18. Isothermal compressibilities of mixtures of cyclohexane with other hydrocarbons at 298.2 K [164].

Cyclohexane and hexane

Mol fraction cyclohexane	Compressibility $\times 10^{10}$ ($m^2\ N^{-1}$) Estimated	Found
0	16.7	16.7
0.1818	15.6	15.7
0.2397	15.2	15.4
0.2935	14.9	15.0
0.3767	14.4	14.6
0.4630	13.9	14.1
0.5086	13.7	13.9
0.5803	13.3	13.4
0.6181	13.1	13.3
0.6819	12.8	13.0
0.7922	12.2	12.3
0.8613	11.9	11.9
1	11.2	11.2

Cyclohexane and decane

Mol fraction cyclohexane	Compressibility $\times 10^{10}$ ($m^2\ N^{-1}$) Estimated	Found
0	11.0	11.0
0.1732	11.0	11.0
0.2769	11.0	11.1
0.3545	11.0	11.1
0.4350	11.0	11.1
0.5070	11.0	11.1
0.5850	11.1	11.1
0.6162	11.1	11.1
0.7044	11.1	11.2
0.7722	11.1	11.2
0.8691	11.2	11.2
1	11.2	11.2

Cyclohexane and tetradecane

Mol fraction cyclohexane	Compressibility $\times 10^{10}$ ($m^2\ N^{-1}$) Estimated	Found
0	9.1	9.1
0.1193	9.2	9.3
0.1584	9.3	9.3
0.2269	9.3	9.4
0.2832	9.4	9.5
0.3484	9.5	9.5
0.4345	9.6	9.7
0.4919	9.7	9.8
0.5761	9.8	9.9
0.6761	10.	10.2
0.7570	10.2	10.3
0.8681	10.6	10.6
1	11.2	11.2

Table 19. Estimated volumes (with volumes before mixing in brackets) of mixtures of 2,2-dimethylpropane (component 1) and cyclohexane (component 2) at 273.2 K.

Mol fraction x_1 2,2-dimethylpropane	Volume (m³) per mol of solution × 10⁵			Volume fraction y_1		Excess volume (m³) × 10⁵	
	2,2-Dimethylpropane $x_1 V (x_1 V_0)$	Cyclohexane $(1-x_1)V'((1-x_1)V'_0)$	Solution	Estimated	Taken	Estimated	Found [165]
0	0 (0)	10.557 (10.557)	10.557 (10.557)	0	(0)	0	0
0.4242	4.5510 (5.0067)	6.4229 (6.0787)	10.974 (11.086)	0.415	(0.452)	−0.112	−0.105
0.5333	5.8105 (6.2945)	5.2868 (4.9269)	11.097 (11.221)	0.524	(0.561)	−0.124	−0.116
0.7387	8.3071 (8.7188)	3.0552 (2.4585)	11.362 (11.477)	0.731	(0.760)	−0.115	−0.095
1.0000	11.8029 (11.8029)	0 (0)	11.803 (11.803)	1	(1)	0	0

2,2-dimethylpropane and cyclohexane are compared with the values calculated from equations (39) and (40). Experimental values [165] of V_0 and V'_0 were used for the calculation of B and the characteristic volumes of 2,2-dimethylpropane (8.132×10^{-5} m^3 mol^{-1}) and the cyclohexane (8.4550×10^{-5} m^3 mol^{-1}) were calculated from the factors given in Table 4.

It is clear from equation (34) that in order to bring two liquids to the same compressibility, the more compressible liquid has to be compressed and the less compressible one expanded. This means that the volume fractions in the mixture must differ from the volume fractions before the mixing. Also, the excess volume, which is the difference between considerably larger terms for the components, should always be negative, i.e. there should be a contraction when unassociated liquids are mixed. However, when unassociated liquids are mixed there is usually an expansion, not a contraction. It would seem that some factor has been overlooked. This factor is probably the attraction between residual charges on the atoms of the molecules. Other things being equal, the attraction between molecules with atoms at the same bond length will be somewhat greater than between those with other bonded atoms. In the mixing of molecules containing a dipole, when two opposite charges come together, the best chance of the charges at the other end coming close is when the dipoles are the same lengths. This is shown diagrammatically in Fig. 9. This attraction between dipoles will be low for molecules with small residual charges, especially if one end of the dipoles is buried in the molecule so that it is not easily accessible to other charges. This is shown by examples when there is a contraction with the mixing of unassociated liquids. The largest contractions among some such examples [165] are for mixtures of 2,2-dimethylpropane and cyclohexane. In Table 19, the estimated excess volumes for mixtures of 2,2-dimethylpropane and cyclohexane at 273.2 K are less than those observed [165].

(d) MOLECULAR VOLUMES AND SOLUBILITIES OF UNASSOCIATED COMPOUNDS

When the estimation of the properties of unassociated liquids were discussed earlier, three kinds of properties or combinations of properties were noted:

(1) There were properties like P_x and γ_x which apparently are constant for all unassociated liquids under all conditions except near the point of transition from liquid to gas or to solid.

(2) Most properties vary with temperature. These properties are functions of the characteristic temperature and often, of the characteristic volume as well.

(3) Properties such as the parachor, which vary from one compound to another but which do not depend upon temperature. These properties are functions of the characteristic volume.

The values of the van der Waals constants are usually obtained from measurements made near the critical point and are not too accurate. Both constants

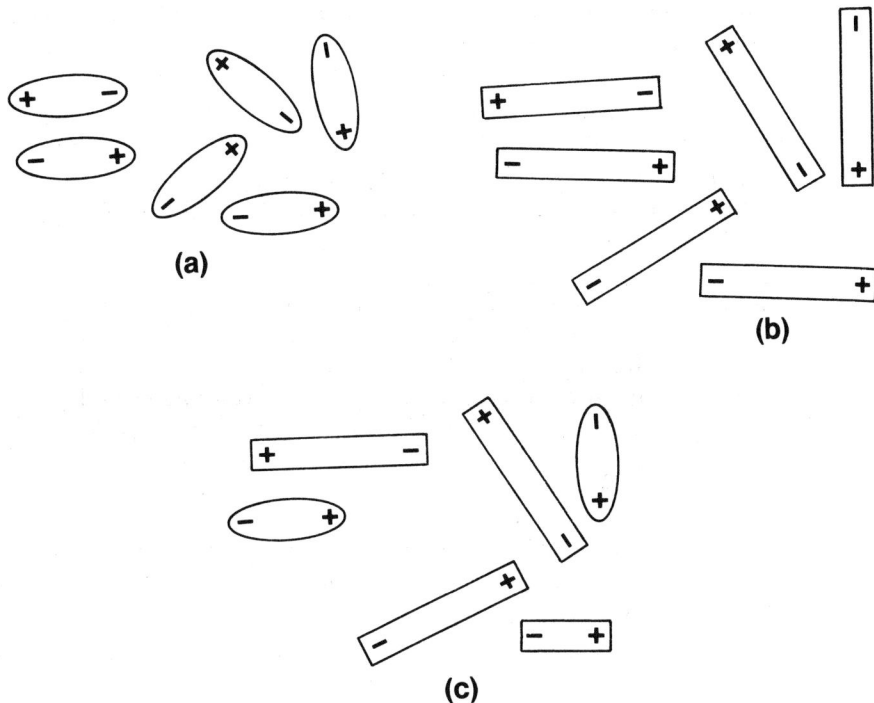

Fig. 9. Representation of mixtures of molecules with dipoles. (a) All molecules short; (b) all all molecules long; (c) mixture of long and short molecules.

belong to the third class just mentioned: that is, they do not depend on temperature but do vary from one compound to another. It would therefore be expected that both constants would be functions of the characteristic volume. van Laar [166] found that both b and $\sqrt{a}$ could be estimated from atomic factors. This suggests that both these constants might be proportional to the characteristic volumes for unassociated liquids. It has been proposed [57] already that $b = 1.84\,V_x$. van Arkel and de Groot [167] observed that $\sqrt{a}/b$ was constant for the inert gases and for halogens (in compounds) and van Liempt [168] found that $\sqrt{a}$ was proportional to b for homopolar compounds.

According to equation (27), the pressure is equal to the difference between a repulsion and an attraction, which at a given temperature equals $1/C\kappa$. This attraction is a measure of the stress required to cause cavitation in a liquid [85]. The term in the van der Waals equation (16) to account for attraction is a/V^2. McGowan [169] equated these measures of the attractive terms at the absolute zero with C equal to 9 and obtained the relationship

$$a^{1/2} = \frac{P_x^{1/2}\,V_x}{3} \tag{41}$$

Further, from equation (17), if $1/V_g$ is neglected, the internal latent heat of vaporisation $\Delta H^v = a/V$ so that

$$(\Delta H^v)^{1/2} V^{1/2} = a^{1/2} = \frac{P_x^{1/2} V_x}{3} \qquad (42)$$

In Table 20, some values of $\sqrt{a}/V_x$ and $\sqrt{\Delta H V}/V_x$ are given (every fourth compound is taken from a larger table [169] of values). It will be seen that these are around $P_x^{1/2}/3$ (= 2.22×10^4 N$^{1/2}$ m^{-1}). The factors from Table 4 have been used to give the characteristic volumes. The constant P_x equals 4.455×10^9 N m^{-2}: it has been called the characteristic pressure and has been used [23] in a number of relationships (for example (5) and (9)) for the estimation of the properties of liquids. The internal latent heat of evaporation ΔH^v is, as explained in Chapter 4, section (a), the latent heat of evaporation ΔH minus the work done by the vapour when it expands. This work can be taken as approximately equal to RT.

Table 20. Relationships between characteristic volumes, van der Waals attraction constants and cohesive energy densities.

Compound	$\dfrac{\delta V}{V_x} = \dfrac{\sqrt{\Delta H^v V}}{V_x}$	$\dfrac{\sqrt{a}}{V_x}$
Propane	1.99×10^4	1.65×10^4
Pentane	2.05×10^4	2.37×10^4
Cyclohexane	2.16×10^4	2.73×10^4
m-Xylene	2.23×10^4	3.08×10^4
Chloroform	2.50×10^4	2.49×10^4
1,2-Dibromomethane	2.50×10^4	1.91×10^4
Chlorobenzene	2.37×10^4	3.07×10^4

From equation (42)

$$\Delta H^v = P_x V_x^2 /(9V) \qquad (43)$$

and this with equation (4) gives

$$\Delta H^v = \frac{P_x V_x}{9} \left(\frac{T_x - T}{T_x} \right)^{0.3} \qquad (44)$$

which resembles equation (45) which was put forward by Watson [170]

$$\Delta H_1^v / \Delta H_2^v = \left(\frac{T_c - T_1}{T_c - T_2} \right)^{0.38} \qquad (45)$$

ΔH_1^{v} and ΔH_2^{v} are the latent heats at T_1 and T_2 respectively and T_c is the critical temperature.

From equation (42) $\sqrt{\Delta H^{\mathrm{v}} V}$ should be proportional to the characteristic volume, which can be obtained by the addition of factors. Einstein [171, 172] suggested that $\sqrt{\Delta H V}$ would be additive and Scatchard [173] pointed out that $\sqrt{\Delta H^{\mathrm{v}} V}$ was linear with the number of carbon atoms in homologous series. Small [174] gave a list of what he calls 'molecular attraction constants', which may be used to estimate $\sqrt{\Delta H^{\mathrm{v}} V}$ for unassociated compounds. Other sets of these constants have been proposed by Hoy [175] and by van Krevelen and Hoftyzer [176]. These constants have been compared [169] with values caculated from V_{x} with equation (42): it will be seen from Table 21 that most of them are close to $P_{\mathrm{x}}^{1/2} V_{\mathrm{x}}/3$. Molecular attraction constants have been much used for the estimation of cohesive energy densities and solubility parameters, particularly in studies of plastics and paints. These quantities can now be written:

$$\text{cohesive energy density} = \Delta H^{\mathrm{v}}/V = P_{\mathrm{x}} V_{\mathrm{x}}^2/9V^2 \tag{46}$$

$$\text{solubility parameter} = \left(\frac{\Delta H^{\mathrm{v}}}{V}\right)^{1/2} = \frac{P_{\mathrm{x}}^{1/2} V_{\mathrm{x}}}{3V} \tag{47}$$

If $a^{1/2}/b$ is a constant, the equation (21) will always give a zero value for ΔH^{M}. The important equation is therefore (22) in which $a^{1/2}/b$ is replaced by $a^{1/2}/V$ which is proportional to V_{x}/V, as indeed is δ. The 'regular solution' equation is often used for the comparison of different solvents for one solute. It is found that the solubilities are more or less in the same order as the values of δ. These values of δ are often obtained from the internal heat of evaporation corrected for temperature and the molecule volume. It is more convenient to use, instead of δ, the readily available ratio of characteristic volume to molecular volume. Both the cohesive density and the work of compression treatments of solubility show that the solubility (as measured by the volume fraction) should be a function of $V_{\mathrm{x}}/V{:}V$ is $M/\rho_1 - \rho_{\mathrm{g}}$ which is usually close to M/ρ_1. Table 22 gives values of V_{x}/V for some liquids. These values may be useful in choice of a solvent. For example, ethylene dibromide has a value of $V_{\mathrm{x}}/V = 0.855$ at 298 K. It has a boiling point of 404 K which is convenient for most purposes, does not give strong interactions, and is sufficiently volatile to be easily removed. It was used [178] for recrystallisation of 2,9-dibromo-3,8-dimethoxy-5a,10b-diphenyl-coumarano-2',3',2,3-coumaran and of 2,4,7,9-tetrabromo-3,8-dimethoxy-5a, 10b-diphenylcoumarano-2',3',2,3-coumaran after the more common solvents proved to be unsuitable.

It is desirable [185, 186] that solubilities should be related to the properties of the pure liquids under similar conditions rather than to properties of dilute gases at very different densities and temperatures. The equation (32) does relate solubilities to properties of the liquids at the temperature of the solution. As soon as a solution becomes concentrated, its properties will differ appreciably from those of the solvent; for this reason, the equation, in which it is assumed

Table 21. Molecular attraction constants ($N^{1/2}$ m²).

Group	Constituents	Small [174]	Hoy [175]	van Krevelen and Hoftyzer [176]	$\dfrac{P_x^{1/2} V_x}{3}$
CH_3	C+3H+3.5 bonds	0.44	0.30	0.42	0.43
CH_2	C+2H+3 bonds	0.27	0.27	0.28	0.31
$-\overset{\mid}{\underset{\mid}{C}}-$	C+2 bonds	−0.19	0.07	0	0.07
$CH_2=$	C+2H+2.5 bonds	0.39	0.26	—	0.39
$C\equiv C$	2C+2 bonds	0.45	—	—	0.44
Phenyl	6C+5H+11.5 bonds	1.50	—	1.52	1.47
Naphthyl	10C+7H+18.5 bonds	2.34	—	—	2.29
O (ethers)	O+1 bond	0.14	0.24	0.26	0.13
CO (ketones)	C+O+2 bonds	0.56	0.54	0.69	0.35
COO (esters)	C+2O+3 bonds	0.63	0.67	0.51	0.48
CN	C+N+1.5 bonds	0.84	0.73	0.98	0.46
NCO	C+N+O+2.5 bonds	—	0.73	—	0.60
F	F+0.5 bond	—	0.08	0.16	0.16
Cl (single)	Cl+0.5 bond	0.55	0.42	0.47	0.39
Br (single)	Br+0.5 bond	0.70	0.53	0.61	0.51
I (single)	I+0.5 bond	0.87	—	—	0.70
CF_2	C+2F+3 bonds	0.31	—	—	0.39
S	S+1 bond	0.46	0.43	0.46	0.36

Table 22. Ratios of characteristic volumes (V_x) to molecular volumes [177] (V) at 298.2 K and characteristic temperatures.

Compound	V_x/V	T_x/K
Perfluoroheptane [179]	0.609	369
Perfluoromethylcyclohexane [179–182]	0.630	379
Diethyl ether	0.698	427
Hexafluorobenzene [183]	0.709	437
n-Hexane	0.726	454
Silicon tetrachloride	0.732	461
Acetone	0.739	469
n-Heptane	0.743	474
1,1-Dichloroethane	0.750	483
Octamethylcyclotetrasiloxane [184]	0.751	484
n-Octane	0.756	491
Methanol	0.757	493
3-Methylheptane	0.759	496
trans-1,2-Dichloroethylene	0.761	498
Carbon tetrachloride	0.762	500
Chloroform	0.764	503
Ethanol	0.765	504
n-Nonane	0.766	506
Isopropanol	0.767	508
Methylcyclohexane	0.771	514
n-Decane	0.774	519
Cyclohexane	0.775	520
cis-1,2-Dichloroethylene	0.778	526
Fluorobenzene	0.778	526
Butanol	0.795	557
n-Tetradecane	0.796	559
1,2-Dichloroethane	0.799	566
Benzene	0.801	570
Toluene	0.802	572
m-Xylene	0.808	586
Carbon disulphide	0.809	588
1-Decanol	0.810	590
1-Octanol	0.820	616
Chlorobenzene	0.821	619
Bromobenzene	0.844	690
Cyclohexanol	0.853	725

Table 22 (cont'd)

Compound	V_x/V	T_x/K
Ethylene dibromide	0.855	733
Nitrobenzene	0.867	788
Iodobenzene	0.871	808
Bromoform	0.881	865
Aniline	0.891	933
Water	0.926	1320

that the solution has the same properties as the solvent, could only be expected to apply to saturated solutions which are dilute, and unassociated liquids do not form dilute saturated solutions near room temperature. Gases and solids do give dilute solutions in many solvents and the equation (32) can be modified for use with these. How this can be done will be described below.

(e) THE DISTRIBUTION LAW

The following explanation of this law is given by Lewis [187]. If a gas is dissolved in a solvent, the number of molecules passing from the liquid to the space above the solvent, in a given time, is equal to the number passing in the opposite direction. If the quantity of gas in the gas phase is doubled, then (in the simplest case) the quantity dissolved must also be doubled in order that the number of gas molecules passing from the gas phase to the solution shall be equal to the number passing in the opposite direction. Now, at constant volume, double the quanity of gas in the gas phase means double the pressure. This has caused the concentration of gas in the solvent to be doubled. In other words, the concentration of dissolved gas is proportional to the gas pressure. This particular case of the distribution law is called Henry's law, after Henry [188] who in 1803 observed that the volume of nitrogen, oxygen, hydrogen sulphide, carbon dioxide or nitrous oxide absorbed by 100 cubic inches of water at 60°F varied approximately as the pressure of that gas above the solution (see Gerrard [189]). Henry wrote: 'Under equal circumstances of temperature, water takes up, in all cases, the same volume of condensed gas as of gas under ordinary pressure. But, as the spaces occupied by every gas are inversely as the compressing force, it follows that water takes up, of gas condensed by one, two or more additional atmospheres, a quantity which, ordinarily compressed, would be equal to twice, thrice and etc. the volume absorbed under the common pressure of the atmosphere.'

The first example of the partition law was given by Berthelot and Jungfleisch [190]. They studied the partition of bromine and iodine between water and carbon disulphide and found that even when the concentrations varied for each halogen, the ratio of the concentrations in the two phases remained constant. Thus

$$\frac{\text{Conc of halogen in carbon disulphide}}{\text{Conc of halogen in water}} = \text{a constant at a given temperature}$$

Nernst [191] generalised the law and showed how it could be applied to study dissociation and association. The distribution law as stated by Nernst is: 'When a solute distributes itself between two non-miscible solvents, there exists for each molecular species, at a given temperature a constant ratio of distribution between the two solvents and this ratio is independent of any other molecular species which may be present'.

Acetic acid exists in the vapour and in unassociated solvents largely as a dimer. In water, the monomer is stabilised by interaction with water and the acid is predominately in this form but ionised slightly. In Table 23 the values of Herz and Fischer [192] for partition of acetic acid between water and benzene are given. If a monomer is the species largely present in one solvent, and in the second solvent associated molecules A_n are formed, and if a' is the fraction of these associated molecules which dissociates into simple molecules, then the concentration of associated molecules $= (1 - a')c$ and the concentration of unassociated molecules $= nac$. According to the law of mass action for the equilibrium $A_n \rightleftharpoons nA$

$$\frac{(a'c)^n}{(1 - a')c} = \text{a constant } K$$

Table 23. Partition of acetic acid between benzene and water [192].

Concentrations (mol m^{-3})			
Benzene layer (B)	Aqueous layer (W)	B/W	$\sqrt{\text{B/W}}$
15.9	579.3	0.0274	0.0069
26.1	855.7	0.0305	0.0060
55.4	1382.1	0.0401	0.0054
107.5	2054.3	0.0523	0.0052
158.0	2586.7	0.0610	0.0049
192.8	2892.6	0.0666	0.0048
255.9	3298.4	0.0776	0.0048
500.7	4976.4	0.1006	0.0045
758.6	6366.0	0.1191	0.0043
905.3	6997.4	0.1294	0.0043

When a' is small, i.e. when the degree of association is large, it can be neglected compared with unity and then $c = K^n\sqrt{c}$. In other words, the concentration of simple molecules is proportional to $\sqrt[n]{c}$ and the partition coefficient becomes $C_1/\sqrt[n]{C_2}$. For the stronger solutions of acetic acid, the acid is largely dimerised in benzene and n is two.

The following quotation from Lewis [193] shows the importance of the distribution law. 'We owe to van't Hoff the discovery of the close connection between the behaviour of gases and the behaviour of substances in the dissolved state. The thermodynamic proof of the applicability of the gas law expansion $PV = RT$ to the osmotic pressure—concentration relations of a dissolved substance cannot be done *simply* on thermodynamic grounds. It is necessary to assume the truth of the experimental law discovered by Henry, namely, that the concentration of gas dissolved in a liquid is proportional to the pressure of the gas at the given temperature.' This is not always appreciated.

(f) CONCENTRATION UNITS

In all the early, and many later, studies of the distribution law (see previous section), concentrations were expressed as molarities, i.e. mol per unit volumes of solutions. Other measures of concentration have, however, been used and it is of interest to consider the relationships between different measures. In the following discussion, any volume change which takes place on solution is ignored. Volume changes are considered in Chapter 4, section (c).

If C is the concentration expressed as a molarity, i.e. mol per unit volume of solution, then the volume fraction y, volume of solute per unit volume of solution, is given by

$$y = CV \tag{48}$$

where V is the molecular volume of the liquid solute (estimated from other properties and temperatures if necessary).

The volume of solute per unit volume of solvent is

$$\frac{CV}{1-CV} \tag{49}$$

The mol of solute per unit volume of solvent is

$$\frac{C}{1-CV} \tag{50}$$

The mass of solute per unit volume of solvent is

$$\frac{CM}{1-CV} \tag{51}$$

where M is the mass of one mol of solute.

The mass of solute per unit mass of solvent is

$$\frac{CM}{\rho'(1-CV)} \tag{52}$$

where ρ' is the density of the pure solvent.

The molal concentration, which is the mol of solute per unit mass of solvent is

$$\frac{C}{\rho'(1-CV)} \tag{53}$$

Gerrard [194] has pointed out that the molality does not equal the molarity but that the ratio of the two units at infinite dilution (i.e. when $C = 0$) equals the density, ρ' of the liquid. The ratio molar/molal falls as the concentrations increase and when the solution is so strong that it is nearly pure solute (i.e. when CV approaches unity), the molal concentration tends to infinity. In the same way the expressions (49), (50), (51) and (52) also tend to infinity when the solution is very concentrated. So does the mol ratio which is

$$\frac{CV^*}{(1-CV)} \tag{54}$$

where V^* is the molecular volume of the pure solvent. In Chapters 4, section (b) and 5, section (a), equation (32), based on volume fractions (or molar concentrations), is given for the estimations of solubilities. This equation can be applied over the whole range from dilute solutions to pure liquid solute. The fact is that partition coefficients (J), ratios of concentrations of a compound in an unassociated liquid and in water, do not usually differ greatly from the ratio of C_L, the concentration of the pure liquid in itself, to C_S, the concentration of the saturated solution in water. In Table 24, the logarithms of partition coefficients between ether and water from Collander [228] are compared with values of $\log_{10}(C_L/C_S)$ for compounds also given in reference [38], Tables II and III.

Table 24. Comparison of partition coefficients (J) between ether and water and the ratios of the concentration of compounds in their pure liquid state (C_L) to the concentration of a saturated solution in water at about 295 K.

Compound	$\text{Log}_{10} J$ [228]	$\text{Log}_{10}(C_L/C_S)$
Methyl acetate	0.4	0.5
Ethyl acetate	0.9	1.1
1-Butanol	0.9	1.1
Ethyl iodide	2.4	2.6

There seems to be little justification for the use of molal concentrations or other measures of concentrations based on per unit mass or per unit volume of solvent.

Yet another measure sometimes used for concentrations is the mol fraction x

$$x = \frac{CV^*}{1 + C(V^* - V)} \qquad (55)$$

CV is the volume fraction (see (48)) and cannot be greater than one and so if CV^* is large the mol fraction will tend to unity. For sufficiently dilute solutions and solutions with V^* close in value to V, the mol fraction will approach CV^*. Lindenberg and Massin [195] expressed partition coefficients as ratios of mol fractions and for phenol between water and benzene; nitrobenzene; and arachis oil, gave 11.1; 50.9; and 346 respectively. It looks from this as if phenol is particularly soluble in arachis oil but this is not so. When these partition coefficients are converted to ratios of concentrations, the figures are 2.2, 9.0 and 5.9 respectively (the molecular mass of arachis oil was taken as 0.95 kg mol^{-1} and the density as 960 kg m^{-3}); the value for arachis oil falls between the values for benzene and nitrobenzene. The question of the units to be used for concentrations has been considered by several workers and they conclude that molarity is best [196 198].

It follows from equation (13) of Hammick and Andrew [110] that V_X, the characteristic volume of the mixture

$$V_X = x_A V_X^A + x_B V_X^B \qquad (56)$$

The use of these expressions may be illustrated as follows. In Chapter 4, section (d), it was shown (47) that the solubility parameter $\delta = 2.2 \times 10^4 \, V_X/V$ where V is the molar volume, M/ρ. From equations (48), (50), (53) and (56), the solubility parameter δ_M for a mixture of two unassociated liquids A and B, if there is no volume change or interaction on mixing,

$$\delta_M = 2.2 \times 10^4 \, V_X^M/V^M = 2.2 \times 10^4 \left[\frac{Y_A \rho_A}{M_A} V_X^A + \frac{Y_B \rho_B}{M_B} V_X^B \right]$$

$$= Y_A \delta_A + Y_B \delta_B \qquad (57)$$

The equation (57) was proposed by Smith, Walkley and Hildebrand [199]. An alternative to (57) is (58)

$$\delta_M = 2.2 \times 10^4 \, (V_X^A [A] + V_X^B [B]) \qquad (58)$$

This could be used when there is a volume change on mixing.

From equation (44), $\Delta H^V = 4.8 \times 10^8 \, V_X^2/V$ and if this equation is used for a mixture in the same way that (58) was obtained for δ_M from (44):

$$\Delta H_M^V = 4.8 \times 10^8 \, (V_X^A [A] + V_X^B [B]) (x_A V_X^A + x_B V_X^B) \qquad (59)$$

This seems to be a new relationship. Usually both ΔH_M^V and the composition change during distillation of a mixture but equation (59) may be useful for the estimation of the (internal) latent heat of evaporation of azeotropes consisting of unassociated liquids giving no interactions. Here ΔH_M^V refers to 298 K.

(g) SOLUBILITIES OF GASES, VAPOURS AND SOLIDS

A solid below the melting point will have a lower vapour pressure p_s than that p of the (super-cooled) liquid at the same temperature and will therefore be less soluble than this liquid by a factor which can be taken as p_s/p. In the same way, the solution of an unsaturated vapour at pressure P will have a concentration equal to the concentration of the solution of the saturated vapour reduced by the factor P/p. In equation (30), C_L has to be multiplied by these factors to give what is often called 'the ideal solubility' C_i of the vapour or solid.

According to the phase rule, a system of one component existing in two phases has one degree of freedom: the pressure and temperature can vary but not independently. If a liquid and its vapour are in equilibrium (vapour) pressure p and temperature T and also at $p + \partial p$ and $T + \partial T$, then since in both cases equilibrium exists, the changes ΔG of Gibbs free energy are equal for both liquid and gas phases so that

$$-S_g \partial T + V_g \partial P = -S_L \partial T + V_L \partial P$$

or

$$(S_g - S_L)\partial T = (V_g - V_L)\partial P.$$

The difference between the (molar) entropies equals the molar heat of vaporisation (ΔH_e) divided by the temperature and hence, providing liquid is present, the vapour pressure is independent of the volume of the vapour:

$$\frac{dp}{dT} = \frac{\Delta H_e}{T(V_g - V_L)} \tag{60}$$

Equation (60) is known as the Clapeyron equation and has been written

$$d(\log_e p) = \frac{-\Delta HT}{p(V_g - V_L)} \ d\left(\frac{1}{T}\right) \tag{61}$$

Equation (61) can be integrated if it is assumed that

$$\frac{\Delta HT}{p(V_g - V_L)}$$

is a constant B; this assumption is nearer the truth than the assumption that either ΔH or $p(V_g - V_L)/T$ is a constant. The integrated equation is

$$\log_e p = A - \frac{B}{T} \tag{62}$$

Provided the temperature is considerably below the critical temperature, V_L can be neglected compared with V_g and if, in addition, the vapour is assumed to behave like a perfect gas, $V_g = RT/p$ and then $B = \Delta H/R$. At the boiling point T_{B1} the vapour pressure is atmospheric and according to Trouton's law [200], at the boiling point $\Delta H/T_B$ is approximately constant ($87 \text{ J mol}^{-1} \text{ K}^{-1}$).

Littlewood [201] has combined (62) with Trouton's Rule and $B = \Delta H/R$ to give

$$\log_{10} p(\text{N m}^{-2}) = 9.8 - 4.8\, T_{\text{B}/\text{T}} \tag{63}$$

The approximate equation (62) with $B = \Delta H/R$ can be applied to the solid as well as to the liquid. At the melting point T_{M}, the values of p for the solid and liquid are equal so that

$$A_{\text{s}} - \frac{\Delta H_{\text{s}}}{RT_{\text{M}}} = A_{\text{L}} - \frac{\Delta H_{\text{L}}}{RT_{\text{M}}}$$

Equation (62) applied to solid and liquid at temperature T gives

$$\log p_{\text{s}} - \log p = A_{\text{s}} - A_{\text{L}} - \frac{\Delta H_{\text{s}}}{RT} + \frac{\Delta H_{\text{L}}}{RT}$$

$$= \frac{\Delta H_{\text{s}}}{RT_{\text{M}}} - \frac{\Delta H_{\text{L}}}{RT_{\text{M}}} - \frac{\Delta H_{\text{s}}}{RT} + \frac{\Delta H_{\text{L}}}{RT}$$

But the latent heat of fusion $\Delta H_{\text{f}} = \Delta H_{\text{s}} - \Delta H_{\text{L}}$ and so

$$\log_{\text{e}} (C_{\text{L}}/C_{\text{i}}) = \log_{\text{e}} (p/p_{\text{s}}) = \frac{\Delta H_{\text{f}}}{R}\left(\frac{1}{T} - \frac{1}{T_{\text{M}}}\right) \tag{64}$$

The latent heat of fusion is usually available at the melting point T_{m} and a correction is required to correct to temperature T. The corrected equation is

$$RT\log_{\text{e}} (C_{\text{L}}/C_{\text{i}}) = (\Delta H_{\text{f}} - \Delta C_{\text{p}} T_{\text{m}})\left(1 - \frac{T}{T_{\text{M}}}\right) - \frac{\Delta C_{\text{p}}}{T}\log_{\text{e}} \frac{T_{\text{m}}}{T} \tag{65}$$

ΔC_{p} equals $C_{\text{p}}^{\text{l}} - C_{\text{p}}^{\text{S}}$, the difference between the specific heat of the liquid and that of the solid. The corrected equation contains two large terms which give a small difference and are not of much practical value. Fortunately, partition coefficients and other ratios of solubilities can be estimated without the use of ideal solubilities.

The solubilities of solid iodine in a number of solvents at 298.2 K have been given [202, 203]. Benesi and Hildebrand [203] extrapolated the molecular volume given for liquid iodine down to 298.2 and give a value of 5.9×10^{-5} m³ mol⁻¹ so that $V_{\text{x}}/V_0 = 1.06$, which is impossibly high and probably means that liquid iodine is not simply I_2 (one bond) but contains species I_n ($n - 1$ bonds). However, the value of $V_{\text{x}}/V_0 = 1.06$ was used, together with those given in Table 22 for solvents, with equation (32) to estimate the values of $\log_{10} C_{\text{s}}$ given in Table 25; the results are compared with experimental figures which have been converted to mol m⁻³ on the assumption that there is no volume change on solution. Solubilities for sulphur have been listed by Hildebrand and Scott [204] and these (mol m⁻³ on the assumption that solution involves no volume change)

Table 25. Solubilities of iodine at 298.2 K.

Solvent	Estimated $\log_{10} C_s$ (C_s in mol m^{-3})	Found [202, 203]
Perfluoroheptane	−0.8	−0.1
n-Hexane	1.2	1.5
Silicon tetrachloride	1.3	1.6
n-Heptane	1.3	1.7
2,2,4-Trimethylpentane	1.1	1.6
1,1-Dichloroethane	1.5	1.3
Octamethylcyclotetrasiloxane [135]	1.5	1.5
trans-1,2-Dichloroethylene	1.7	2.3
Carbon tetrachloride	1.7	2.1
Chloroform	1.7	2.5
cis-1,2-Dichloroethylene	1.9	2.3
Benzene	2.1	2.7
1,2-Dichloroethane	2.1	2.4
Carbon disulphide	2.6	3.0
Ethylene dibromide	2.8	3.0
Bromoform	2.9	3.0
Ideal	3.6	3.6

are given in Table 26. Hildebrand and Jenks [205] used 1.35×10^{-4} m^3 mol^{-1} as the molecular volume of liquid sulphur at 298.2 K. From this figure and 0.282, which these authors took for the mol fraction of the ideal solution, C_i equals 2080 mol m^{-3}. The estimated solubilities from these figures, the characteristic molecular volume of S_8 (eight bonds), the ratios of characteristic molecular volume to molecular volume for the solvents (Table 22) and the equation (32) are given in Table 26.

Hildebrand and Scott [135] have pointed out that a difficulty in any theory of solubility is that it must deal with small differences between large quantities. This is the case when equation (32) is used and in view of this, the agreement with experimental values is quite encouraging. Small changes in characteristic molecular volumes and molecular volumes have a large effect upon the solubilities estimated. Also, there is evidence that solvents and solutes may interact where this has not previously been suspected. The observed solubilities of sulphur in ether and in carbon disulphide are considerably higher than the estimated ones and so these two solvents may complex with sulphur. Smith and Walkley [206] have suggested that carbon disulphide does complex with sulphur and also that iodine complexes with benzene. Hildebrand and Scott [207] found that iodine not only complexes with benzene but it also seems to form weak complexes with bromoform, the two dichloroethanes, and the two dichloro-

Table 26. Solubilities of sulphur at 298.2 K.

| Solvent | Solubility (mol m^{-3}) | |
	Estimated	Found [204]
Diethyl ether	4.8	28
n-Heptane	27	9
Carbon tetrachloride	52	51
Chloroform	57	70
Benzene	146	71
Ethylene dichloride	163	40
Toluene	178	69
m-Xylene	210	67
Carbon disulphide	212	2550
Ethylene dibromide	625	229
Iodobenzene	834	148
Ideal	2080	2080

ethenes, although the solutions of iodine in these solvents are violet and not the brown colour which indicates strong complex formation. Octamethylcyclotetrasiloxane does not complex with iodine. Since the internal latent heats per unit volume of octamethylcyclotetrasiloxane and perfluoroheptane are nearly the same, these solvents would be expected from treatment of solubilities based on solubility parameters to be completely miscible and to dissolve other compounds to about the same extent. However, the two solvents are not completely miscible [208] and Shinoda and Hildebrand [209] found that iodine was much more soluble in octamethylcyclotetrasiloxane than in perfluoroheptane (see Table 25). Ross and Hildebrand [185] point out that octamethylcyclotetrasiloxane resembles carbon tetrachloride in its solvent properties. At 298.2 K the ratio of the characteristic volume to molecular volume V_x/V is 0.751 for octamethyl-cyclotetrasiloxane and 0.782 for carbon tetrachloride but only 0.609 for perfluoroheptane.

Hildebrand [135] calculated what he calls the ideal solubility (as a mol fraction x) of a gas from the vapour pressure (or pressure itself) at a given temperature from the approximate Raoult's law equation

$$x = P/p$$

P is the vapour pressure over the solution and p, the saturation vapour pressure, for a gas is obtained from the plots of $\log p_0$ against $1/T$ (equation (62)) for the liquid extrapolated, if necessary, beyond the critical point to the desired temperature.

The ratio V_x/V drops as the temperature rises, so that for many unassociated organic liquids at their boiling points (V_x/V) is around 0.7 and at the critical point the ratio is only about 0.26. Thus for a permanent gas (V_x/V) must be so small compared with (V_x'/V') for the solvent that in equation (32), the terms

$$\frac{1}{8}\left(\frac{V_x}{V}\right)^5$$

and

$$\frac{1}{9}\left(\frac{V_x}{V}\right)^6\left(\frac{V'}{V_x'}\right)$$

may, as a first approximation, be neglected compared to the second term

$$\frac{1}{72}\left(\frac{V_x'}{V'}\right)^8\left(\frac{V}{V_x}\right)^3$$

The logarithms of the solubilities of a permanent gas do give straight lines when plotted against $(V_x'/V')^8$ for solvents. This has already been illustrated for argon [163]. The logarithms of Ostwald coefficients [210–216], L (the ratio of concentration of gas in the solution and in the gas space) for argon in 17 solvents at 298.2 K were plotted against $(V_x'/V')^8$. The points fell near a straight line corresponding to (66)

$$-\log_{10}L = 2.532\,(V_x'/V')^8 + 0.162\ (N = 0.994) \tag{66}$$

In Fig. 10, values of $\log_{10}L$ for argon are plotted against $(V_x'/V')^8$ and as well as unassociated liquids, water and alcohols are among the solvents. It will be seen that the points for these associated solvents fall close to the line. It would therefore seem that equation (32) can be used for the solution of compounds in associated and unassociated solvents provided the solutions are dilute. A small concentration of an inert compound might be expected to have little effect upon association of a solvent. The equation (32) would not, however, be expected to apply when the associated liquids is the solute because in a dilute solution, the association would almost certainly be reduced and might disappear altogether. No allowance has been made here for the reduction in solubilities caused by the break-up of association when holes are made to accommodate the argon molecules. These molecules are small and so the term for hole formation would probably be negligible compared with the effect of the difference in compressibility. The term for hole-formation (see next section) would have to be included in the estimation of larger molecules in such associated liquids as water and methanol if large molecules were being disolved in them. It is interesting that compounds with a high content of fluorine have low values of V_x/V and are therefore good solvents for gases. In future, this property may find important applications. Emulsions of perfluorinated hydrocarbons in water have been studies as carriers for oxygen and carbon dioxide in place of blood in living animals and this subject has been reviewed recently [216]. The perfluorinated compounds, because their V_x/V values are so low compared with most other compounds, will be less soluble and less likely to show physical toxicity.

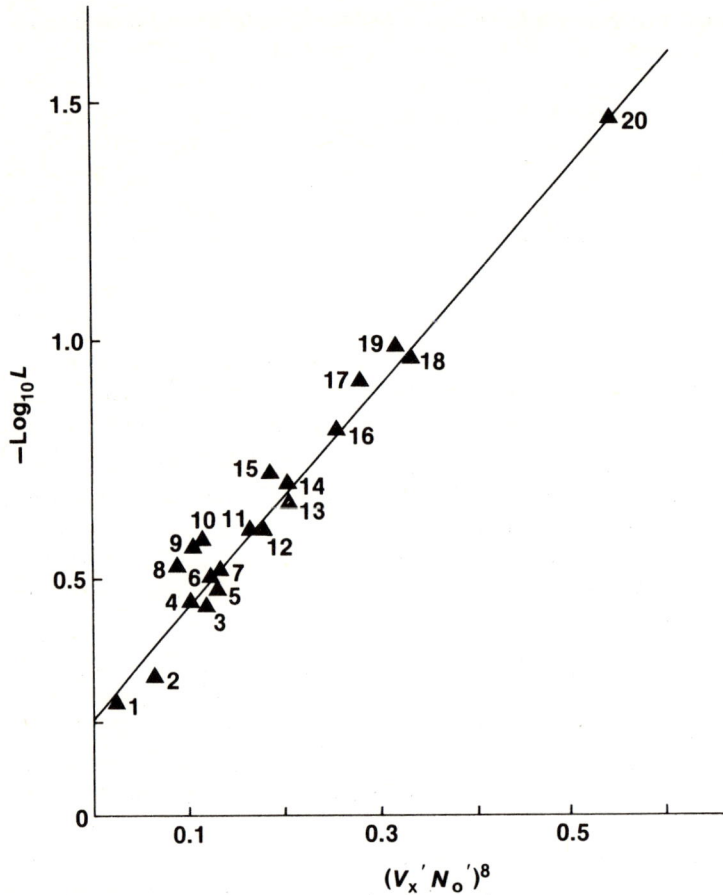

Fig. 10. Solubilities of argon at 298.2 K. Relationship between Ostwald coefficients (L) and $(V_x'/V')^8$ for solvent. Solvents are: (1) perfluoromethylcyclohexane; (2) hexafluorobenzene; (3) methylcyclohexane; (4) n-octane; (5) cyclohexane; (6) n-decane; (7) fluorobenzene; (8) acetone; (9) methanol; (10) ethanol; (11) benzene; (12) toluene; (13) 1-octanol; (14) chlorobenzene; (15) 1-decanol; (16) bromobenzene; (17) cyclohexanol; (18) iodobenzene; (19) nitrobenzene; (20) water.

Equation (32), repeated here,

$$RT \log_e (C_s/C_L) = P_x V_x \left[\frac{1}{8} \left(\frac{V_x}{V} \right)^5 - \frac{1}{72} \left(\frac{V_x'}{V'} \right)^8 \left(\frac{V}{V_x} \right)^3 \right.$$

$$\left. - \frac{1}{9} \left(\frac{V_x}{V} \right)^6 \left(\frac{V'}{V_x'} \right) \right] \tag{32}$$

shows that the solubility depends on the characteristic volume of the solute V_x as well as on the ratio V_x/V_0. However, as long as the solution is dilute, the solubility does not depend on V_X', the characteristic volume of the solvent, but only on the ratio V_X'/V'. Polymers, and other substances with molecules of large size, behave normally as solvents: V_X'/V' can be worked out from the molecular mass M' and the characteristic volume V_X' of the units making up the polymer and the density. It is often more convenient to find T_X' and use (see equation (5)) $(1 - T/T_X')^{2.4}$ instead of $(V_X'/V')^8$. For polyolefines T_X has been given [23, 85] as 800 K and so from equation (66) for T equal to 298.2 K

$$-\log_{10} L = 2.532 \left(1 - \frac{298.2}{800}\right)^{2.4} + 0.162 = 0.989$$

Michaels and Bixler (216] give $-\log_{10} L$ for argon in amorphous polyethylene as 0.987, which is closer to the value calculated than might have been expected. However, polymers will only dissolve if the expression in brackets on the right of the equation is very small, so that this expression multiplied by the large characteristic volume V_X gives not too large a (negative) value of $\log C_S/C_L$.

(h) ESTIMATION OF CHARACTERISTIC TEMPERATURE AND SOLUBILITIES BY COMPUTER

In Chapter 2, methods have been given for the estimation of many of the properties of a compound from two constants — the characteristic volume V_X and the characteristic temperature T_X. It is usually necessary to measure some properties to find T_X and these T_X values will vary somewhat. The T_X value will be chosen for some estimation after the values listed have been weighted in favour of those considered to be most accurate and those derived from properties and under conditions nearest to those for which the T_X value will be used.

For polymers, although values of the characteristic volume V_X and the mass per mol M are not usually available, the ratio V_X/M can readily be calculated from the values for the unit making up the structure. For poly(ethene), the unit $(-CH_2 CH_2)_n$ (two carbons, four hydrogens and six bonds) gives $V_X = (2.818 \times 10^{-5})_n$ m^3 mol^{-1} and $M = (2.8054 \times 10^{-2})_n$ kg mol^{-1}. These figures can be used with formula (4) to find T_X from the liquid density. The formulae (5) and (6) can be used to give T_X directly from surface tensions or isothermal compressibilities of the liquid. In Table 27, the densities and surface tensions given by Schonhorn and Sharpe [217] and the isothermal compressibilities given by Cogswell [218] have been used to find values for the characteristic temperature of liquid poly(ethene). These values are around 800 K which was taken [23, 85] for the characteristic temperature of polyethylene: the range is 760–816 K. Values of each property have been estimated for T_X equal to 760, 800 and 816 K.

In Appendices I and II, there are programs in BASIC to be used on a computer for the calculation of values of T_X from properties of liquids and for the estimation from T_X of properties of unassociated liquids. Another program in

Table 27. Estimation of properties of poly(ethene).

Property	T (K)	Value found (SI units)	T_x from property	Estimated values of property with T equal to		
				760	800	816
Density	411.2	793	774	788	802	807
	425.2	788	786	778	793	798
	439.2	781	792	769	784	790
	466.2	762	791	749	766	772
Surface tension	411.2	0.0274	805	0.0254	0.0272	0.0279
	425.2	0.0264	809	0.0242	0.0260	0.0267
	439.2	0.0253	810	0.0230	0.0248	0.0256
	466.2	0.0233	814	0.0207	0.0226	0.0234
Isothermal compressibility	423.2	9.7×10^{-10}	760	9.7×10^{-10}	8.7×10^{-10}	8.4×10^{-10}
	543.2	16.1×10^{-10}	816	21.4×10^{-10}	17.4×10^{-10}	16.1×10^{-10}

Appendix II is given for the estimation of solubilities in unassociated liquids and in Appendix III, there are values of some properties for use with this program. In these programs SI units are used. Estimated solubilities can be expressed in a variety of ways, since densities of the solutions can be calculated from the characteristic volumes and characteristic temperatures of the components if it is assumed that there is no volume change on solution. For the estimation of the solubilities of solids, melting points and latent heats of fusion are required. When the solute is a liquid, in place of the melting point, any temperature below that for the solubility can be entered with any value for the latent heat of fusion because these figures will then be ignored. If the solute and solvent are given the same characteristic volume and characteristic temperature, the solubility given by the program will be an estimate of the ideal solubility of a solid or the concentration of a liquid in its own liquid phase.

In Table 28 the solubilities of anthracene measured by Mahieu [219] are compared with the values estimated with the aid of the program in Appendix II and the values for properties given in Appendix III. The solubilities estimated are of the right order but on the whole the agreement is rather poor.

Table 28. Solubilities of anthracene in some unassociated liquids [219].

Solvent (temperature)	Solubility (kg per kg solvent)	
	Experimental	Found
Hexane (298.2)	3.1×10^{-3}	2.6×10^{-3}
Cyclohexane (313.2)	6.5×10^{-3}	9.3×10^{-3}
1,1'-Oxybis-ethane		
(diethyl ether) (298.2)	8.5×10^{-3}	1.1×10^{-3}
2-Propanone (acetone)		
(298.2)	1.33×10^{-2}	2.9×10^{-3}
Bromobenzene (298.2)	1.37×10^{-2}	7.0×10^{-3}
Nitrobenzene (298.2)	1.51×10^{-2}	9.9×10^{-3}
Chloroform (298.2)	1.62×10^{-2}	2.4×10^{-3}
Chlorobenzene (298.2)	1.64×10^{-2}	7.6×10^{-3}
Benzene (298.2)	1.70×10^{-2}	7.6×10^{-3}
Carbon disulphide (298.2)	2.03×10^{-2}	5.8×10^{-3}
Carbon disulphide (313.2)	3.14×10^{-2}	9.9×10^{-3}

Equation (32) and the program in Appendix II are based on the work required to change the compressibility of the solute until it equals the compressibility of the solvent. The work should, however, be that required to bring the compressibilities of solute and solvent to that of the solution and equation (32) will only apply to dilute solutions.

The T_X values for most of the unassociated organic solvents fall within a narrow range, as has already been noted, they are nearly all completely miscible with each other. Further, the solubility of a given solid in them does not vary greatly. Since the solubilities of liquids and solids in associated liquids show wide variation, clearly some new factor has to be considered in these cases. This factor is the break-up of the association which results when molecules are dissolved in the associated liquid and will be considered in the next chapter.

(i) CHARACTERISTIC VOLUMES AND MUTUAL SOLUBILITIES OF UNASSOCIATED LIQUIDS

Equation (4) can be used to replace values of V_X/V in equation (32) by T/T_X to give (67).

$$\frac{-\log_e(C_S/C_L)}{V_X} = \frac{P_X}{RT}\left(1 - \frac{T}{T_X}\right)^{1.5}$$

$$\left[\frac{\left(1 - \dfrac{T}{T_X'}\right)^{2.4}}{\dfrac{1}{2}\left(1 - \dfrac{T}{T_X}\right)^{2.4}} + \frac{\left(1 - \dfrac{T}{T_X}\right)^{0.3}}{9\left(1 - \dfrac{T}{T_X'}\right)^{0.3}} - \frac{1}{8}\right]$$

$$(67)$$

Provided the values of

$$1 - \frac{T}{T_X}$$

are not too small (less than 0.2), the expression on the right hand side of equation (67) is altered by only a small amount if the values of T_X and T_X' are reversed (see Table 29). Since C_S/C_L = the volume fraction y (see equation 52) this means that

$$\frac{\log y}{\log y'} = \text{approximately } \frac{V_X}{V_X'} \tag{68}$$

i.e. for two unassociated liquids, which when mixed give dilute solutions in two phases, the ratio of logarithms of the volume fractions of the minor component in each layer equals approximately the ratio of the respective characteristic volumes.

From equation (68), it is clear that compounds with very high characteristic volumes, of which polymers are an important class, will usually have low solubilities unless they give specific interactions with the solvent. However, such compounds should behave normally as solvents although they will usually have high characteristic temperatures. Polymers consist of a mixture of species with a

Table 29. Estimation of $-(\log_e y)/V_x$ from equation (68).

A	B	Estimated $-(\log_e y)/V_x$	
		with T_x = A and T'_x = B	with T_x = B and T'_x = A
1 200	1 100	48	48
1 200	1 000	235	234
1 100	1 000	70	70
1 200	900	664	656
1 100	900	353	350
1 000	900	108	107
1 200	800	1 525	1 498
1 100	800	1 026	1 011
1 000	800	555	549
900	800	173	172
1 200	700	3 208	3 125
1 100	700	2 455	2 398
1 000	700	1 681	1 648
900	700	930	916
800	700	298	295
1 200	600	6 593	6 349
1 100	600	5 471	5 202
1 000	600	4 259	4 125
900	600	2 978	2 897
800	600	1 692	1 656
700	600	561	553
1 200	500	14 064	13 339
1 100	500	12 356	11 721
1 000	500	10 407	9 912
900	500	8 268	7 900
800	500	5 932	5 695
700	500	3 484	3 369
600	500	1 209	1 183
1 200	400	34 868	32 767
1 100	400	31 829	29 894
1 000	400	28 361	26 627
900	400	24 393	22 897
800	400	19 847	18 638
700	400	14 681	13 811
600	400	8 984	8 494
500	400	3 312	3 175
450	400	1 047	1 019

range of molecular volumes and it is not easy to find examples to test the relationship (68). Apelblat [220] has studied the mutual solubilities of methyl diphenyl phosphate ($V_x = 1.9701 \times 10^{-4}$ m^3 mol^{-1}) and some n-alkanes over a range of temperatures. He gives his results as mol fractions and does not give the densities which are required to convert these mol fractions to concentrations and volume fractions. He does dive [221] a density $\rho_1 = 1225.8$ km m^{-3} at 298.15 K and $d\rho_1/dT = -0.85$ kg m^{-3} K^{-1} for methyl diphenyl phosphate. On the assumption that there is no volume change when the liquids are mixed, densities of the solutions have been worked out from these figures; densities of n-decane are given by Rossini *et al.* [222] and of the other hydrocarbons by Timmermanns [42, 177]. In Table 30, values are given of $(\log y)/\log y')$ at various temperatures for the two phases from hydrocarbons and methyl diphenyl phosphate. These values are rather higher than the ratios of the characteristic volumes but the agreement with equation (68) is quite encouraging. It is also probably that methyl diphenyl phosphate is a somewhat associated liquid.

Table 30. Values of $(\log y/\log y')$ for the two phases from hydrocarbons and methyl diphenyl phosphate at various temperatures (y is the volume fraction of methyl diphenyl phosphate in the hydrocarbon and y' is the volume fraction for the hydrocarbon in methyl diphenyl phosphate).

	$(\log y/\log y')$				
T (K)	Pentane	Hexane	Heptane	Octane	Decane
263.15	2.57	2.19	1.90	1.68	1.36
273.15	2.58	2.19	1.90	1.68	1.36
283.15	2.58	2.19	1.90	1.68	1.36
293.15	2.58	2.19	1.90	1.68	1.36
303.15	2.58	2.19	1.90	1.68	1.36
313.15	2.58	2.20	1.91	1.68	1.36
323.15	2.58	2.20	1.91	1.69	1.37
333.15	2.58	2.20	1.91	1.69	1.37
343.15	2.58	2.20	1.91	1.69	1.37
353.15	2.57	2.20	1.91	1.69	1.37
363.15	2.57	2.20	1.91	1.69	1.37
373.15	2.56	2.20	1.92	1.69	1.37
Ratio of characteristic volumes	2.42	2.07	1.80	1.59	1.30

5

Specific Interactions and Associated Liquids

(a) THE PROCESS OF SOLUTION

The process of solution of a compound can be considered to occur in two stages. First, holes have to be made in the solvent to accommodate the molecules of the compound and this will require work. Next, the molecules of the compound have to be placed in the holes. Since most non-interacting unassociated liquids mix in all proportions, very little overall energy change must occur when solution takes place. The work required for making the holes will therefore be compensated by the work regained when the holes are filled. If the liquid is associated, i.e. there are specific interactions between the molecules because some special structure exists, extra work will be required to make the holes and this will not be recovered when non-interacting molecules are used to fill the holes, e.g. in such associated liquids as water, salt solutions, molten salts and mercury.

Solubilities of gases were treated more or less on the above lines by Eley [223, 224]. He states that differences between individual organic solvents is too small to justify consideration. Also the energy change, and entropy change, when gas molecules are placed in the cavities are about the same for all solvents including water. The difference in behaviour between water and unassociated liquids is to be accounted for by ΔE_c the internal energy changed involved in the formation of the cavities. Eley used the relationship

$$\Delta E_c = T \frac{\alpha}{\kappa} \bar{V}$$

where T is the temperature, α the coefficient of thermal expansion, κ the iso-thermal compressibility of the solvent and $\bar{V}$ the partial molar volume of the solute in the solvent. McGowan [38] used the parachor V_p as proportional to the molecular volume of the cavities and, since the other factors affected solubility in water were independent of the solute, wrote for these cases where there were no specific interactions. Here V_p has been replaced by the characteristic volume V_x:

$$-\log_{10}(C_s/C_L) = kV_x \qquad (69)$$

where C_s is the solubility, C_L is the concentration of the liquid in its own liquid phase (or the ideal solubility of a solid) and k is a constant at a given temperature. The equation was tested on a large number of non-interacting compounds by Deno and Berkheimer [225]. Every fifth compound on their list has been used for Table 31. For the three solids, partition between benzene and water was used.

It has sometimes been assumed (for example, in discussion of hydro-phobicity) that there are specific attractive forces between molecules in unassociated organic liquids. However, the fact that the solubilities of a wide variety of hydrocarbons and other compounds can be estimated by means of the equation just given shows that this is not so. Actually, the energies arising from van der Waals, or London, forces are practically the same for hydrocarbon–hydrocarbon interactions as for hydrocarbon–water interactions. Deno and Berkheimer [226] explain this cancelling out of energies arising from London dispersion forces as follows:

'Let us consider a molecule such as benzene immersed first in water and then in hexane. The energy arising from London forces [227] between two small spherical molecules in the gas phase is given by

$$E = -\frac{3\alpha_1'\alpha_2'}{2r^6} \frac{I_1 I_2}{(I_1 + I_2)}$$

The polarizability α' and the ionization potential I for benzene are common factors for the equation applied to either benzene–water or benzene–hexane. The ionization potential for water and hexane are 12.5 and 10.5 eV. Although the absolute difference between these two numbers may seem large, the percent difference is small when used in the equation, so that only small energy differences arise from differences in ionization potential. The relative invariance of ionization potential is characteristic of compounds of C, H, O and N, and these are of primary interest in organic chemistry. When elements such as sulphur, iodine, etc. are introduced, their effect is overshadowed by the mass of hydrocarbon, so that, on the average, the effective ionization potential for inter-molecular attractions is that of a typical hydrocarbon.

The electronic polarizabilities of water and hexane are 3.70 and 29.8 cm^3 mole^{-1}. These values initially seem much different but what governs interaction energies in solution is the polarizability per unit volume of the solvents. These values are 0.21 and 0.23, for water and hexane respectively. The London

Table 31. Characteristic volumes and solubilities of some non-interacting compounds [225] in water at 298.2 K.

Compound	V_x (m^3 mol^{-1})	Log C_L	Log C_s	$\dfrac{\text{Log}(C_L/C_s)}{V_x}$
Benzene	7.164×10^{-5}	4.05	1.36	3.75×10^4
1,3-Dimethylbenzene	9.982×10^{-5}	3.91	0.24	3.65×10^4
Butylbenzene	1.280×10^{-4}	3.80	−0.94	3.70×10^4
Diphenylmethane	1.4651×10^{-4}	3.78	−1.06	3.30×10^4
2,4-Diphenyl-4-methyl-2-pentene	2.1266×10^{-4}	3.62	−3.98	3.57×10^4
Octane	1.2362×10^{-4}	3.79	−0.91	3.80×10^4
trans-1,2-Diphenylethylene (s)	1.5630×10^{-4}	3.31	−2.93	3.99×10^4
Phenanthrene (s)	1.4544×10^{-4}	2.69	−2.05	3.26×10^4
Benz[b] anthracene (s)	1.8234×10^{-4}	1.23	−5.27	3.56×10^4
Tetrachloromethane	7.391×10^{-5}	4.02	0.70	4.49×10^4
1,1,1-Trichloroethane	7.575×10^{-5}	4.00	0.99	3.97×10^4
2-Chloropropane	6.537×10^{-5}	4.04	1.59	3.75×10^4
1-chloro-2-methylpropane	7.946×10^{-5}	3.97	1.00	3.74×10^4
Dibromomethane	5.995×10^{-5}	4.16	1.82	3.90×10^4
1,1,2,2-Tetrabromoethane	1.0904×10^{-4}	3.93	0.27	3.36×10^4
1-Bromo-2-methylpropane	8.472×10^{-5}	3.96	0.57	4.00×10^4
1-Iodopropane	7.885×10^{-5}	4.09	1.40	3.41×10^4
Chlorobenzene	8.388×10^{-5}	3.98	0.56	4.08×10^4

dispersion forces will nearly cancel, and this result can be generalized to most systems of interest in organic chemistry.'

Quite apart from the dispersion forces cancelling for many compounds, there is some evidence that whilst the London equation describes the attraction between molecules in imperfect gases, it does not hold for liquids [23].

(b) INTERACTIONS BETWEEN SOLVENT AND SOLUTE

For liquids which give interactions in one or both phases, an interaction term E was introduced [38] so that equation (69) became (70)

$$-\log_{10}(C_s/C_L) = kV_x - E \tag{70}$$

This equation has been used for solubilities C_s in water of many liquid compounds with one interacting group, and E was taken [38] to be 1.75 but the value varies considerably. For partition coefficients J between water and an organic liquid, equation (1) is modified to (71) which corresponds with (70)

$$-\log_{10} J = kV_x - E \tag{71}$$

Collander [228, 229] has listed the partition coefficients for many organic compounds between water and ether. In Table 32, his results for the compounds with one interacting group are shown, with the omission of acidic and basic compounds.

Table 32. Specific interaction terms for partitions between diethyl ether and water [228, 229].

Compound	T (K)	Partition coefficient	V_x (m^3 mol^{-1})	$36\,000\,V_x - \log_{10} J$
Methanol	293.2	0.14	3.082×10^{-5}	1.92
Ethanol	292.2	0.26	4.491×10^{-5}	2.20
n-Propanol	295.2	1.9	5.900×10^{-5}	1.84
n-Butanol	291.2	7.7		1.74
iso-Butanol	293.2	6.9		1.79
s-Butanol	293.2	4.5	7.309×10^{-5}	1.98
t-Butanol	293.2	2.2		2.29
Diethyl ether	293.2	10		1.63
Methyl acetate	293.2	2.7	6.057×10^{-5}	1.75
Ethyl acetate	293.2	8.5	7.466×10^{-5}	1.76
Formaldehyde	293.2	0.11	2.652×10^{-5}	1.91
Propionaldehyde	292.2	2.0	5.470×10^{-5}	1.67
Acetone	293.2	0.62	5.470×10^{-5}	2.18
Formamide	294.2	0.0014	3.650×10^{-5}	4.17
Acetamide	295.2	0.0025	5.059×10^{-5}	4.42

Table 32 (cont'd)

Compound	T (K)	Partition Coefficient J	V_x (m^3 mol^{-1})	$36\,000\,V_x - \log_{10} J$
Chloracetamide	293.2	0.096	6.283×10^{-5}	3.28
Propionamide	296.2	0.013	6.468×10^{-5}	4.21
n-Butyramide	296.2	0.058	7.877×10^{-5}	4.07
Acetonitrile	293.2	0.60	4.042×10^{-5}	1.68
Butyronitrile	294.2	10	6.860×10^{-5}	1.47
Phenol	292.2	44	7.751×10^{-5}	1.15
Acetanilide	288.2	3.0	9.728×10^{-5}	3.02

The equation given above in the form $\log_{10} J = 36\,000\,V_x - E$ (J = concentration in non-aqueous phase ÷ concentration in aqueous phase) has been applied [230] to the estimation of partition coefficients measured by Flynn [231] for hydrocortisone and prednisolone derivatives between ether and water. Except for a few cases when the interacting groups were close together, the interaction term for each carbonyl, hydroxyl and ester group was taken as 1.9, i.e. the interaction made the compound 80 times more soluble in the aqueous phase than it would otherwise have been. The substitution of fluoride for hydrogen appeared to give a small negative interaction (-0.15). The agreement between the estimated partition coefficients and the experimental ones was satisfactory.

The analysis of data on partitioning between water and organic solvents carried out by Dunn and Wold [232] gives support to the views expressed above. They conclude that there are two fundamental factors which determine the partition coefficient. One factor is associated with the chain length, in homologous series (molecular volume) and the second appears to be the result of dipolar interactions of solute and solvent.

The most interaction takes place between a compound in solution, Y, and solvent, S. One product is usually present in much greater quantity than any others over a range of concentrations and one can write

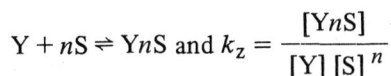

$$Y + nS \rightleftharpoons YnS \text{ and } k_z = \frac{[YnS]}{[Y][S]^n}$$

so that the apparent concentration of $[Y] = [Y] + [YnS] = [Y] + k_z[Y][S]^n$. The number of times this apparent concentration is greater than $[Y]$ is $1 + k_z[S]^n$.

Hydroxyl groups seem to be of special importance in giving rise to interactions and if $\Sigma[ROH]_1$ and $\Sigma[ROH]_2$ are the total concentration of hydroxyl in two phases which are in equilibrium (i.e. in a partition), it can often be stated that

$$E = \log_{10} \frac{1 + k_z(\Sigma\,[ROH]_1)^n}{1 + k_z(\Sigma\,[ROH]_2)^n} \tag{72}$$

Further, $k_z(\Sigma\,[ROH]_1$ and $k_z(\Sigma\,[ROH]_2$ are seldom of the order of one. If they are both much smaller than one, $E = \log_{10} 1 = 0$ which means there is no appreciable interaction. When the terms involving concentration are both large compared with one

$$E = \log_{10} \frac{(\Sigma\,[ROH]_1)^n}{(\Sigma\,[ROH]_2)^n} = n \log_{10} \frac{\Sigma\,[ROH]_1}{\Sigma\,[ROH]_2} \tag{73}$$

When ether is in equilibrium with water at 298.2 K, the upper layer consists of 9504 mol m^{-3} ether and 588 mol m^{-3} water and the lower layer consists of 51 330 mol m^{-3} water and 802 mol m^{-3} ether [233]. The logarithm of the ratio of the concentration of water in the two phases $\log_{10}(51\,330/588)$ equals 1.94, close to the figure used for all the interactions in Table 32. This suggests that it is the water which gives rise to the strong interactions, making $k_z[H_2O]$ (since $n = 1$) large compared with one in both phases.

The interaction between ethers and water has been studied by ultrasonics and the results [234] show that each ether oxygen is associated with one molecule of water: i.e. $n = 1$ here also.

The influence of water content of solvent on partition coefficients has been noted by Dryssen and Hay [235]. It has already been mentioned that carboxylic acids are largely dimeric in the vapour and in solvents with which they do not interact. Dryssen and Hay have found that di-n-butyl phosphate dimerises in most solvents. They measured the dimerisation constants K_z and the partition coefficients J between the solvents and dilute nitric acid (100 mol m^{-3}), and found that if $\log K_z$ was plotted against $\log J$ the points fell fairly well on a line of slope -2. Also, $\log J$ gave approximately a straight line when plotted against $\log$ (water content of solvent).

For a single compound (characteristic volume V_x) the partition coefficients J_1 and J_2 between two pairs of solvents will be from equation (71)

$$\log_{10} J_1 = k_1 V_x + E_1$$

$$\log_{10} J_2 = k_2 V_x + E_2$$

if V_x is eliminated, these give

$$\log_{10} J_1 = (k_1/k_2)\,(\log_{10} x_2) + E_1 - (k_1/k_2)\,(E_2) \tag{74}$$

This equation resembles (75), which was suggested by Smith [33–36] and Collander [229, 236]

$$\log_{10} J_1 = \underline{a}\,\log_{10} J_2 + \underline{b} \tag{75}$$

where $\underline{a}$ and $\underline{b}$ are constants. In Smith's, and many other examples, $k_1 = k_2$ approximately so that $\underline{a} = 1$ and the ratio $J_1/J_2 = $ a constant. An example of this is given in Table 3.

The equation (75) was examined for partitions between water and many organic liquids by Leo, Hansch and Elkins [237]. They found that the constants a and b did not correlate with the dipole moments, the dielectric constants, the solubility parameters or the molar attraction constants of the organic liquids. However, the constants were related to the solubilities of water in these organic liquids. A comparison of equations (74) and (75) shows that $a = k_1/k_2$ and in the following two sections, it is shown that k values depend largely on the concentration of water in the non-aqueous layers. Also, it has just been shown that when the hydroxyl concentration of the non-aqueous layer is high, the interactions depend on this concentration. The findings of Leo, Hansch and Elkins give support to these conclusions. For the solvents giving non-aqueous layers with considerably more water than 1-octanol (the standard), values of a were less than one, and values of b were positive. On the other than, when the non-aqueous layer contained less water than that of 1-octanol, a was nearly always greater than one and b was either close to zero or, more often, negative. Currie, Lough, Silver and Holmes [238] have compared partitions for the system cyclohexane–water with those for 1-octanol–water and found excellent agreement provided there were no interacting groups. Many of the compounds used in the examples discussed by Leo, Hansch and Elkins [237] were carboxylic acids or amines, since partition coefficients for these are easy to measure. These compounds, however, can give particularly strong interactions and show peculiarities, e.g. dimerisation of acids and solvation of amines. Such considerations may have led Leo, Hansch and Elkins to suggest that separate versions of equation (75) should be used for partitioning of hydrogen donors and of hydrogen acceptors with those solvents which dissolve the smaller amounts of water.

Mention should be made of the attempt of Dolezalek [239] to correlate departures from ideality in solutions, solely on the assumption that there were chemical equilibria between like molecules (association) and unlike pairs of molecules (solvation). He applied the method to the system acetone–chloroform, which has been studied by Zawidski [240], who gave the partial pressures over solutions. The results could be explained with:

$$\frac{[CHCl_3 . CH_3 COCH_3]}{[CHCl_3][CH_3COCH_3]} = 1.25 \times 10^{-3} \text{ mol}^{-1} \text{ m}^3$$

Dolezalek and Schulze [241], for the system chloroform–ether, gave.

$$\frac{[CHCl_3 . (C_2H_5)_2O]}{[CHCl_3][(C_2H_5)_2O]} = k_p$$

T (K)	293.15	306.4	333.15	353.15	373.15
k_p(mol^{-1} m^3)	2.96×10^{-3}	2.36×10^{-3}	1.0×10^{-3}	8×10^{-4}	7.1×10^{-4}

They were able to obtain satisfactory values for the total pressure over solutions to compare with those measured by Kohnstamm and van Dalfsen [242].

In the discussion given above, no allowance has been made for the fact that solvents such as water and alcohols are associated. The association can be described by $mS \rightleftharpoons S_m$ so that:

$$k_m = [S_m]/[S]^m \text{ and } [S] = (S/k)^{1/m} \tag{76}$$

If all the solvent can be considered to be associated as S_m, then $[ROH] = m[S_m]$ and the equation (74), which took no account of association ($\underline{m}$ was taken as equal to one), can be modified to

$$E = \log_{10} \frac{(\Sigma[ROH]_1)^{n/m}}{(\Sigma[ROH]_2)^{n/m}} = \frac{n}{m} \log_{10} \frac{\Sigma[ROH]_1}{\Sigma[ROH]_2} \tag{77}$$

It has been pointed out above that n/m is about one for hydroxyl, carbonyl, ester and aliphatic either groups. This means (see (77)) that roughly as many solvent molecules ($\underline{n}$) are involved in the interactions with these groups as the number ($\underline{m}$) of solvent molecules associating with one another. The interactions for phenols and phenolic ethers, like anisole, are about half [38, 48] those for the hydroxyl carbonyl and ester groups and so for the former $\underline{n}$ would seem to be about half $\underline{m}$.

There is some uncertainty about the degree of association ($\underline{m}$) in water and alcohols. Equations (4), (5) and (9) have been combined [23] to give a relationship between viscosity and isothermal compressibility. When this relationship was applied to methanol and ethanol, the results suggested that these compounds were trimers in the liquid state. Ibbotson and Moore [243] have studied solutions of ethanol in carbon tetrachloride. They consider that monomer, linear dimer and trimer and cyclic tetramer are present and give association constants for the last three species as 9.5×10^{-4} mol^{-1} m^3, 9.5×10^{-5} mol^{-2} m^6 and 6.5×10^{-7} mol^{-3} m^9. The compositions of the solutions shown in Fig. 11 were worked out from these constants. The results of Kunst, van Duijn and Bordewijk [244] suggest that a tetramer is the main species present in concentrated solutions of 3-ethyl-pentanol-3 in carbon tetrachloride. Salamon, Liszi and Ratkovics [245] consider the average degree of association in pure 1-pentanol and 1-heptanol is four. These and other results point to a value for $\underline{m}$ of around three or four in the pure liquid and very concentrated solutions. In Fig. 12, values of $\log_{10}$ (vapour pressure) for n-hexanol and its unassociated isomer di-n-propyl ether have been plotted against the reciprocal of the temperature. At 298 K, p_s for di-n-propyl ether is about eight times that of n-hexanol, but the differences between the vapour pressures decrease with rise of temperature.

In Table 33, examples are given of the use of equation (71) for the estimation of solubilities. This table is adapted from one given previously [38]: the parachor has been replaced by the characteristic volume and SI units are used so that concentrations are now in mol m^{-3}. The agreement between $\log_{10} C_s$ and

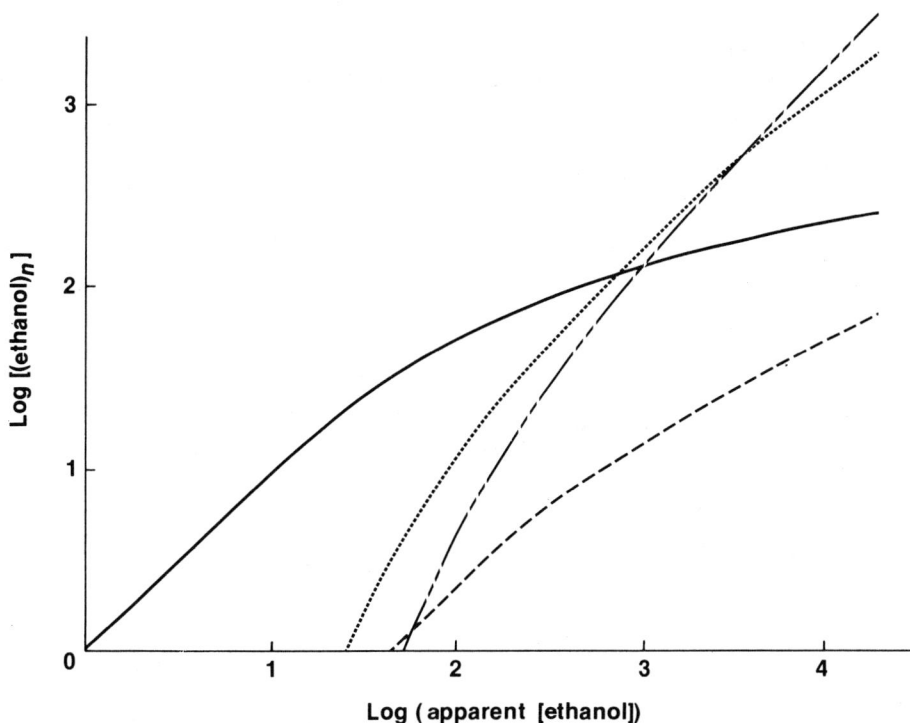

Fig. 11. Composition of ethanol solutions in carbon tetrachloride [245]. —— Monomer ($n = 1$); ----- linear dimer ($n = 2$); ..... linear trimer ($n = 3$); —--—- cyclic tetramer ($n = 4$).

$\log_{10} C_L + 1.75 - 38\,000\,V_x$ is quite good. All the compounds are liquids and all have one group giving interaction. The same value (1.75) for E was found to account for the interaction of the group in an ester, ether, ketone, alcohol or phenol. This is not unexpected for the ester, ether and carbonyl group since these do not associated appreciably in the pure liquid, but it is perhaps surprising that for alcohols and phenols, which are associated in the liquid state, the same interaction term can be used. In partitions, from say ether to water, there is no problem because the major component (solvent) in both phases is the same. It might be possible to improve the estimates of solubilities of compounds if in equation (71) allowance could be made for association of compounds when this occurs in the pure liquid.

No allowance in equation (71) has been made for any effect on the solubilities in water arising from differences in the compressibilities of compounds, and the accuracy of the estimates might be improved if any influence of this on k were taken into account. Provided the aqueous solution was dilute so that its compressibility differed little from that of water, equation (32), which was used to estimate the solubility of one unassociated liquid in another, might be served to correct for compressibility differences. This, however, is by no means certain. The idea does receive some support from the fact (see Fig. 10) that the solubilities of argon in unassociated and in associated liquids fall on the same line.

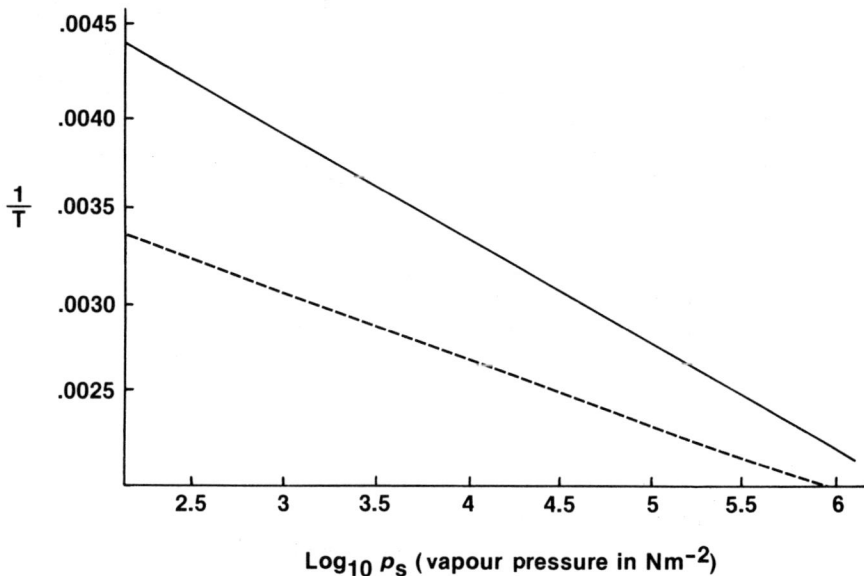

Fig. 12. Comparison of vapour pressures of hexanol and di-n-propyl ether (1,1´-oxybis-propane). —— 1,1´-Oxybispropane; - - - - - - hexanol.

Table 33. Estimation of solubilities C_s (mol m^{-3}) of liquids in water.

Compound	$Log_{10} C_L$	$-38\,000\ V_x$ $+ \log_{10} C_L + 1.75$	$Log_{10} C_s$
Acetic acid, butyl ester	3.88	1.7	2.3
Acetic acid, ethyl ester	4.01	2.9	2.9
Acetic acid, methyl ester	4.10	3.5	3.6
Acetic acid, propyl ester	3.94	2.3	2.3
Benzaldehyde	4.00	2.4	2.5
Benzoic acid, ethyl ester	3.84	0.9	0.7
Benzyl alcohol	3.99	2.2	2.5
Butanoic acid, ethyl ester	3.89	1.7	1.6
1-Butanol	4.04	3.0	3.0
Butanone-2,	4.05	3.2	3.5
Butanone-2,3-methyl-	3.98	2.6	2.8
Cyclohexanol	3.98	2.3	2.5

Table 33. (contd.)

Compound	$\mathrm{Log}_{10}\,C_L$	$-38\,000\,V_x$ $+\,\mathrm{Log}_{10}\,C_L + 1.75$	$\mathrm{Log}_{10}\,C_s$
Ethanone, 1-phenyl-	3.93	1.8	1.7
Ethyl ether	3.98	2.9	2.9
Formic acid, ethyl ester	4.10	3.5	3.1
1-Heptanol	3.85	1.2	1.2
2-Heptanone	3.86	1.4	1.6
3-Heptanone	3.86	1.4	1.5
Hexanoic acid, ethyl ester	3.78	0.5	0.6
1-Hexanol	3.90	1.8	1.8
2-Hexanone	3.92	2.0	2.2
3-Hexanone	3.92	2.0	2.2
Octanoic acid, ethyl ester	3.70	−0.6	−0.4
1-Octanol	3.80	0.6	0.6
1-Pentanol	3.97	2.4	2.4
2-Pentanone	3.97	2.5	2.8
2-Pentanone, 3-methyl-	3.91	2.0	2.3
2-Pentanone, 4-methyl-	3.90	2.0	2.3
3-Pentanone	3.98	2.6	2.7
3-Pentanone, 2,4-dimethyl-	3.85	1.4	1.7
3-Pentanone, 2-methyl-	3.92	2.0	2.2
Phenol, 4-butyl-	3.81	0.4	0.4
Phenol, 2-methyl-	3.99	2.2	2.4
Phenol, 3-methyl-	3.98	2.2	2.3
Phenol, 2-methyl-5- (1-methylethyl)-	3.81	0.4	0.8

(c) SOLVENTS OTHER THAN WATER

For some series of organic acids and bases, Smith [35] found that the logarithms of the partition coefficients between the two phases formed by the mixing of glycerol and acetone gave straight lines when plotted against the molecular volumes.

Deno and Berkheimer [225] suggested that the equation (70)

$$-\log_{10}\,(C_s/C_L) = kV_x - E \tag{70}$$

could be used for solubilities of non-electrolytes in associated liquids other than water if appropriate changes were made for the constants. An example they gave was the solubilities of alkanes [246] in liquid sulphur dioxide at 244.2 K. It will be seen from Table 34 that k is approximately constant at 1×10^4 mol m^{-3}. If

Table 34. Solubilities [246] of alkanes in sulphur dioxide at 244.2 K.

Alkane	V_x (m^3 mol^{-1})	$Log_{10} C_L$	$Log_{10} C$	$k = \dfrac{1}{V_x} (log_{10} C_L - log_{10} C)$
Butane	6.723×10^{-5}	4.02	3.38	0.95×10^4
Hexane	9.541×10^{-5}	3.89	2.99	0.94×10^4
Heptane	10.951×10^{-5}	3.85	2.70	1.05×10^4
Nonane	13.769×10^{-5}	3.75	2.40	0.98×10^4
Decane	15.178×10^{-5}	3.72	2.01	1.13×10^4

Concentrations in mol m^{-3}.

equation (32) is used to estimate these solubilities, the results suggest that sulphur dioxide and the hydrocarbons would be miscible. The fact that this is not so supports the view that sulphur dioxide is an associated liquid. De Ligny, Denessen and Alfenaar [247] found that free energies for transfer of a number of compounds between N-methylformamide and water gave a straight line if plotted against the van der Waals volumes, which were calculated as described by Bondi [83, 84] and which are roughly equal to 0.7 V_x (see Chapter 2, section (f)). Molal concentrations were used but the densities of water and N-methyl-formamide are so close that for dilute solutions these can be taken as molar concentrations and the logarithm of the ratios ($log_{10} J$) of the solubilities in N-methylformamide and in water worked out. These are compared in Table 35 with the characteristic volumes. None of the compounds would be expected to give specific interactions and it will be seen that $log_{10} J$ is approximately equal to 32 000 V_x. This gives k in equation (70) as 36 000 − 32 000, i.e. 4000 mol m^{-3}. Box, de Ligny and Alfenaar [248] noted that $log_{10} J$ from solubilities in methanol and water also gave a straight line when plotted against V_w. Ratios of solubilities in methanol and in unassociated liquids, as well as other evidence, suggest a figure of 5900 for the k of methanol at 298.2 K. Ethanol has a smaller value for k of about 3070.

It has been found (J.C. McGowan and J. Burgess, unpublished results) that equation (70) can be written in the more generalized form (78):

$$-log_{10} (C_S/C_L) + \text{interaction terms}$$
$$= V_x (0.65[H_2 O] + 0.24[CH_3 OH] + 0.18[C_2 H_5 OH]) \qquad (78)$$

so that it applies not only to water, methanol and ethanol but to mixtures of these liquids. Terms for other associated liquids can be added to the right hand side of equation (78) if required.

It has been stated above that n equals one, in the interaction term, for partition of each carbonyl, hydroxyl and ester group between water and ether. The results of Bonner [249] for the partition of ether in phases containing water and ethanol (Table 36) shows that $\underline{n}$ for the interaction of the ether group itself

Table 35. Ratios (x) of solubilities in N-methylformamide and water [247] at 298.2 K.

Compound	V_x (m^3 mol^{-1})	$\text{Log}_{10} J$	$(\text{Log}_{10} J)/V_x$
CH_4	2.495×10^{-5}	0.789	31 600
$C(CH_3)_4$	8.131×10^{-5}	2.458	30 200
$Si(CH_3)_4$	9.179×10^{-5}	3.046	33 200
$Ge(CH_3)_4$	9.598×10^{-5}	3.132	32 600
$Sn(CH_3)_4$	1.0431×10^{-4}	3.180	30 500
$C(C_2H_5)_4$	1.3767×10^{-4}	4.442	32 300
$Si(C_2H_5)_4$	1.4815×10^{-4}	4.985	33 600
$Sn(C_2H_5)_4$	1.6067×10^{-4}	5.045	31 400

Average 31 900

is also one: i.e. the interaction term equals the logarithm of the ratio of hydroxyl concentrations in the two phases. The symbol Δ is used to denote the difference between concentrations and here it refers to the two phases.

Another example of the use of equation (78) is given in Table 37. The compositions (weight %) [250] were used, of phases in equilibrium, for the systems n-octane—water—ethanol and n-nonane—water—ethanol. The densities of the phases can be obtained (by the use of proportional parts) from density figures for various compositions and then the concentrations of the components in the phases can be worked out. These compositions are given in the table and the ratios of the hydrocarbon concentrations in the two phases at equilibrium are compared with the values calculated from

$$\log_{10} \frac{[\text{hydrocarbon}]_1}{[\text{hydrocarbon}]_2} = V_x \left(0.65\Delta[H_2O] + 0.18\Delta[C_2H_5OH] \right)$$

There is no interaction term. All the experimental values for the ratios are higher than the calculated ones but the agreement between the two sets of figures is reasonable.

The treatment given above relates solubilities to molecular volumes multiplied by a term with the units of pressure (or reciprocal of compressibility). Some workers [251—253] have used estimates of the surface area of molecules to correlate and to predict partition coefficients and solubilities. The area is of course related to the volume and the surface tension is related to the isothermal compressibility [45] (see equations (5) and (6)) and it is not too easy to choose between the two treatments. However, a major disadvantage of surface area is that it is not too easy to define and a variety of methods exist for its estimation based on molecular models [253] or atomic radii [64]. Leo, Hansch and Jow [254] agree that molecular size primarily determines the partition coefficients between 1-octanol and water for unassociated compounds giving no interactions.

Table 36. The system diethyl ether/ethanol/water [249].

Conc (mol m^{-3}) in lower layer			Conc (mol m^{-3}) in upper layer			$V_x(0.65\Delta[H_2O] + 0.18\Delta[C_2H_5OH])$	$Log_{10}\dfrac{[ether]_2}{[ether]_1} + log_{10}\dfrac{(\Sigma[ROH]_1)}{(\Sigma[ROH]_2)}$
Ether	Water	Ethanol	Ether	Water	Ethanol		
1 827	32 066	5 212	7 878	3 584	3 438	1.38	0.64 + 0.72 = 1.36
2 162	29 560	5 288	6 994	5 372	4 039	1.17	0.51 + 0.57 = 1.08
2 874	24 725	5 396	5 935	10 425	4 825	0.69	0.32 + 0.30 = 0.62
3 370	22 099	5 392	5 233	13 200	5 048	0.43	0.19 + 0.18 = 0.37

Table 37. Compositions (mol m^{-3}) of equilibrium phases.

(a) System n-octane–water–ethanol ($V_x = 1.2360 \times 10^{-4}$ m^3 mol^{-1} for n-octane)

Octane Density (kg m^{-3})	Water	Ethanol	n-Octane	Aqueous Density (kg m^{-3})	Water	Ethanol	n-Octane	Calc.	Found
699	0	0	6 119	860	14 100	12 770	150	26.2	40.6
702	0	427	5 980	821	7 840	13 615	460	8.4	13.0
703	39	702	5 865	810	5 620	13 540	745	5.4	7.9
705	78	1 132	5 700	788	3 150	12 620	1 310	3.2	4.4
713	198	2 848	5 060	756	1 340	9 650	2 515	1.7	2.0
718	319	3 647	4 760	747	1 040	8 350	3 010	1.45	1.6
727	444	4 703	4 400	739	820	7 090	3 480	1.2	1.3

(b) System n-nonane–water–ethanol ($V_x = 1.3769 \times 10^{-4}$ m^3 mol^{-1} for n-nonane)

Nonane Density (kg m^{-3})	Water	Ethanol	n-Nonane	Aqueous Density (kg m^{-3})	Water	Ethanol	n-Nonane	Calc.	Found
714	0	0	5 570	835	9 270	13 850	230	14.9	23.8
717	0	370	5 460	807	6 090	13 940	430	7.6	12.7
718	40	750	5 320	797	3 670	13 600	810	4.4	6.5
722	80	1 820	4 965	773	1 630	11 440	1 690	2.4	2.9
724	120	2 140	4 860	768	1 360	10 840	1 900	2.1	2.5
726	200	2 900	4 590	760	1 010	9 700	2 300	1.7	2.0
733	285	4 455	4 075	749	665	7 580	3 025	1.3	1.4
734	336	4 700	3 990	748	620	7 370	3 100	1.2	1.3

They expected that it would be the area of the molecules which would be related to the logarithms of the partition coefficients, but they found that molecular areas calculated by several methods gave a poorer correlation than molecular volumes.

(d) CORRECTIONS FOR DIFFERENCES IN COMPRESSIBILITY

So far in this chapter, no allowance has been made for differences in compressibility between solvent and solute. Results for small molecules (argon was used as an example) suggest that the influence of compressibility can be treated in the same way for unassociated and associated solvents. If this is so, the value of k can be split into two parts. For example, for water, k can be considered to be made up of the volume effect which arises from the break-up of the water structure when other molecules are introduced and of the need to bring the solute to the compressibility of water. The solubility of benzene in water at 298.2 K comes to 0.518, as a volume fraction, if calculated from its $T_x = 570$ K and with $T_x = 1320$ K for water. This result can be written

$$-\log_{10}(C_S/C_L) = (V_x \text{ for benzene}) \times (0.072[H_2O])$$

If this is subtracted from the total factor (0.65), the factor for the volume effect is about 0.58. If instead of benzene, hexane ($T_x = 454$) is considered, the compressibility gives 0.127 as a volume fraction, i.e.

$$-\log_{10}(C_S/C_L) = (V_x \text{ for hexane}) \times (0.170[H_2O]).$$

The total effect for hexane is $-\log_{10}(C_S/C_L) = V_x(0.17 + 0.58)$ if 0.58 is used for the volume effect: this seems reasonable since benzene has a value of T_x that is around the average. The equation developed for estimation of solubility can now be written

$$-\log_{10}(C_S/C_L) + \text{interaction terms}$$

$$= (\text{compressibility term}(\log_{10} y) + V_x(0.58[H_2O]$$

$$+ 0.24[CH_3OH] + 0.18[C_2H_5OH]) \quad (79)$$

The compressibility term is calculated as described in equation (32). The coefficients for methanol and ethanol have not been altered because T_x for these solvents are only slightly less than T_x for benzene. The T_x value (1320 K) based on the density of water at 298.2 K has been used. If estimated from the isothermal compressibility at 298.2, T_x comes to only 914 K: this low figure probably arises because the structure of water is altered as the compressibility is measured. In the equation above, the coefficients for the concentrations are: water 0.58, methanol 0.24 and ethanol 0.17. It is of interest that these numbers are roughly proportional (factor about 10^{-5} J m^3) to the concentrations of the liquids (i.e. to the concentration of hydroxyl) in their own liquid state at 298.2 K. These concentrations are: 55 344 for water, 24 547 for methanol and 17 041 mol m^{-3} for ethanol.

(e) MIXED SOLVENTS AND CHROMATOGRAPHY

The equation (78) has been given above for solubilities C_s in mixtures of water, ethanol and methanol

$$-\log_{10}(C_s/C_L) + \text{interaction terms} = V_x(0.65[H_2O]$$
$$+ 0.24[CH_3OH]$$
$$+ 0.18[C_2H_5OH]) \qquad (78)$$

If there are no volume changes on the mixing of the solvents according to equation (52), the concentration of a component [A] in a mixture equals $Y_A[A]_0$ when Y_A is the volume fraction of the component A and $[A_0]$ is its concentration in the pure liquid. If (52) and (78) are combined

$$-\log_{10}(C_s/C_L) + \text{interaction terms}$$
$$= V_x(0.65y_{H_2O}[H_2O]_0 + 0.24y_{CH_3OH}[CH_3OH]_0$$
$$+ 0.18y_{C_2H_5OH}[C_2H_5OH]_0) \qquad (80)$$

For the solubilities in the pure solvents, water, methanol and ethanol, $\log_{10}(C_s/C_L) + $ interaction terms equals $0.65\ V_x[H_2O]_0$, $0.24\ V_x[CH_3OH]_0$ and $0.18\ V_x[C_2H_5OH]_0$ respectively. The equation (80) thus resembles an equation put forward by Kemula and Buchowski [255, 256]. For the effect of change in phase composition on the partition coefficient (J) between a mixture of two solvents A and C and a third B, miscible in all proportions with A but immiscible with C, they gave

$$\log J = y_A \log J_A + y_B \log J_B \qquad (81)$$

where J_A and J_B are the partition coefficients between C and pure A and pure B respectively and y_A and y_B are the volume fractions of composition in the phase of variable composition. Kemula and Buchowski used mixtures of water and methanol. They partitioned o- and p-nitrochlorobenzenes into these from n-heptane and iso-octane, and oestrone and oestradiol-17β from carbon tetrachloride. Equations of the type (79) allow for changes in volume on the mixing and treat interactions separately. They are to be preferred to equations of the type (81). Mixed solvents are much used in chromatography and this subject can now be conveniently discussed.

Consden, Gordon and Martin [257] gave the formula (82) for partition coefficients

$$J = \frac{\text{conc in aqueous phase}}{\text{con in solvent phase}} = A_L/A_s \left(\frac{1}{R_F} - 1\right) \qquad (82)$$

where

$$R_F = \frac{\text{movement of band for compound}}{\text{movement of advancing front of liquid}}$$

A_L = cross-sectional area of the solvent phase

and

A_s = cross-sectional area of the aqueous phase

so

A_L/A_s = ratio of volumes of solvent and aqueous phase in the chromatogram — a constant for a given chromatogram.

The equation applies to thin-layer and paper chromatography when the support is inert. Procházka [258] and others attribute values of k, from the formula, which disagree with those determined directly to absorption through interaction with the support.

Bate-Smith and Westfall [259] proposed that

$$\log_{10}\left(\frac{1}{R_F} - 1\right)$$

be called R_M so that

$$\log_{10} J = \log_{10}(A_L/A_s) + R_M \tag{83}$$

Relationships between R_M and the π of Hansch *et al.* (see Chapter 6, section (i)) [260] and the parachor (or characteristic volume V_x) [261] have been pointed out. Soczewinski and Wachtmeister [262] have used equation (81) in chromatography. They write

$$R_M^m = y_A R_M^A + y_B R_M^B \tag{84}$$

They tested (84) with the partitions of certain phenolic dibenzofurans between di-isopropyl ether or di-n-butyl ether and mixtures of water and dimethyl sulphoxide and the results were in reasonable agreement with those estimated from (84). Soczewinski [263] later gave results for the partitions of α- and β-naphthol and 8-hydroxyquinoline between dipentyl either or decalin and mixtures of dimethyl sulphoxide and diethylene glycol. Equation (84) has also been used successfully [260] for partitioning of alkyltritylamines between paraffin and mixtures of acetone and water. Equation (81) has been applied to partitions of substances from the gas phase into binary liquid mixtures [264, 265] and has been found to give good results for a wide variety of systems. Reasons for deviations from what is required by equation (81) have been discussed [266, 267]: these deviations are usually small.

In gas—liquid chromatography, the substance is carried down the column in a gaseous moving phase and the stationary phase is a non-volatile liquid held on a solid. Mixtures are separated and pass out as distinct zones because compounds are carried along the column at different rates. Under set conditions a constant volume of gas is required to pass a given amount of a compound along a column. This volume per gram of liquid in the stationary phase corrected for drop of pressure along the column and reduced to 273.2 K is called the 'specific retention volume' V_g and is related to the partition coefficient L (which corresponds to the Ostwald solubility coefficient of the gas in the liquid of the stationary phase) by the relationship (85)

$$V_g = \frac{273.2L}{\rho_L T} \qquad (85)$$

ρ_L is the density of the liquid forming the stationary phase, at the temperature of the experiment T. The partition coefficient L equals the concentration of the compound in this liquid divided by that in the gas.

Gas–liquid chromatography can yield useful information about specific interactions [268–270]. Littlewood [268] measured specific retention volumes of many compounds in six hexadecyl derivatives. It is of interest to compare the values of V_g he gives for the solvents 1-chlorohexadecane and 1-hexadecanol. The characteristic temperatures derived from the densities ($T_x = 618$ K for 1-chlorohexadecane and 662 for 1-hexadecanol) are not far apart so that any corrections required for the effect of compressibility will be about equal for the solvents. For the 15 hydrocarbons and six alkyl halides studied L values were calculated from the specific retention volumes and densities at 333.2 K by means of equation (85). The ratios (L for 1-chlorohexadecane)/(L for 1-hexadecanol) varied from 1.27 for 1-pentene to 1.49 for n-heptane with an average value for all these compounds was 1.38. The alcohols gave quite different values for this ratio of L values: methanol (0.25); ethanol (0.19); n-propanol (0.21), n-butanol (0.22).

Martire and Riedl [270] measured specific retention volumes of a number of compounds in n-heptadecane, di-n-octyl ether and di-n-octyl ketone. Since L values give partition coefficients between liquid and vapour, the ratios of L values will give effectively the partition coefficient for the compound between the liquids used as stationary phases. Table 38 gives some effective partition coefficients derived from the results of Martire and Riedl. As a result of their experiments these authors concluded that di-n-octyl ether and di-n-octyl ketone both formed 1:1 complexes with alcohols and they were able to suggest equilibrium constants for the formation of these complexes.

Table 38. Effective partition coefficients between n-heptadecane and (a) di-n-octyl ether and (b) di-n-octyl ketone at 323.2 K.

Compound	(a) $\dfrac{(L \text{ for n-heptadecane})}{(L \text{ for di-n-octyl ether})}$	(b) $\dfrac{(L \text{ for n-heptadecane})}{(L \text{ for di-n-octyl ketone}}$
n-Pentane	0.99	1.16
Isopentane	0.98	1.15
n-Hexane	0.99	1.18
2-Methylpentane	0.99	1.18

Table 38. (continued)

Compound	(a) $\dfrac{(L \text{ for n-heptadecane})}{(L \text{ for di-n-octyl ether})}$	(b) $\dfrac{(L \text{ for n-heptadecane})}{(L \text{ for di-n-octyl ketone})}$
3-Methylpentane	0.99	1.18
2,2-Dimethylbutane	1.00	1.17
2,3-Dimethylbutane	1.00	1.16
n-Heptane	1.01	1.21
3-Methylhexane	1.00	1.20
2,4-Dimethylpentane	1.00	1.19
Methanol	0.25	0.14
Ethanol	0.31	0.17
1-Propanol	0.32	0.19
2-Propanol	0.38	0.21
1-Butanol	0.34	0.19
2-Methyl-1-propanol	0.33	0.19
2-Butanol	0.41	0.25
2-Methyl-2-propanol	0.47	0.26

(f) SOLUBILITIES IN SOLUTIONS OF SALTS

The effects of dissolved salts on the properties of water have been studied for many years. Tammann [271–273] suggested that the effect of dissolved salts on a solvent should be compared with the external pressure required to produce the same effect. He showed that thermal expansion, compressibility and many other properties of salt solutions could be correlated with these external pressures. He noted [272] that, in general, the higher the molecular volume of the salt, the smaller the effect on the properties of the solvent. This work was continued by Euler [274], Geffeken [275] and others. The volume contractions when salts were dissolved in water were correlated with the lowering of the solubilities in water of compounds such as ethyl acetate [274] and ether [276]. These contractions were worked out from the densities of the solvent and the solid salts. Tammann [277] also proposed the equation (86) for the effect of pressure (P) on the solubility of a solid (molecular mass M and density ρ) in a phase (solid or liquid) with compressibility (κ)

$$RT \log_e S_p/S = - M \kappa P^2 / 6 \rho \qquad (86)$$

where S is the solubility at low pressure (e.g. atmospheric) and S_p that at pressure P.

Setschenow [278, 279] studied the solubilities of carbon dioxide in aqueous solutions of salts and found equation (87) to hold

$$\log S_0/S_m = \underline{k}_s C_s \qquad (87)$$

Here S_m and S_0 are the solubilities of the non-electrolyte in salt solution and in pure water respectively. The equation (87) has since been found [274, 280–282] to hold for the solubilities of many non-electrolytes besides carbon dioxide and the constant $\underline{k}_s$ can be positive or negative since there may be 'salting in' as well as 'salting out' of non-electrolytes. Deno and Spink [280] noted the resemblance between the Setschenow equation (87) and equation (70)

$$\log_{10} C_s/C_L = -kV_x + E \tag{70}$$

for the solubility of non-electrolytes in water. They pointed out that if both equations applied to salt solutions, k_s and V_x are the only properties which vary with change of non-electrolyte, so that if E could be taken as constant, k_s should be proportional to V_x. Deno and Spink found that for 41 out of 57 values on a list [281] of k_s values for non-electrolytes, including those which had E not equal to zero, the values of k_s/V_x were within 50% of the value for benzene.

McDevit and Long [282, 283] assumed that non-electrolytes merely occupy volume and that the excess work required to introduce the non-electrolyte into the solution of electrolyte was proportional to the volume change which occurs when the (liquid) salt is mixed with water. They gave equation (88) for the Setschenow constant $\underline{k}_s$.

$$\underline{k}_s = \frac{\bar{V}_i^0(V_s - \bar{V}_s^0)}{2.3026\,\kappa RT} \tag{88}$$

Here $\bar{V}_i^0$ is the partial molar volume of the non-electrolyte at infinite dilution, $\bar{V}_s^0$ is the partial molar volume of the electrolyte at infinite dilution, V_s is the (estimated) molecular volume of pure (liquid) electrolyte and κ is the isothermal compressibility of the solvent (i.e. water). Estimates have been made [284] of the molecular volumes V_s of pure liquid salts but these are not too reliable. However, McDevit and Long suggested that in place of V_s, the variation of 'effective pressure' P_e exerted by the salt with concentration could be used. This idea of 'effective pressure' was based on the Tait equation.

Tait [285–290] studied the compressibility of water and solutions of salts and ethanol. He suggested that the average compressibility for an increase in pressure from atmospheric to P was given by

$$\frac{C^*}{L^* + P}.$$

The constant C^* did not alter when a salt was dissolved in the water and the constant L^* at a given temperature was proportional to the weight of salt dissolved in 100 parts of water. Hayward [291] has pointed out that Tait's equation can be written

$$\frac{V_0 - V}{PV_0} = \frac{C^*}{L^* + P} \tag{89}$$

where V_0 is the volume under one atmosphere and V that under the additional pressure P. Tammann [271, 292] replaced the average compressibility

$$\frac{V_0 - V}{PV_0}$$

by

$$\frac{1}{V_0} \cdot \frac{\mathrm{d}V}{\mathrm{d}P}$$

which gives equation (90). Hayward observes that many others have since repeated this error and he discusses the advantages of

$$-\frac{1}{V_0}\left(\frac{\mathrm{d}V}{\mathrm{d}P}\right)_T = \frac{C^*}{L^* + P} \tag{90}$$

$$-\frac{1}{V}\left(\frac{\mathrm{d}V}{\mathrm{d}P}\right)_T = \frac{C}{L + P} \tag{91}$$

Neece and Squire [293] have discussed the Tait equation and its relationship with the attractive and repulsive forces between molecules in solids, liquids and gases. Unless the pressure is very high, it does not matter much whether equation (90) or (91) is used, in fact

$$C^* = \frac{1}{V_0} \cdot \frac{C}{1 + C}$$

and

$$B^* + P = \frac{B + P}{1 + C}.$$

The equation (91) is equivalent to (26) and has been discussed in Chapter 4, section (b).

Gibson [294, 295] applied equation (90) to solutions of salts. He divided the constant L^* into the value of L^* for water itself plus P_e which he called 'the effective pressure' exerted by the salt. Gibson considered that P_e was proportional to the produce of the concentration of the salt and the concentration of the solvent (water) in the solution. McDevit and Long [282] substituted the value of

$$\frac{\mathrm{d}P_e}{\mathrm{d}C_s}$$

as C_s tends to zero, for $(V_s - \vec{V}_s^0)/\kappa$ in their equation (88) and gave (92)

$$k_s = \frac{V_i^0}{2.3026\,RT} \frac{\mathrm{d}P_e}{\mathrm{d}C_s} \tag{92}$$

Equation (92) does not require the molecular volume V_s, of the liquid electrolyte, which is difficult to estimate. McDevit and Long used equations (88) and (92) to calculate $\underline{k}_s$ values for benzene and most of the values they obtained were about twice the experimental ones. They attributed this to the fact that no correction had been made for the sizes of the ions and non-electrolyte.

Blandamer, Burgess and McGowan [296] have suggested that the solubilities S_0 and S of non-electrolytes in water and in salt solutions respectively can be related to the characteristic volumes V_x of the non-electrolytes by the equation (93)

$$-\log_{10} S_0/S_m + \text{interaction terms (if any)}$$

$$= V_x(0.65[H_2O]_0 - 0.65[H_2O]_w - 1.35I) \tag{93}$$

This implies that high volume effects of salts can be attributed solely to the charges on the ions and that, apart from this, the salt acts as an inert diluent. The concentration of water $[H_2O]_0$ refers to the solution of non-electrolyte in water and $[H_2O]_w$ to the salt solution. The term I is the ionality (or ional concentration) of the salt present: it equals

$$\sum_j C_j z_j^2$$

where C_j is the molar concentration (mol m^{-3}) of each ion present and z_j is the charge on that ion. The term I has already been used [297–299] and this divided by the salt concentration is the partial molar volume of salt in the solution ($\bar{V}_2$). Further, $I/[\text{salt}] = \Sigma z^2$ (the sum of the squares of the charges on the ions making up the salt) and so

$$\underline{k}_s = V_x(1.35\Sigma z^2 - 36\,000\,\bar{V}_s^\circ) \tag{94}$$

In Table 39, the $\underline{k}_s$ values for benzene ($V_x = 7.164 \times 10^{-5}\,m^3\,mol^{-1}$) given by equation (94) with partial molar volumes at infinite dilution [108] for electrolytes shown in Tables 12 and 13 have been compared with experimental values of $\underline{k}_s$ listed by Deno and Spink [280]. Values of $\underline{k}_s$ for quaternary ammonium bromides, but not chlorides, are given, and these have been used.

For nitrobenzene [300], trinitrotriamminecobalt [301], bis(2,2'-bipyridyl)-dicyanoiron(II) [296], dicyanobis(5-nitro-1,10-phenanthroline)iron(III) [296] and various other non-electrolytes, the estimated lines for plots of log S_0/S_m against [salt] have to be rotated clockwise about the origin to fit with the experiment. Deno and Spink [280] have attributed these increases in solubility to direct interaction between the added salts and the non-electrolytes. If the salt and non-electrolyte form a 1.1 complex

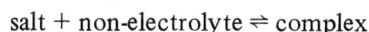

$$\text{salt} + \text{non-electrolyte} \rightleftharpoons \text{complex}$$

then

$$\frac{[\text{complex}]}{[\text{salt}][\text{non-electrolyte}]} = k_0$$

Therefore apparent solubility = [salt] + [complex] = [salt] $(1 + k_0$ [complex]). The solubility is apparently increased by a factor of $1 + k_0$ [complex].

Table 39. Setschenow constants k_s for benzene [280] and partial molecular volumes [108] $\bar{V}_s^\circ$ at infinite dilution in water.

Electrolyte	k_s (m³ mol⁻¹)	7.164×10^{-5} $(1.35 \, \Sigma z^2 - 36\,000 \, \bar{V}_s^\circ)$
NaCl	2.0×10^{-4}	1.5×10^{-4}
KCl	1.7×10^{-4}	1.2×10^{-4}
KBr	1.2×10^{-4}	1.1×10^{-4}
RbCl	1.4×10^{-4}	1.1×10^{-4}
Na₂SO₄	5.5×10^{-4}	5.5×10^{-4}
LiCl	1.4×10^{-4}	1.5×10^{-4}
NaOH	2.6×10^{-4}	2.1×10^{-4}
NH₄Cl	1.0×10^{-4}	1.0×10^{-4}
BaCl₂	3.3×10^{-4}	5.2×10^{-4}
$(CH_3)_4$NBr	-1.5×10^{-4}	-1.0×10^{-4}
$(C_2H_5)_4$NBr	-2.5×10^{-4}	-2.5×10^{-4}
$(n-C_3H_7)_4$NBr	-4.1×10^{-4}	-4.2×10^{-4}

(g) SOLUBILITIES OF SALTS

It is possible to treat the solubilities of electrolytes in the same way as non-electrolytes but the electrolytes give higher interactions. Rothmund [302] suggested the following relationship for solubilities of salts in water containing non-electrolytes

$$\log S_w - \log S_0 = k_R C_s \qquad (95)$$

This bears a resemblance to the Setschenow equation; S_w and S_0 are the solubilities of the salt in the solution of the non-electrolyte and in pure water respectively. McGowan [303] found that k_R was proportional to the characteristic volume V_x' of the non-electrolyte and so

$$\log S_w - \log S_0 = k_R' \, V_x' \, C_s \qquad (96)$$

This equation was found by Burgess, Morton and McGowan [304] to account satisfactorily for the solubilities of caesium hexachlororhenate(IV), hexabromorhenate(IV) and tetraoxorhenate(VII) in alcohol–water mixtures.

The equations (95) and (96) only hold if the salt is not appreciably soluble in the non-electrolyte and if there are no specific interactions between the salt and the non-electrolyte.

An alternative treatment has been proposed [310] for the solubilities of salts in mixtures of water, methanol and ethanol

$$-\log_{10} \frac{S}{C_{\mathrm{L}}} + \text{interaction terms}$$

$$= \frac{V_{\mathrm{x}}}{N} (0.65[\mathrm{H_2O}] + 0.24[\mathrm{CH_3OH}] + 0.18[\mathrm{C_2H_5OH}]$$

$$+ 1.35I) \tag{97}$$

Equation (97) has been applied to solubilities of salts in mixtures of water and alcohols. For the time being, corrections for differences in compressibilities have been ignored. The interaction terms might be expected to equal n times the logarithms of the difference between the total hydroxyl content of the solvents. In Fig. 13, values of $\log_{10}[\text{salt}] + V_{\mathrm{x}}/2(0.65[\mathrm{H_2O}] + 0.24[\mathrm{CH_3OH}] + 0.18[\mathrm{C_2H_5OH}] + 2.7[\text{salt}])$ have been plotted against the total hydroxyl contents $\log_{10}([\mathrm{H_2O}] + [\mathrm{CH_3OH}] + [\mathrm{C_2H_5OH}])$ for saturated solutions of some 1:1 electrolytes in solvent mixtures at 298.2 K. The points for potassium perchlorate [305–308] and caesium perchlorate [306–308] will be seen to give points near lines of slope 6, and these points are for the complete range from pure water to pure alcohols. On the other hand, values for the solubilities of potassium chloride [309], tetramethylammonium perchlorate [306] and tectra-(n-propyl)ammonium perchlorate [306] will be seen to give points near lines of slope 8. It will be noted above that V_{x} has been divided by N, the number of particles into which the salt ionises. For one ion

$$\log_{10} S^{\mathrm{I}} = -kV_{\mathrm{x}}^{\mathrm{I}} + \text{other terms}$$

then for a second ion

$$\log_{10} S^{\mathrm{II}} = -kV_{\mathrm{x}}^{\mathrm{II}} + \text{other terms}$$

and so on for the other ions, so that $\log_{10} S^{\mathrm{I}} + \log_{10} S^{\mathrm{II}} + $ similar terms for other ions into which the salt ionises $= \log_{10}[\text{solubility product}] = -kV_{\mathrm{x}}$ (for salt) + other terms.

But log [solubility

$$= \frac{1}{N} \log [\text{solubility product}]$$

$$= \frac{-kV_{\mathrm{x}}}{N} + \frac{\text{other terms}}{N} \tag{98}$$

The treatment, which has just been described for the solubilities of salts, can be used for internal salts. McGowan and Mellors [310] plotted values of $\log_{10}$ [solubility] $+ V_{\mathrm{x}}(0.65[\mathrm{H_2O}] + 0.18[\mathrm{C_2H_5OH}] + 2.7[\text{amino acid}]$ against $\log \Sigma[\mathrm{ROH}]$ for those amino acids which contain $-\mathrm{CH}_{\mathrm{NH_3^+}}^{\mathrm{COO^-}}$ as the only group giving interactions, and found that the points fell on straight lines of slope 12. This is illustrated for DL-alanine [311,312] and DL-α-aminobutyric acid [311] in Fig. 14. (The lines in this figure have been drawn with slopes 12.) The high

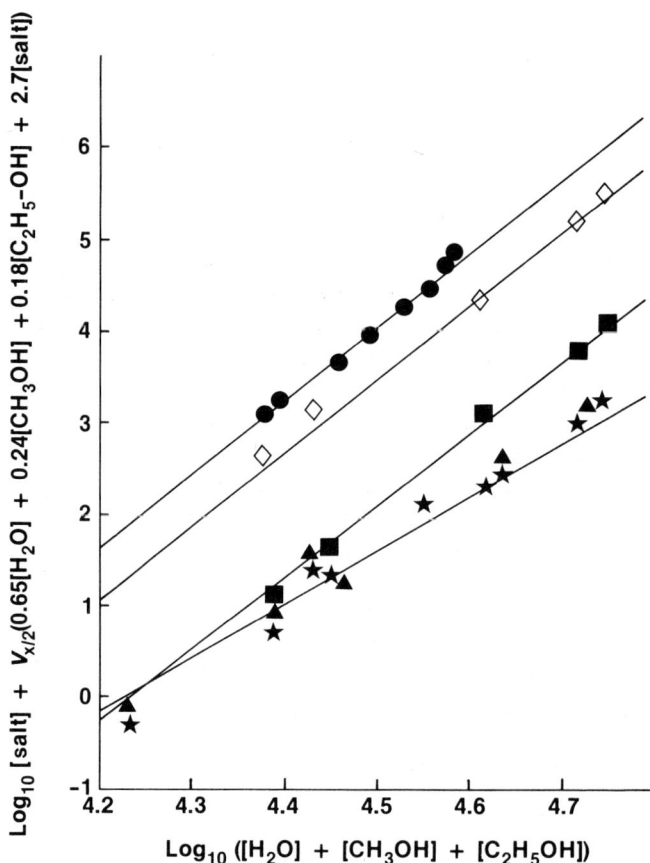

Fig. 13. Solubilities of salts in mixtures of water, methanol and ethanol. ● Potassium chloride; ▲ potassium perchlorate; ★ caesium perchlorate; ■ tetramethylammonium perchlorate; ◇ tetra(n-propyl)ammonium perchlorate.

for the number of hydroxyl groups which appear to be involved in these interactions and those for salts are comparable with those reported for salts elsewhere [313]. The solvent associated with the process of solution does not appear to be combined but may take up a preferred orientation around the ions. There is evidence [314, 315] that the hydroxyl groups of water, methanol and ethanol are equally effective for interactions.

Hollenberg and Ifft [316] have deduced hydration numbers from comparisons of the near infra-red spectra of the aqueous solutions with that of water. For glycine they give 10.5 molecules of water at 293 K dropping to 8.1 at 313 K. The corresponding values for L-isoleucine are 19.6 and 11.1. A method based on the velocity of ultrasonic waves through solutions in water and ethanol gave 4.4 for the hydration of glycine [317]. The difference between the partial molar volumes of amino acids, which are internal salts, and isomeric compounds without ionic charges has been related [318–320] to the number of water

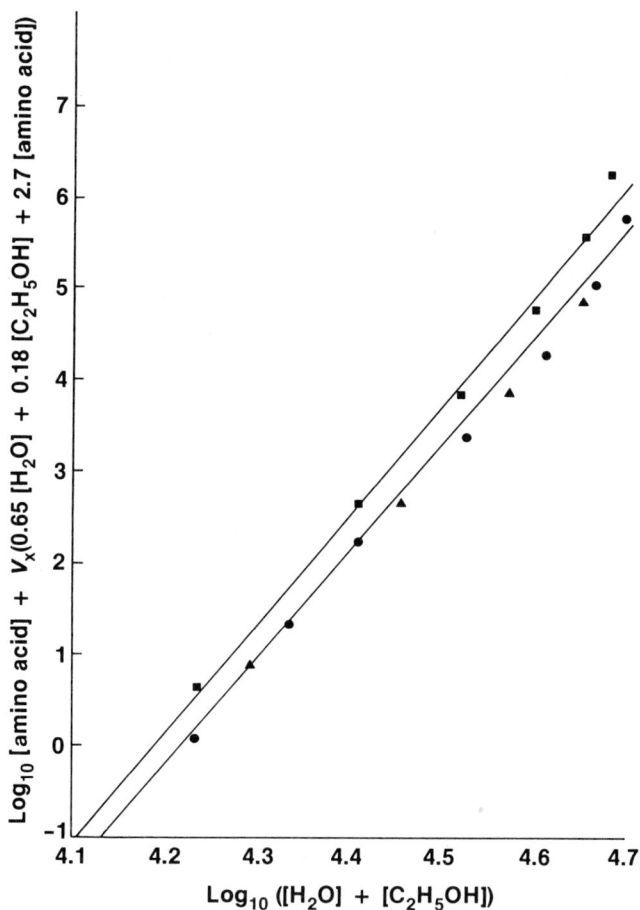

Fig. 14. Solubilities of amino acids in mixtures of water and ethanol. ● DL-Alanine [311]; ▲ DL-alanine [312]; ■ DL-α-aminobutyric acid [311].

molecules involved in the hydration of the amino acid. The value found is about 4.3 but this is for the difference between the two isomers and does not include the water which solvates the isomeric compound (e.g. a hydroxy-amide).

Equation (71) relates the partition coefficient J to the characteristic volume V_X of the compound being partitioned and the interaction E. If $E(1)$ is the interaction given by a single group so that $E = E(1) \times n$, then n, the number of groups in the compound involved in the interaction, is given by (99).

$$n = \frac{-\log_{10} J + kV_X}{E(1)} \tag{99}$$

Collander [228] gave partition coefficients between water and ether for α-alanine ($V_X = 7.055 \times 10^{-5}$ m³ mol⁻¹), 2-aminobutanoic acid ($V_X = 8.464 \times 10^{-5}$ m³ mol⁻¹) and leucine ($V_X = 1.1282 \times 10^{-4}$ m³ mol⁻¹). For partitions between water and ether, the values are given (see Chapter 5, section (b)), were $k = 36\,000$ mol m^{-3} and $E(1) = 1.9$. Equation (99) with these figures gives $n = 4.4$, 4.5 and 5.3 for α-alanine, 2-aminobutanoic acid and leucine respectively.

However, difficulties can arise in the use of equations (97) and (98) to obtain values for n and V_X. Values so obtained may be quite misleading. The interaction term $n \log_{10} \Sigma [\text{ROH}]$, n times the logarithm of the total hydroxyl content, and the value of $0.65[\text{H}_2\text{O}] + 0.24[\text{CH}_3\text{OH}] + 0.18[\text{C}_2\text{H}_5\text{OH}]$ are both dependent upon solvent composition. In Fig. 15, $\log_{10}(\Sigma[\text{ROH}])$ has been plotted against $0.65[\text{H}_2\text{O}] + 0.24[\text{CH}_3\text{OH}]$ and $0.65[\text{H}_2\text{O}] + 0.18[\text{C}_2\text{H}_5\text{OH}]$ for mixtures of

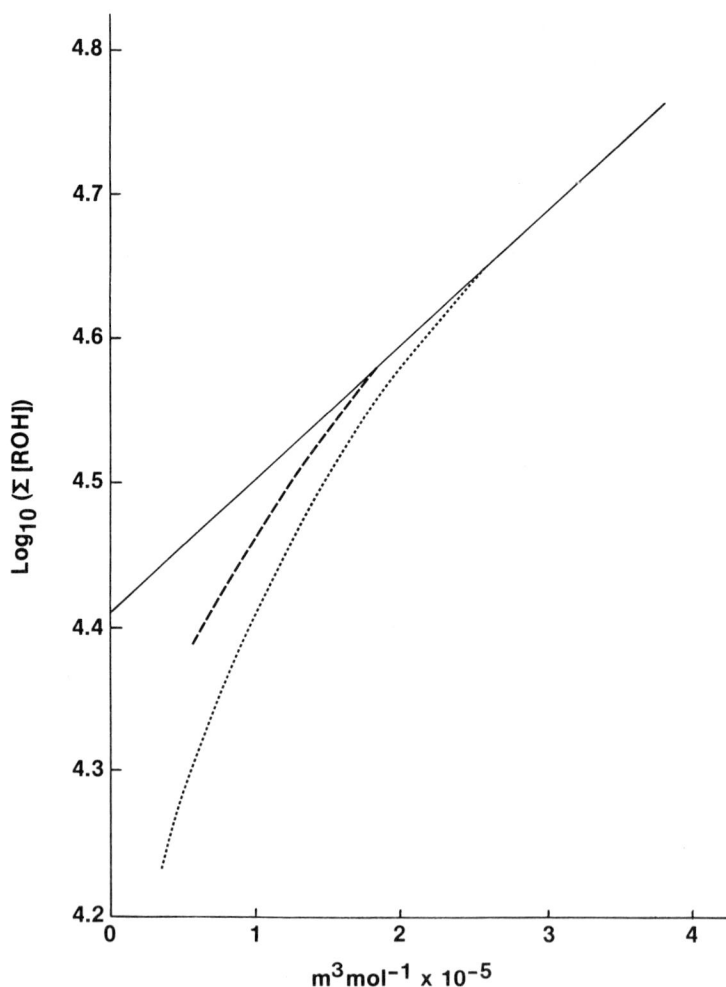

Fig. 15. Solvent composition and equations (97) and (98). - - - - - - $0.65[\text{H}_2\text{O}] + 0.24[\text{CH}_3\text{OH}]$; . . . . $0.65[\text{H}_2\text{O}] + 0.18[\text{C}_2\text{H}_5\text{OH}]$.

water and methanol and ethanol respectively. It can be seen that if the alcohol content is not too high (up to 50% methanol and 30% ethanol by volume) the curves lie close to the straight line drawn on Fig. 15 with slope 1.1×10^4. Thus if the solubility is low, experimental points plotted as in Figs 13 and 14 will fall near a straight line of slope 1.1×10^4 V_x/N until the alcohol concentration becomes high. However, even when the solubility is high, plots suggested by equations (97) and (98) may still be unreliable because $\log_{10} S$ is a function of solubility S and the ionality I for a given electrolyte is proportional to the solubility. It is always necessary to be cautious when equations contain terms which are not independent. Some aspects only of the solvation of ions are discussed here. This subject is treated at length by Burgess [321].

'Hydrophobicity' has been described [322] as a 'hazy concept subject to various surprisingly unsatisfactory explanations'. However, Tanford and Nozaki [324] have defined clearly what they mean by hydrophobicity as the free energy of transfer of the compound, from solution in ethanol, to solution in water. It has been shown [310] that equation (79) can be used to derive hydrophobicities defined in this way. On the subject of hydrophobicity the following three 'laws' of Colacicco [323] are of interest.

1st Law: water is structured around the polar groups and not around the hydrophobic groups of bimodal molecules.

2nd Law: the hydrophobic bond does not exist.

3rd Law: the alternative to the non-existent hydrophobic bond is the hydrophilic bond.

More recently, it has been suggested [325–327] that changes in the entropy of the solvent water contribute nothing to the entropy of solution. Cramer [328, 329] finds little evidence for hydrophobic effects at all. He suggests that the central issue should be 'Are there any experimental data which require a hydrophobic effect?' instead of 'Can the experimental data be manipulated so as to allow postulation of a hydrophobic effect?' Most of the difficulties with the concept of hydrophobicity have arisen from lack of appreciation of the effects of specific interactions and molecular volumes on solubilities in associated solvents. The concept of the hydrophobic bond has been criticised by Hildebrand [330, 331].

(h) SALTS AND UNASSOCIATED LIQUIDS

Deno and Berkheimer [226] give the solubilities of tetra(n-alkyl)ammonium perchlorates in water and in ethanol at 298.2 K. The curves for two of these salts in Fig. 13 suggest that $\underline{n}$ will be equal to 8 and so

$$\log_{10} \frac{[\text{salt in ethanol}]}{[\text{salt in water}]} + 8 \log_{10} \frac{[\text{H}_2\text{O}]_0}{[\text{C}_2\text{H}_5\text{OH}]_0}$$

should equal $V_X/2(0.65[H_2O]_0 - 0.18[C_2H_5OH]_0)$. The comparison is made in Table 40 and the agreement is reasonable. The solubilities of the salts in benzene were also measured and tetra(n-pentyl)ammonium perchlorate and tetra(n-hexyl)ammonium perchlorate were found to be more soluble in benzene than in water. The authors pointed out that if it is desired to conduct a reaction in a hydrocarbon solvent using a small inorganic ion, solubility can be achieved by the use of a salt with a large counter ion, preferably spherical to minimise micelle formation. Such salts generally have low lattice energies so that the absolute solubilities will be reasonably high. Two important developments based on these principles are phase-transfer catalysis and paired-ion chromatography. Phase-transfer catalysis has been reviewed by Dehmlow [332]. One example given is the reaction of 1-chloro-octane with aqueous sodium cyanide. This can be accomplished with 99% yield in less than 2 hours if 1.3 mol % of tributyl-(hexadecyl)phosphonium bromide is present. Without the catalyst, no 1-cyano-octane is formed even if the reagents are boiled together for 2 weeks. Among the advantages of phase-transfer catalysis are low cost and simplicity.

Table 40. Characteristic volumes and the ratio of the solubilities [226] for tetra(n-alkyl)ammonium perchlorates in water and ethanol.

Salt	$Log_{10} \dfrac{[\text{salt in ethanol}]}{[\text{salt in water}]}$	V_X $(m^3\ mol^{-1})$	$\dfrac{1.645 \times 10^{-4}}{V_X - 4.093}$
$(CH_3)_4N\ ClO_4$	-1.93	1.2378×10^{-4}	-2.06
$(C_2H_5)_4N\ ClO_4$	-1.27	1.8014×10^{-4}	-1.13
$(C_3H_7)_4N\ ClO_4$	-0.14	2.4756×10^{-4}	-0.02
$(C_5H_{11})_4N\ ClO_4$	1.74	3.8240×10^{-4}	2.20
$(C_6H_{13})_4N\ ClO_4$	2.82	4.4982×10^{-4}	3.31

Davies [333] has studied the diffusion of salts from water to nitrobenzene. He found that, at a given temperature, equation (100) was obeyed

$$\frac{1}{A} \times \frac{dn}{dt} = k'_f C_1 - k'_R C_2 \tag{100}$$

dn/dt is the diffusion rate (mol s^{-1}),
A is the area through which diffusion occurs,
C_1 is the concentration of salt in the aqueous phase,
C_2 is the concentration of salt in the organic (nitrobenzene) phase,
k'_f and k'_R are the forward and reverse permeability constants.

Davies also measured the partition coefficients for the salts between water and nitrobenzene. He found that a plot of log k'_f against log (partition coefficient) gave a straight line of unit slope. The reverse permeability constants (k'_R), unlike the forward constants (k_f'), were nearly the same for all the salts and did not depend upon the partition coefficients. Davies further found that monolayers of lipid and protein had no effects on the rates of diffusion in either direction. Davies explains these results with the aid of a diagram (Fig. 16). Salts are usually much more soluble in water than in nitrobenzene and there is a large energy barrier to be overcome on passage from the water to the organic liquid; this is largely made up of the partition coefficient free energy. For diffusion in the other direction from nitrobenzene to water, there is only a small energy barrier, which does not involve the partition coefficient, and once the salt is in the water, the large barrier has to be surmounted for passage back again.

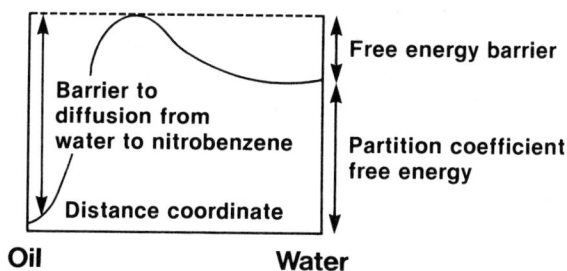

Fig. 16. Energy barriers and diffusion.

Nitrobenzene can be used as an ion exchange membrane. Eisenman [334, 335] showed that nitrobenzene with 5% oleic acid in solution could be used in a cation-selective electrode; nitrobenzene can be used in an anion-selective electrode if the oleic acid is replaced by dodecylamine.

Nitrobenzene is an interesting solvent. The partitioning of nitrobenzene between benzene and water suggests [336] that nitrobenzene in benzene is partially associated to a dimer. Solubilities in aqueous salt solutions [300] (see Chapter 5, section (f)) indicate that nitrobenzene interacts directly with salts. Iwamoto, Ito and Yamamoto [337] measured the partition coefficients for quaternary ammonium iodides between several solvents and water at 298.2 K. Their results for the partition coefficients between nitrobenzene and water are plotted against the characteristic volumes on Fig. 17; the results can also be expressed as $\log_{10}$ (partition coefficient) $= 3.92 - 15\,170\,V_x$ ($n = 5$: $r = 0.9985$). Points from similar measurements of Davies [333] and from solubility measurements of Walden [338] are shown in Fig. 17. Davies also measured partition coefficients for alkali metal iodides; the points for these do not fall on the same line as the quaternary ammonium iodides.

Danil de Namor and Hill [339] have measured the solubilities of many 1:1 electrolytes in nitrobenzene at 298.2 K. They corrected for ion-pair association and worked out the free energies of transfer for the salts from water to nitro-benzene. From the results the ratios of the solubilities of the dissociated salts in water and nitrobenzene can be worked out, and for all 33 salts

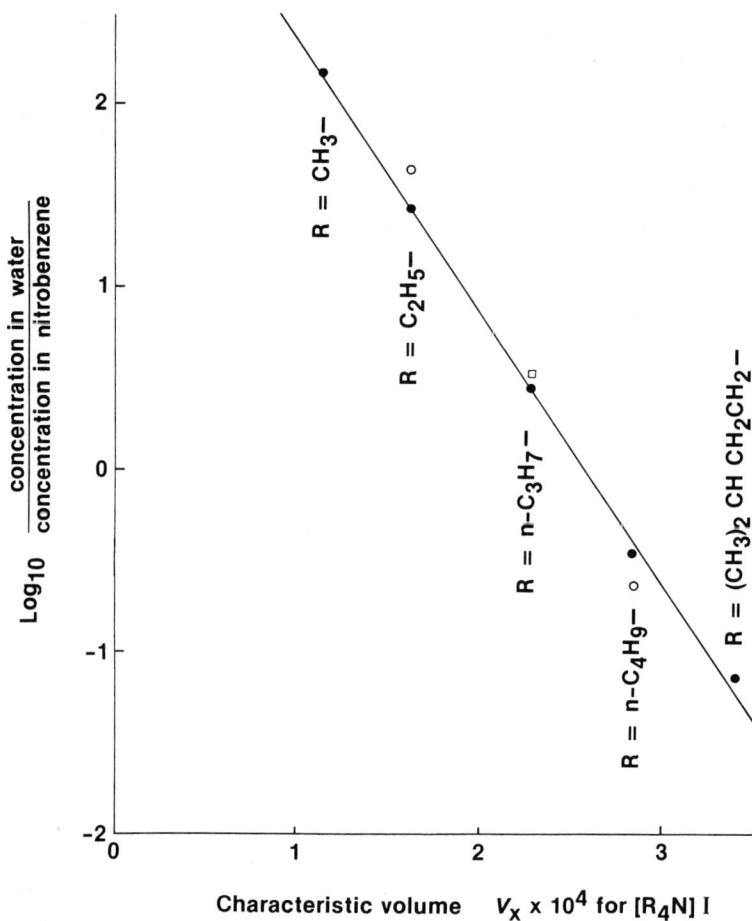

Fig. 17. Partition coefficients of tetra-alkylammonium iodides between nitrobenzene and water at 298.2 K. ● Iwamoto, Ito and Yamamoto [337]; ○ Davies [333]; □ Walden [338].

$$\log_{10} \frac{\text{solubility in water}}{\text{solubility in nitrobenzene}} = 5.268 - 22\,000\,V_x$$

$$(r = 0.971)$$

Abraham and Danil de Namor [340] had earlier studied the transfer of 1:1 electrolytes between water and the isomeric dichloroethanes. For the 24 salts tested with 1,2-dichloroethane

$$\log_{10} \frac{\text{solubility in water}}{\text{solubility in 1,2-dichloroethane}} = 6.360 - 21\,300\,V_x$$

$$(r = 0.973)$$

For 22 salts with 1,1-dichloroethane

$$\log_{10} \frac{\text{solubility in water}}{\text{solubility in 1,1-dichloroethane}} = 6.830 - 20\,400\, V_x$$

$$(r = 0.979)$$

Further results were given [341] for transfer to 1:1 electrolytes between water and 1-propanol. A few ammonium salts were studied. These salts were not used in the experiments described above and they did not fit in with the correlation of the other 27 salts.

$$\log_{10} \frac{\text{solubility in water}}{\text{solubility in 1-propanol}} = 4.29 - 14\,900\, V_x$$

$$(r = 0.992)$$

These results illustrate that characteristic volume is the important factor in the determination of the ratios of solubility in water to that in anhydrous organic solvents.

Paired-ion chromatography has been the subject of several reviews [342, 343]. Ions can be extracted from aqueous solutions into organic solvents if suitable counter-ions are used. An ion pair is considered to be formed in the organic solvent

$$Q^+_{aq} + X^-_{aq} \rightleftharpoons QX_{org}$$

E_{QX}, the extraction constant, $= [QX]\,[Q^+]^{-1}\,[X^-]^{-1}$.

Some figures taken from the reviews are given in the Table 41. The tetra-butylammonium ion is often used as a counter-ion for anions in paired-ion chromatography and it will be seen from section (a) of Table 41 that the values of $\log E$ for some of its salts are in the same order as V_x for the anions (given in brackets). Picrate is an effective counter-ion for many cations. Choline(2-hydroxy-ethyl-trimethylammonium) picrate is about as well extracted as trimethylethylammonium picrate by 1-pentanol and ethyl acetate. These solvents can interact with hydroxyl; chloroform gives much less interaction and trimethylethylammonium picrate is about 30 times more readily extracted than choline picrate by this solvent. The last section of Table 41 shows that some alkaloids and drugs are effective counter-ions. It seems likely that many bio-logically active compounds which contain large ions are physically toxic. In Table 42, the doses [344, 345] of N,N-dialkyl-1-n-decyl-3(carbamoyl)-piperidinium bromides required to give 50% inhibition of choline esterase are compared with the partition coefficients [345] of the salts between water and benzene and the characteristic volumes calculated for the bases. The figures in each column are in exactly the same order.

The partition coefficient, which is the ratio of concentrations of a compound in two phases, equals the ratio of the volume fractions of the compound in these phases (from equation (50)). In equation (70) for the estimation of solubilities

Table 41. Extraction constants for salts of large ions with chloroform as the organic solvent.

Ion	$\text{Log}E_{QX}$
(a) Tetrabutylammonium as counter-ion	
Cl^-	-0.11 $(V_X = 2.10 \times 10^{-5}\ m^3\ mol^{-1})$
Br^-	1.29 $(V_X = 2.62 \times 10^{-5}\ m^3\ mol^{-1})$
NO_3^-	1.39 $(V_X = 3.20 \times 10^{-5}\ m^3\ mol^{-1})$
I	3.01 $(V_X = 3.45 \times 10^{-5}\ m^3\ mol^{-1})$
ClO_4^-	3.48 $(V_X = 4.44 \times 10^{-5}\ m^3\ mol^{-1})$
Picrate	5.91 $(V_X = 12.76 \times 10^{-5}\ m^3\ mol^{-1})$
(b) Picrate as counter-ion	
$C_2H_5N(CH_3)_3^+$	0.04
$HOCH_2CH_2N(CH_3)_3^+$	-1.45
(c) Chloride as counter-ion	
Codeine	-1.12
Papaverine	1.96
Methadone	2.24
Chlorpromazine	2.45

of liquids, C_s/C_L equals the volume fraction in the solution. A correction is required if the solute is not a liquid and C_L is replaced by what is called the ideal solubility. A factor is used which reduces C_L to the solubility predicted for the compound in its own liquid phase. The methods by which this is done are described in Chapter 4. In addition to phase changes, other factors affecting solubilities and partition coefficients are differences in compressibility, characteristic volume, interactions and the presence of electric charges. These have now been discussed. These seem to be the main factors but there may be others. It might be expected that the term involving the electrical charges would include the dielectric constant but this does not seem to be required for the examples given above. It may be that any effect of dielectric constant is largely cancelled by some other factor.

In industry and elsewhere, estimates of solubilities and partition coefficients are often required and the treatment given above should prove helpful. Physical toxicity, which has been mentioned, will now be considered in more detail.

Table 42. Inhibition [344] of cholinesterase by N,N-dialkyl-1-n-decyl-3(carbamoyl)piperidinium bromides.

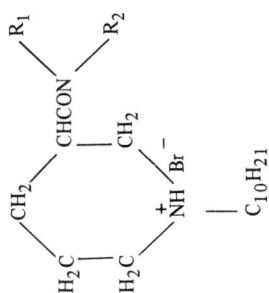

Substituents	Formula of base	V_x ($m^3 mol^{-1}$) for base	Dose to give 50% choline esterase inhibition ($mol\, m^{-3}$)	Partition coefficient of bromide between water and benzene [345]
Dimethyl	$C_{18}H_{36}ON_2$ (57 bonds)	2.7515×10^{-4}	0.027	0.20
Pentamethylene	$C_{20}H_{38}ON_2$ (62 bonds)	2.925×10^{-4}	0.00766	0.49
Diethyl	$C_{20}H_{40}ON_2$ (63 bonds)	3.033×10^{-4}	0.00527	1.58
Hexamethylene	$C_{21}H_{40}ON_2$ (65 bonds)	3.066×10^{-4}	0.00318	1.81
Di-n-propyl	$C_{22}H_{44}ON_2$ (69 bonds)	3.315×10^{-4}	0.00105	7.26

6

Physical Toxicity

(a) PHYSICAL TOXICITY AND LIVING CELLS

Physically toxic compounds affect all living cells. In small doses they stimulate cells and an increase in respiration may be observed [346]. This stimulation probably arises from an uncoupling of oxidative phosphorylation. At larger doses of the physically toxic compound, there is inhibition of many biological processes. Anaesthesia is reversible and complete recovery occurs if the exposure to the compound is terminated, though prolonged anaesthesia may be fatal [347].

Physically toxic compounds not only cause narcosis but they also affect cell division. It is the effects in plants which have been studied most thoroughly. The most characteristic of these effects is c-mitosis (i.e. colchicine-mitosis because the effects resemble those produced by colchicine), which is interference with the orientation of the mitotic spindle that forms in the normal metaphase stage of cell division. Levan [348] describes full c-mitosis as complete inactivation of the spindle. The chromosomes are scattered at random over the cell and form characteristic c-pairs. After division of the chromosomes, one single tetraploid nucleus is often formed. When roots, or other plant organs are treated with a substance causing c-mitosis, a characteristic swelling called a c-tumour is produced. In a normal root, the cells grow mainly in a longitudinal direction but in a c-tumour they grow roughly equally in all directions and this shows up as a tumour. Growth, for at least 24 hours, is necessary for the c-tumour to appear and so, if the compound is especially toxic, no tumours may be seen. Most compounds are toxic at high enough concentrations and, just as there is a correlation between c-mitosis and water solubility, there is a correlation between the toxic concentration and solubility in water but toxicity requires higher concentrations. Levan and Östergren [349, 350] pointed out that the c-mitotic activity of compounds was related to their physical properties. In an important paper, Östergren [351] reviews the subject of c-mitotic activity and lists compounds known to show it. He describes tests in which he used *Allium cepa* and *Pisum sativum*. Some substances are inactive because the solubilities are so low that what would be expected to be a toxic dose cannot be attained: this had been noted earlier for narcotic effects [352]. The reason for the inactivity was demonstrated by the following method used earlier by Overton [11] for narcotics. The compound which is inactive is used with the addition, at a concentration which is just too weak to give an effect, of a fully effective compound. The result is often that an effect is found for the combination although separately each would be too weak to be effective. An illustration of the fact that compounds which are insufficiently soluble to give a certain full biological effect (e.g. no growth) may still give a milder effect (e.g. retardation of growth) and can in combinations contribute towards giving the full effect, is provided by the work of Bateman [353]. He found that saturated solutions of diphenyl, acenaphthene and durene were insufficiently soluble to inhibit growth of the fungus *Fomes annosus*. The percentage retardations of growth for saturated solutions were:

acenaphthene	82.6%
diphenyl	84.0%
durene	95.6%

A mixture of acenaphthene and diphenyl gave 96.6% retardation. A mixture of the three compounds was used and no visible growth was found after 21 days. However, the fungus was not dead because after removal of the hydrocarbons by the aeration, it started to grow again and after 3 days the rate of growth was the same as that on the control medium. Miller, Paton, Smith and Smith [354] found that perfluorinated propane (C_3F_8) did not produce anaesthesia even at saturated vapour pressure but it could contribute something of the order of 40% of the normal anaesthetic dose if mixed with nitrous oxide.

Östergren [351] found that nitrous oxide at ordinary pressure produced c-mitosis in *Pisum sativum* but not in *Allium* root. He suggested that at higher pressures nitrous oxide would affect *Allium* and later it was found [32] that nitrous oxide at 6 atmospheres gave full polyploidy of *Allium* and so did nitrogen at 80 atmospheres. In Table 43, some figures for the concentrations required to inhibit mitosis are given together with the ratio of these concentrations to the concentrations of saturated solutions of the compounds in water. The results are taken from a list [346]; the values for acenaphthene and naphthalene are from Levan and Östergren [349] who used *Allium*, and the other values are those of Gavaudan, Poussel and Dodé [355] who worked with *Triticum*. It is of interest that treatment of yeasts with camphor has produced giant varieties which were probably polypoids [356, 357].

Table 43. Concentrations required for inhibitions of mitosis and ratios of these
to concentrations of saturated solutions [32, 346, 349].

Compound	Concentration of inhibition of mitosis $(mol\ m^{-3})$	Ratio	$\dfrac{toxic\ concentration}{concentration\ of\ saturated\ solution}$
Acenaphthene	0.005		0.20
Naphthalene	0.078		0.24
Ethyl benzoate	0.6		0.23
Chlorobenzene	1.0		0.28
Benzene	6.4		0.33
Chloroform	8.3		0.10
Diethyl ether	200		0.20

The effects of narcotics on the development of animal cells have received less
study than those effects for plants. Fühner [358] found that when the eggs of
the sea urchin *Strongylocentrotus lividus* were treated with sufficiently high
concentrations of alcohols, the larvae formed from the eggs had rudimentary
skeletons. His results for the normal alcohols are given in Table 44. The interpretation of results like these will be discussed in the next chapter, but it is of
interest to note that $33\ 000\ V_x + \log_{10} C_t$ is nearly a constant (3.99). The interaction which has been given to an alcohol with the biophase is -1.2 and
therefore the toxic concentration in the biophase is $3.99 - 1.2$, around 2.8
$mol\ m^{-3}$, which is the figure obtained for the mitosis of *Allium cepa* (see Table
47). Alcohols with more than eight carbon atoms had no effect upon the
development of the eggs of the sea urchin. Either these alcohols diffused into the
eggs too slowly or they were too insoluble in the biophase to reach the dose
necessary for toxicity.

Table 44. Effect of alcohols on the development of eggs of the sea urchin
Strongylocentrotus lividus at room temperature (288–291 K).

Alcohol	Toxic concentration [358] $(C_t)\ (mol\ m^{-3})$	V_x $(m^3\ mol^{-1})$	$33\ 000\ V_x + \log_{10} C_t$
Methanol	719	3.082×10^{-5}	3.81
Ethanol	408	4.491×10^{-5}	4.09
n-Propanol	136	5.900×10^{-5}	3.95
n-Butanol	45.4	7.309×10^{-5}	4.07
n-Heptanol	1.72	1.1536×10^{-4}	4.06
n-Octanol	0.51	1.2945×10^{-4}	3.98

Corman [359] found that urethane and a number of its derivatives inhibited cell division of fertilised eggs of the sea urchin. Urethane has been found [360–366] to induce pulmonary tumours in mice. It is not known, however, whether these effects are given specifically by urethanes or by physically toxic compounds in general.

When winter approaches the larvae of the sugar-beet web worm, *Loxostege sticticalis*, enter into a dormant prepupal stage and remain like this until the following spring. High temperatures do not break the dormancy but if the temperature is gradually lowered to below freezing, pupation occurs. The dormant period (prepupal diapause) is greatly reduced by exposure to xylene, carbon tetrachloride, diethyl ether and ethylene dichloride [367].

Yasuda-Yasaki, Namiki-Kanie and Hachisuka [368] tested a variety of compounds for inhibition of the germination of *Bacillus subtilis* PCI219 spores under the influence of the initiator L-alanine. The inhibition was reversed when the spores were washed. Among the compounds used were 20 alcohols, and $\log I_{50}$ for these correlated well with the logarithms of the partition coefficients between water and 1-octanol. Above 1-decanol there was a 'cut-off' and a saturated solution of 1-dodecanol would only give 10% inhibition of the germination initiated by L-alanine.

(b) PHYSICAL TOXICITY AND ENZYMES

Examples are found in which physically toxic substances inhibit the activity of enzymes. McLennan and Elliott [369] studied the effects of narcotic drugs on acetylcholine synthesis in brain cortex slices. They found the synthesis was accelerated by very low doses, and inhibited at higher concentrations. The concentrations of narcotics which produce inhibition *in vitro* were roughly equal to the concentrations estimated for narcosis *in vivo*. Other examples like this one often refer to systems in which many components besides the enzyme and the substrate are present. Schreiner [370, 371] and coworkers, however, claim to have inhibited the following five purified enzymes: catechol oxidase, lipooxygenase, acetyl cholinesterase, α-chymotrypsin and leucine amino-peptidase by krypton, xenon, sulphur hexafluoride and nitrous oxide — all of which produce narcosis in animals. The action of physically toxic compounds on enzymes is discussed in Chapter 7.

(c) ESTIMATION OF PHYSICAL TOXICITIES

It has been found that values of the logarithm of the toxic dose of a physically toxic compound ($\log_{10} C_t$) for a given biological effect can be made up from factors, which can be derived from equation (44), which is similar to the one (70) already given for partitions

$$-\log_{10} C_t + \log_{10} C_B = kV_x - E \qquad (101)$$

Here k is a constant, C_t is the toxic concentration in water, C_B is the toxic (constant) concentration in the biophase, V_x is the characteristic volume and E is the sum of the interaction terms. The values of k ($33\,000$ mol m^{-3}) and E (-1.2) for hydroxyl, keto, ether and ester groups show that the biophase is associated and probably contains considerable quantities of water. The nature of the biophase will be discussed in the next chapter. Equation (101) has been used to correlate toxicity and enzyme inhibition data [372] and to predict the toxicities of aqueous solutions to fish [373]. An additional example is given Table 45 based on the toxicities to bluegill (*Lepomis machochirus*) [374].

Table 45. Concentrations (mol m^{-3}) for acute toxicities of hydrocarbons and their chlorinated derivatives to bluegill (*Lepomis machochirus*) after 96 hours of exposure at 295 K.

Compound	Formula	Toxic conc C_t found	(C_t) (m^3 mol^{-1}) C_t calculated[a]
Dichloromethane	CH_2Cl_2	2.59	2.32
Tetrachloroethene	C_2Cl_4	0.08	0.17
1,1-Dichloroethene	$C_2H_2Cl_2$	0.76	1.09
1,2-Dichloroethene	$C_2H_2Cl_2$	1.44	1.09
1,1,1,2-Tetrachloroethane	$C_2H_2Cl_4$	0.12	0.12
1,1,2,2-Tetrachloroethane	$C_2H_2Cl_4$	0.13	0.12
1,3-Dichloropropene	$C_3H_4Cl_2$	0.06	0.37
1,2-Dichlorobenzene	$C_6H_4Cl_2$	0.04	0.06
1,3-Dichlorobenzene	$C_6H_4Cl_2$	0.03	0.06
Toluene	C_7H_8	0.14	0.14
1-Chloronaphthalene	$C_{10}H_7Cl$	0.01	0.01

a C_t calculated from equation (101) using $\log_{10} C_t = -33\,000\,V_x + 2.0$.

In Table 46, a set of factors, based on the values of k and E just given, with $E = -0.6$ for phenols and phenol ethers, are listed to replace those published many years ago [47].

Table 46. Factors (f) for the calculation of physical toxicities C_t in aqueous solutions from $\log_{10} C_B = \log_{10} C_t + \Sigma f$.

Ethane	1.30	Benzene	2.42
Thiophene	2.12	Other hydrocarbons	$33\,000\,V_x$ (with V_x in m^3 mol^{-1})

Substitution of CH by	N	-1.34
	C–OH (alcoholic)	-1.00
	C–CHO	-0.67

Table 46. (continued)

Ethane 1.30	Benzene	2.42
Thiophene 2.12	Other hydrocarbons	33 000 V_X (with V_X in m^3 mol^{-1})

	C–OH (phenolic)	−0.40
	C–F	+0.06
	C–Cl	+0.40
	C–CH$_3$	+0.464
	C–Br	+0.58
	C–NO$_2$	+0.58
	C–I	+0.85
	C–C$_6$H$_5$	+2.08
Substitution of C–C by	C–O–C (aliphatic)	−0.98
	C–C–C $\overset{\|}{O}$	−0.66
	C–C–O–C $\overset{\|}{O}$	−0.47
	C–O–C (phenolic)	−0.40
	C–CH$_2$–C	+0.464
	C–S–C	0.54
Substitution of C=C by	CH–CH	0.143

A table of values for $\log_{10} C_B$ (a constant for a given biological effect) was also given. In the earlier work, it was assumed that the biophase was an unassociated liquid with a compressibility near that, say, of benzene. However, this does not seem to be correct. The biophase resembles a polymeric liquid and is somewhat associated. No appreciable correction appears to be required for compressibilities in equation (101).

In Table 47, values of $\log_{10} C_B$ have been revised and some additional ones given: C_B is now in mol m^{-3}.

The factors given in Table 46 may be useful for the investigation of biological activities which might be physical. Evans, James and Luscombe [393] consider that the action of many compounds giving carminative activity is physical. They studied the effects of a variety of compounds on the inhibition of the response to carbachol (carbamylcholine chloride, H$_2$NCOO(CH$_2$)$_2$N$^+$(CH$_3$)$_3$Cl$^-$) of guinea pig isolated ileum at 303 K, and give C_t, the concentrations required to inhibit the response by 50%. Incidentally, some of the concentrations were above the solubilities of the compounds: these were obtained by extrapolation from concentrations giving responses less than 50%. Such hypothetical figures for C_t may be misleading and are best avoided. The equation (101) can be written

Table 47. Values of $\log_{10} C_B$ for various biological effects (C_B in mol m^{-3})

Biological effect	Conditions	$\log_{10} C_B$	Reference	Code	Number of results
Kill *Staphylococcus aureus*	5 min at 310 K	4.4	[375]	A	8
Kill *Staphylococcus aureus*	10 min at 293 K	4.3	[376, 377]	B	22
Kill *Staphylococcus aureus*	10 min at 293 K	4.3	[378]	C	12
Kill *Staphylococcus aureus*	10 min at 293 K	4.1	[379—381]	D	22
Kill *Staphylococcus aureus*	10 min at 310 K	4.1	[380—385]	E	38
Kill *Salmonella typhosa*	10 min at 293 K	4.1	[376, 377]	F	62
Kill *Salmonella typhosa*	10 min at 293 K	4.1	[386]	G	11
Kill *Candida albicans*	10 min at 310 K	4.1	[381, 385]	H	16
Kill *Mycobacterium tuberculosis*	10 min at 310 K	4.1	[381, 385]	I	16
Kill *Staphylococcus aureus*	15 min at 310 K	4.1	[387]	J	10
Kill *Candida tropicalis*	30 min at 298 K	4.0	[388]	K	25
Kill *Salmonella typhosa*	10 min at 293 K	4.0	[379—381]	L	23
Kill *Salmonella typhosa*	15 min at 293 K	4.0	[389]	M	9
Kill *Salmonella typhosa*	15 min at 293 K	3.9	[387]	N	10
Kill *Sporotrichum* species	30 min at 298 K	3.9	[388]	O	7
Kill *Salmonella typhosa*	10 min at 310 K	3.8	[380—385]	P	37
Kill *Salmonella typhosa*	15 min at 310 K	3.8	[389]	Q	9
Kill *Aphis rumicis*	At room temp.	3.8	[390]	R	20
Kill fungus 'Madison 517'		3.6	[391, 392]	S	56
Kill *Escherichia coli*	24 h at 310 K	3.6	[389]	T	5
Kill grain weevils	5 h at 298 K	3.4	[24, 30]		
Kill *Escherichia coli*	48 h at 310 K	3.2	[420, 421]	U	31

Table 47. (continued)

Biological effect	Conditions	$\text{Log}_{10} C_B$	Reference	Code	Number of results
Kill wireworms	17 h at 288 K	3.2	[4]		
Kill *Pseudomonas aeruginosa*	48 h at 310 K	3.1	[421]	V	26
Inhibit lysophosphatidylcholine acyltransferase		2.9	[50, 398]		
Inhibit mitosis of *Triticum*		2.9	[346]	W	14
Inhibit growth of *Fomes annosus*		2.8	[353]	X	15
Inhibit mitosis of *Allium cepa*		2.8	[349–351]	Y	52
Reduce haemolysis of erythrocytes by 50%		2.7	[50, 398]		
Narcotise tadpoles		2.7	[11]	Z	91
Narcotise mice		2.6	[6]		
Narcotise human beings		2.6	[422, 423]		
Safe concentration giving no toxic symptoms		1.5	[424]		

$$\log_{10} C_B - \log_{10} C_t = \Sigma f \tag{102}$$

where Σf is the sum of the factors (from Table 46). In Table 48, values of Σf and $3.8 - \log_{10} C_t$, with C_t in mol m^{-3}, are compared. In most cases, there is good agreement between the figures, and Evans, James and Luscombe appear to be right to attribute the carminative action to 'physical toxicity'. However, 3.8 is a high figure for $\log_{10} C_B$. It will be seen from Table 47 that this value of $\log_{10} C_B$ is equal to the value which would kill *Aphis rumicis* and *Salmonella typhosa* (codes P, Q and R). Codes are used to label some of the biological activities measured for aqueous solutions, and in Table 48 these codes are used to label the biological activities for which $\log_{10} C_B - \log_{10} C_t$ are quoted from those given for many compounds [47]. The compounds in the table are those for which $\log_{10} C_B - \log_{10} C_t$ values have been given [47] and C_t measured by Evans, James and Luscombe [393].

Table 48. Physical toxicity and carminative activity.

Compound	Σf	$\log_{10} C_B - \log_{10} C_t$ [47]	Carminative activity [393] $3.8 - \log_{10} C_t$
Acetic acid, n-butyl ester	2.3	S2.4; Z2.1	2.3
Acetic acid, ethyl ester	1.4	S1.5; Z1.3	1.5
Acetic acid, propyl ester	1.8	S1.9; Z1.8	1.8
Camphor	—	Y(3.0)	3.1
Catechol	1.7	E1.9; K1.8; N1.8; P2.1	1.9
o-Cresol	2.6	A2.5; C2.6; D2.4; E2.4; F2.5; H2.5; I2.5; L2.4; P2.5; R2.6; U2.4; V2.3; Z2.7	2.5
m-Cresol	2.6	A2.5; C2.6; D2.4; E2.4; F2.6; H2.5; I2.5; J2.5; L2.4; N2.6; P2.5; R2.6; U2.4; V2.3; Z2.7	2.4
p-Cresol	2.6	A2.5; B2.6; C2.6; D2.4; E2.4; F2.6; H2.5; I2.5; J2.6, L2.4; N2.6; P2.5; R2.6, U2.4; V2.3	
Dibutyl ether	3.3	S3.2	2.1
Diethyl ether	1.3	S1.3; W0.7; Y1.0; Z1.0	1.5
3:4-Dimethylphenol	3.0	D2.7; E2.8; F3.0; H2.9; I2.9; K2.9; L2.8; P2.9	2.8
Dipropyl ether	2.3	I2.9; K2.9; L2.8; P2.9; S2.3	1.9
Eugenol	3.5	Z2.8	3.3
1-Hexanol	2.3	F2.5; S2.5	2.4

Table 48. (continued)

Compound	Σf	$\mathrm{Log}_{10}\,C_B - \log_{10} C_t$ [47]	Carminative activity [393] $3.8 - \log_{10} C_t$
o-Methoxyphenol	2.2	C2.3; E2.1; P2.1; Z2.3	2.2
p-Methoxyphenol	2.2	C2.3; E2.1; L2.2; P2.1	2.2
1-Pentanol	1.8	F2.0; S2.1	2.0
Hydroquinone	1.7	D1.6; E1.8; K1.5; L2.1; N2.2; P1.7; U2.2; V2.6; X1.3	1.8
Resorcinol	1.7	A1.8; D1.8; E1.7; F1.8; G1.7; K1.5; L1.6; N1.6; P1.7	1.9
Thymol	4.0	A3.9; D3.5; F3.8; K3.6; L3.8; O3.7; U3.1; V2.4; Z4.1	3.6

The program in Appendix II may be helpful for the study of the relationship between the concentrations for a given biological effect C_t and characteristic volumes V_x. Correlations are expressed as

$$-\log_{10} C_t = kV_x - (\log_{10} C_B + E)$$

(see equation (101)). The total number of compounds and the correlation coefficient are given. Allowance can be made for interactions of isolated ester, alcohol, aldehyde, ketone and ester groups. Other interactions will be included in the $\log_{10} C_B$ term. When the correlation has been done, the program enables values of C_t to be estimated from V_x for compounds other than those tested.

(d) PHYSICAL TOXICITY IN SYSTEMS CONTAINING AQUEOUS AND NON-AQUEOUS PHASES

The equation (101) has been adapted by McGowan [26] so that it can be used to give the toxicities of physically toxic compounds in systems containing an organic phase as well as water; the treatment was applied to the injection of physically toxic compounds into animals. The usual way to express such doses is in mol per kg (e.g. of body weight), for which the symbol C_t' will be used. If C_w is the toxic concentration in the aqueous phase of the system, equation (101) can still be used with C_w substituted for C_t. In the original simple treatment of physical toxicity it was assumed that all unassociated organic liquids giving no specific interactions had the same value for k and that the biophase was such a liquid. This assumption will be made here. Later, when the nature of the biophase is discussed (Chapter 7), evidence will be given that the biophase is a separate phase which consists of a somewhat associated liquid. If the system consists of $x_x\%$ by weight of aqueous phase (density ρ_w) and $x_f\%$ of non-aqueous phase (density ρ_f)

$$C_t' = \frac{C_w x_w}{100\rho_w} + \frac{C_B x_f}{100\rho_f} \tag{103}$$

and the density of the system

$$\rho_s = \frac{100}{(x_f/\rho_f) + (x_w/\rho_w)} \tag{104}$$

from (101) and (104).

$$C_t' = \frac{C_B x_f}{100\rho_f} + \frac{C_B x_w}{100\rho_w} 10^{-k V_x + E} \tag{105}$$

If the toxic concentration is measured at C_t mol per m^3 system, C_t can be obtained by multiplication of C_t' by the density of the system (ρ_s) from (104)

$$C_t = \frac{C_B x_f \rho_s}{100\rho_f} = \frac{C_B x_w \rho_s}{100\rho_s} 10^{-k V_x + E} \tag{106}$$

$$= C_B \left[\begin{pmatrix} \text{volume fraction} \\ \text{of non-aqueous} \\ \text{phase} \end{pmatrix} + \begin{pmatrix} \text{volume fraction} \\ \text{of aqueous} \\ \text{phase} \end{pmatrix} \times 10^{-k V_x + E} \right] \tag{107}$$

Experiments can usually be made over a large range of C_t and for most of the range only one of the two terms in equation (106) will be of importance. If $kV_x - E$ is high enough, the second term can be neglected and

$$C_t = C_B X \text{ (volume fraction of non-aqueous phase)} = \text{a constant}$$

If $kV_x - E$ is small enough, the compound will be largely dissolved in the aqueous phase. When $kV_x - E$ is zero, $C_t = C_B$. Very often the volume fraction of the aqueous phase is close to unity and then for low values of $kV_x - E$.

$$C_t' = C_B \, 10^{-k V_x + E}$$

approximately. The result is that if the negative logarithm of the toxic concentration, $(-\log C_t)$, is plotted against $kV_x - E$, the points will fall near a straight line of slope 45° cutting the $-\log C_t$ axis at $-\log_{10} C_B$ (the negative logarithm of the toxic concentration in the biophase), when $kV_x - E$ is zero. Then at some point depending on the volume fraction of non-aqueous layer present, the line will turn and for high values of $kV_x - E$, the points will fall near a horizontal line with $-\log C_t = -\log_{10} C_B - \log$ (volume fraction of non-aqueous phase). If there is an appreciable amount of lipid in the system and if the compound is much more soluble in lipid than in water, from equation (105)

$$C'_t = \frac{C_B x_f}{100 \rho_f} = \text{a constant}$$

Mills [394] considers that mammals consist of approximately 66% water (x_x) and 4% lipid (x_p). The following values have been given [395] for $-\log_{10} C'_t$ for doses of hydrocarbons required to kill rats within 24 hours:

toluene	1.7
o-xylene	1.7–1.9
m-xylene	1.7–1.8
p-xylene	1.7–1.8
mesitylene	1.9–2.0
pseudocumene	1.8–2.0

These values are approximately constant and if used in the above equation with ρ_f equal to 0.93, $\log_{10} C_B$ comes to about 2.5, which is reasonable since it was previously found [47] that $\log_{10} C_B$ was 3 for the death of rats in 3 hours. (It should be noted that SI units are now being used and the concentrations given in early papers in mol litre^{-1} have to be multiplied by 1000 to give mol m^{-3}.)

More recently, further results have been given [396] for LD$_{50}$ of compounds required to kill rats by intraperitoneal injection. These give the following $-\log_{10} C'_t$ values:

carbon tetrachloride	2.2
chlorobenzene	2.3
toluene	2.2
benzene	2.5

These values are also apparently constant but correspond to lower doses (C'_t) than those given by Cameron et al. [395]. Variation between different sets of experiments is to be expected.

Measurements have been made [397] of the effects of chlorinated biphenyls and other compounds (see list in caption to Fig. 18) on the activity of the lymphocyte plasma membrane enzyme 5'-nucleotidase in cells from the spleens of mice. In Fig. 18, the $\log_{10}$ (concentration required to produce half-maximal inhibition) (log K_i) is plotted against $36\,000\,V_x - E_B$. The concentrations are in mol m^{-3}. The values of E_B used were 1.2 for alcoholic hydroxyl and -0.35 for chlorine. The points fall near a curve given by

$$K_i = 6.92 \times 10^{-2} + 1780 \times 10^{-(36\,000 V_x - E_B)} \tag{108}$$

If equation (108) is compared with equation (107)

$$\frac{\text{volume of non-aqueous phase}}{\text{volume of aqueous phase}} = 3.89 \times 10^{-5}$$

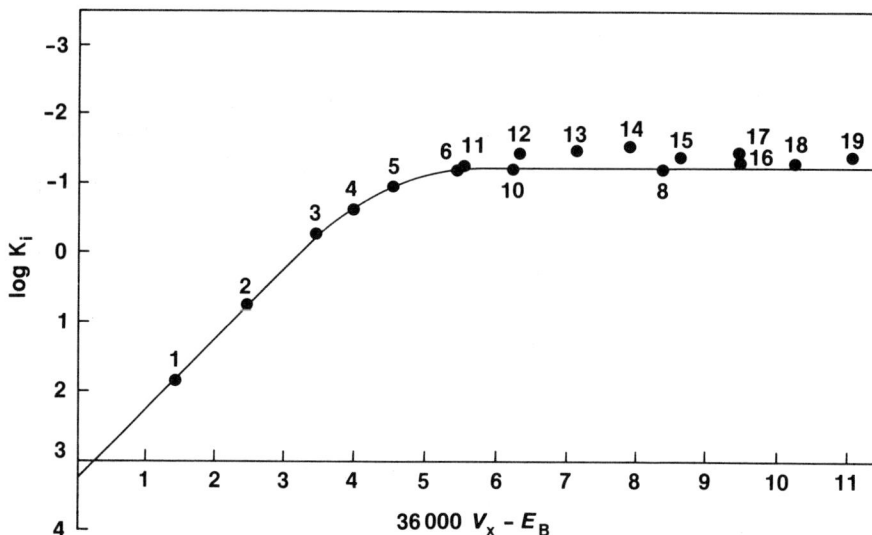

Fig. 18. Inhibition of the lymphocyte plasma membrane 5'-nucleotidase by chlorinated biphenyls and other compounds [397]. (1) Butanol; (2) hexanol; (3) octanol; (4) nonanol; (5) decanol; (6) dodecanol; †(7) tetradecanol; (8) *trans*-retinol; †(9) chloro-octane; (10) chlorodecane; (11) 4-chlorobiphenyl; (12) 2,2'-dichlorobiphenyl (CB); (13) 2,4,5-tri-CB; (14) 2,2',4,5'-tetra-CB; (15) 2,2',3,4,5'-penta-CB; (16) 2,2',3,4,4',5-hexa-CB; (17) 2,2',4,4',5,6'-hexa-CB; (18) 2,2',3,4,4',5,6'-hepta-CB; (19) 2,2',3,4,4',5,6,6'-octa-CB.

† No K_i value was obtained for this compound but an LD_{50} was given.

Also since the volume of the non-aqueous phase is so much smaller than that of the aqueous phase, $\log C_t = \log C_B$ when $-kV_x + E_B$ is zero. Therefore from equation (108), $\log_{10} C_B = 3.25$.

The effects [50, 398, 399] of various compounds on the activity of the synaptosomal enzyme acyl coenzyme-A lysophosphatidylcholine acyl transferase from mouse brain were determined and it was found that

$$K_i = 0.2 + 1000 \times 10^{-(36\,000 V_x - E_B)} \qquad (109)$$

with E_B equal to 1.2 for a carbonyl, ester, aliphatic hydroxyl or aliphatic ether and 0.6 for phenolic hydroxyl or aromatic ether. If this equation is compared with equation (107)

$$\frac{\text{volume of non-aqueous phase}}{\text{volume of aqueous phase}} = 2 \times 10^{-4} \text{ and } \log_{10} C_B = 3.$$

Anaesthetics protect erythrocytes from haemolysis [400]. In Fig. 19, concentrations required to reduce osmotic haemolysis by 50% (AH_{50}) have been used as a measure of physical toxicity. Values given by Roth and Seeman [401] and Greenberg *et al.* [50] are used and the points fall near a curve corresponding to

$$AH_{50}/1000 = 4 \times 10^{-5} + 0.6 10^{-36\,000 V_x + E_B}$$

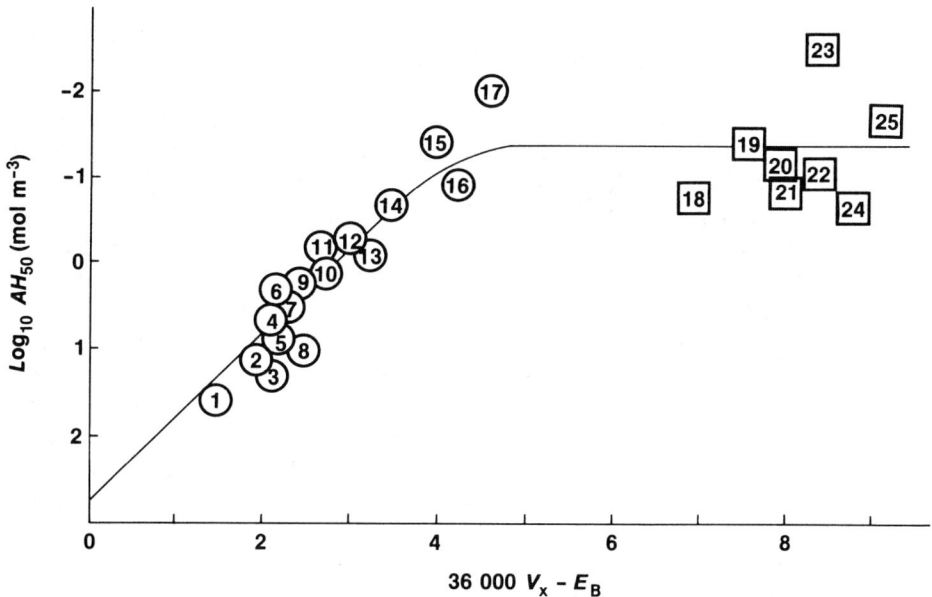

Fig. 19. Anti-haemolytic concentrations (AH_{50}), characteristic volumes (V_x) and interaction terms (E_B). The AH_{50} is the concentration of each compound required to inhibit by 50% the hypotonic lysis of erythrocytes. Compounds in circles are for human erythrocytes, from the work of Roth and Seeman [401]. Compounds in squares are for equine erythrocytes, from Huszar, Greenberg and Mellors [398]. The compounds are: (1) 1-butanol; (2) 1-Pentanol; (3) benzyl alcohol; (4) 4-fluorophenol; (5) phenol; (6) 4-$CO_2 CH_3$-phenol; (7) chloroform; (8) 4-methoxyphenol; (9) 1-hexanol; (10) p-cresol; (11) 4-chlorophenol; (12) 1-heptanol; (13) 3,5-dimethylphenol; (14) 1-octanol; (15) 1-nonanol; (16) 4-t-butylphenol; (17) 1-decanol; (18) 11-hydroxy-Δ^9-tetrahydrocannabinol (THC); (19) cannabinol; (20) Δ^9-THC; (21) Δ^8-THC; (22) synhexyl Δ^9-THC; (23) retinol; (24) cannabidiol; (25) cannabigerol.

All compounds for which E values can be allotted are included. From the results:

$$\frac{\text{volume of non-aqueous phase in system}}{\text{volume of aqueous phase in system}} = \frac{4 \times 10^{-5}}{0.6} = 7 \times 10^{-5}$$

so that in a litre of the liquid there would be less than one-tenth of a millilitre of non-aqueous phase. This volume for the non-aqueous phase of the erythrocyte suspension is consistent with our estimates of the volume of lipids in the erythrocyte membranes and does account for the curve shown in the Fig. 19. If only aqueous phase were present the curve would have a slope of 45° throughout, but it bends and becomes practically horizontal, corresponding to a constant concentration of 4×10^{-2} mol m^{-3} in the system, i.e. in 7×10^{-5} m^3 of non-aqueous phase. Thus C_B is $(4 \times 10^{-2})/(7 \times 10^{-5})$ mol m^{-3} and $\log_{10} C_B$ is 2.8. In the next section, the following values of $\log_{10} C_B$ are given:

for narcosis of tadpoles $\log_{10} C_B = 2.7$
for narcosis of mice or human beings $\log_{10} C_B = 2.6$

It is of interest that all these values for anaesthetic effects are so close. Hyde [402, 403] has used equations similar to these just discussed for systems containing water and non-aqueous phases.

Batelli and Stern [404] carried out some of the earliest studies of the effects of anaesthetics on enzyme activity. They studied the inhibition of succinate dehydrogenase in tissue homogenates of ox diaphragm and sheep liver. The uptakes of oxygen were measured at 288 and 313 K for periods of time in the presence of various concentrations of anaesthetics. Values of $\log_{10} C_t$ for 15–20% inhibition over 30 minutes with muscle tissue at 313 K are plotted in Fig. 20 against $36\,000\,V_x - E$ (with $E = 0.6$ for the two phenols and 1.2 for alcohols and ketones). The line shown has a slope of 45°. The muscle and liver tissue gave very similar results and in each case, the concentration for 15–20% inhibition was about half that required for complete inhibition. Batelli and Stern considered that proteins rather than lipids were involved in the action of anaesthetics. They observed that all the anaesthetics caused 'nucleoproteins' to separate from aqueous solutions. At a certain critical concentration, centrifugation of the liver preparation gave a clear fluid free from 'nucleoprotein' and this critical concentration was usually close to that required for complete inactivation of the succinic acid oxidation.

Modern work on the multiprotein complex (complex II) of the electron transport chain, which reduces succinate and passes electrons to ubiquinone, shows that the complex consists of four polypeptides. The two largest polypeptides form the so-called succinate dehydrogenase can be split off the two smaller polypeptides by certain salts, notably perchlorate [405]. The larger unit is soluble and is composed of two iron—sulphur proteins, one of which is also a flavoprotein [406]. The two smaller polypeptides are rendered insoluble by perchlorate cleavage and form a precipitate [407]. Other enzymic reactions are affected by salts. Hatefi and Hanstein [408] found that a number of salts induced enzymically catalysed lipid oxidation, and that sodium thiocyanate was the most effective of the salts tested.

Chazotte and Vanderkooi [409] studied the inhibition of a number of oxidases by some alcohols and local anaesthetics of the tertiary amine class. They found that low concentrations of many of the compounds activated the enzymes whilst higher doses gave inhibition. Although their experimental methods and conditions are quite different from those of Batelli and Stern, it is of interest to note (Table 49) how well the two sets of results for the inhibition of succinate dehydrogenase compare.

(e) PHYSICAL TOXICITIES WITH SALT SOLUTIONS

Miller [18] suggested that the increase in toxicity of phenol in aqueous solutions of many salts was caused by salting out, i.e. by the rise in chemical potential of

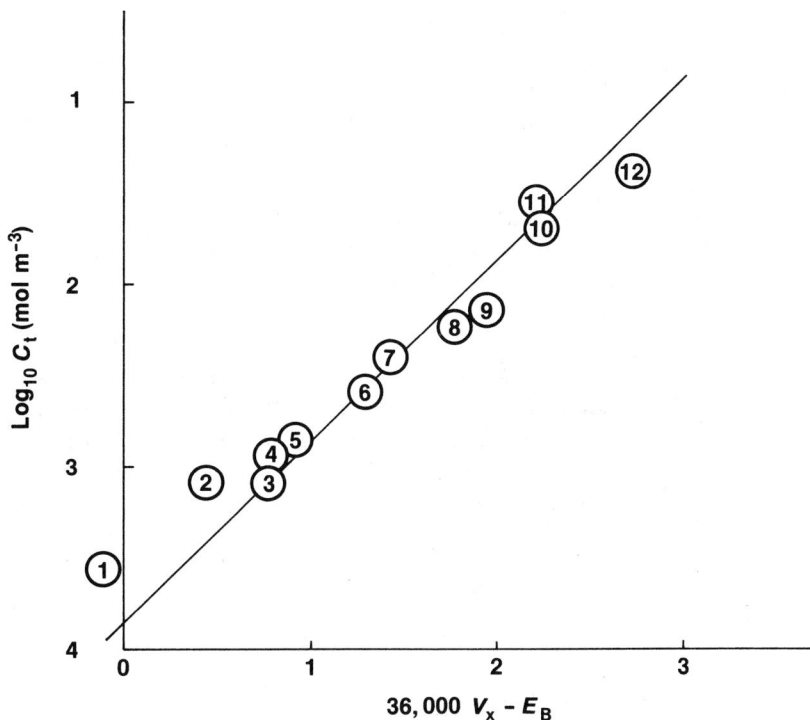

Fig. 20. The inhibition of succinate oxidation in bovine diaphragm homogenates. The concentration needed for 15–20% inhibition (C_t) was measured for 12 compounds [404]. The compounds are: (1) methanol; (2) ethanol; (3) acetone; (4) 2-propen-1-ol; (5) propanol; (6) methyl ethyl ketone; (7) isobutanol; (8) methyl propyl ketone; (9) isopentanol; (10) chloroform; (11) phenol; (12) o-cresol.

the phenol. Experiments undertaken in his laboratory [19, 410, 411] demonstrate this. In Table 50, the number of anthrax spores (*Bacillus anthracis*) alive after treatment [412] with 4% phenol in solutions of salts (all at 1000 mol m^{-3}) are compared with the chemical equivalent of the solutions in which kerosene was used as the organic solvent. The chemical equivalent is the strength of that solution of phenol in water which would give the same concentration in the organic solvent as was given by the salt solution. It is interesting that sodium benzoate, which, of the salts used, has the largest volume, salts phenol into water, whereas all the other salts salt out the phenol. The effect of volume on physical toxicities in sea water is, as expected [26], slightly higher than for water itself. It would be of interest to study the effects of physically toxic substances on those bacteria [413] which can live in 20–30% solutions of sodium, and in lithium chloride solution (0.45 kg per kg water) [414], which is nine times stronger osmotically than saturated brine.

The equation (87) has already been used to predict the effects of salts on partitioning of non-electrolytes between aqueous solutions and an organic phase

Table 49. Inhibition of succinate dehydrogenase by alcohols.

Alcohol	V_x (m³ mol⁻¹)	C_t (mol m⁻¹)					
		Enzyme from ox diaphragm muscle at 313 K [404]		Enzyme from sheep's liver at 3.3 K [404]		50% inhibition at 298 K of enzyme [409]	
		15–20% inhibition	Complete inhibition	15–20% Inhibition	Complete inhibition	From ox heart	From rat liver
Methanol	3.083×10^{-5}	3680	6050	3150	5780	–	–
Ethanol	4.492×10^{-5}	1220	3170	1580	2970	–	–
2-Propen-1-ol	5.471×10^{-5}	890	1640	670	1340	–	–
1-Propanol	5.901×10^{-5}	750	1190	680	1090	–	–
1-Butanol	7.310×10^{-5}	–	–	–	–	420	170
1-Propanol, 2-methyl-	7.310×10^{-5}	250	440	240	410	–	–
1-Pentanol	8.718×10^{-5}	–	–	–	–	125	65
1-Butanol, 3-methyl-	8.718×10^{-5}	140	190	130	180	–	–
Benzyl alcohol	9.160×10^{-5}	–	–	–	–	130	80
1-Hexanol	1.02178×10^{-4}	–	–	–	–	95	45

Table 50. The effects of salts on the partition of phenol between water and kerosene and on the toxicity of 4% solutions towards anthrax spores.

Salt	Chemical equivalent (%) of 4% phenol in water [411]	Number of colonies of B. anthracis [412]
Na benzoate	3.1	1963
None	4.0	1505
KI	5.0	368
NH_4Cl	5.3	336
$NaNO_3$	5.4	422
Na acetate	5.4	804
KBr	5.8	295
LiCl	6.1	253
$NaClO_4$	6.15	280
KCl	6.25	174
NaCl	6.5	131

$$\log_{10}(S_0/S_m) = \underline{k}_s C_s \tag{87}$$

Here S_m and S_0 are the solubilities of the non-electrolyte in the salt solution of concentration C_s, and in water alone respectively. Further, the relationship (94) has been given to relate $\underline{k}_s$ to Σz^2, the sum of the squares of the charges on the ions making up the salt, the characteristic volume V_x of the non-electrolyte and $\bar{V}_s^\circ$, the partial molar volume of the salt in the solution

$$\underline{k}_s = V_x(1.35\,\Sigma z^2 - 36\,000\,\bar{V}_s^\circ) \tag{94}$$

From equation (94), it will be seen that $\underline{k}_s$ can be positive or negative depending on whether $36\,000\,\bar{V}_s^\circ$ is smaller or larger than $1.35\,\Sigma z^2$. The solubility of sodium benzoate in water at 298 K has been given [415] as 2888 mol m^{-3} and the density of this solution is 1155 kg m^{-3}. From these figures and equation (11), $\bar{V}_s^\circ$ for sodium benzoate equals 8.97×10^{-5} n^{-3} m^{-1}. This figure and equation (94) give $\underline{k}_s = -0.53$ and indicate that sodium benzoate would salt-in non-electrolytes.

A few experiments of Bancroft and Rutzler [416] led them to believe that some effects in animals of certain anaesthetics could be reversed by injection of 10% aqueous sodium thiocyanate. Sodium thiocyanate has not a large enough $\bar{V}_s^\circ$ value [103] for one to expect from equation (94) that it would salt-in non-electrolytes and before an explanation is attempted, it is desirable that the results of Bancroft and Rutzler should be repeated and extended.

(f) FURTHER ASPECTS OF PHYSICAL TOXICITY

In order that the preceding equations can be applied, the toxic doses for a certain definite biological effect must be used. Correlations have been found between various measures of biological effect for compounds at a fixed dose [417–419] and parachor (i.e. characteristic volume). In some studies such correlations may prove of value.

The partition coefficient of a compound is equal to the ratio of its solubilities in the two phases, i.e. to the ratio of the volume fractions in the phases (see Chapter 5). In order to produce a certain biological effect, Mullins [25] has suggested it is not that a definite concentration of any inert molecule is needed in the biophase but that a constant volume of the biophase should be occupied. However, at present, it is not easy to decide between these alternatives. The volume fractions corresponding to a fixed concentration are for many compounds nearly proportional to V_x, the characteristic volumes. It is therefore possible by adjustment to k (and sometimes E) to get reasonable agreement with either view.

(g) HYDRATION AND SWEETNESS OF CERTAIN CARBOHYDRATE DERIVATIVES

Collander [229] gives approximate values for the partition coefficients of some carbohydrates between water and ether. In Table 51, values of the hydration number n have been calculated from these with equation (99), and the interaction term E for a hydroxyl group equal to -1.9. It is of interest that not all the oxygen atoms in the carbohydrates give interactions and that n is close to values given in the literature [425, 426] for hydration numbers. Juszkiewicz [425] obtained hydration numbers by a method [317, 427] based on the velocity of ultrasonic waves through solutions in mixtures of water and ethanol. He found that hydration varied slightly as the concentration of carbohydrate increased but this was not enough to affect the value expressed as the nearest whole number. Munton [426] derived hydration from densities and osmotic coefficients. For glucose, the hydration determined by both methods was 5, in agreement with the values of n from the partition coefficient. It looks as if the disaccharides sucrose, maltose (4-O-α-D-glucopyranosyl-D-glucose) and lactose (4-O-α-D-galactopyranosyl-D-glucose) have hydration and n equal to 7, or more likely 8. Rhamnose (6-deoxymannose) and the pentoses, arabinose and xylose have hydration equal to 4. In addition, the hydration of D-ribose has been given as 4 [428]. The hexoses appear to have n equal to 5 and when two hexoses combine to form a disaccharide n seems to be 8. The difference between these values of n is 3 and it is of interest that Juszkiewicz and Potaczek [429] found the hydration of dextran to be about 3 mol of water per mol of hexose unit and to be independent of the molecular weight of the dextran.

In Table 52, values of n, the number of water molecules involved in the interaction, have been calculated with equation (99) for compounds related to

Table 51. Interaction and hydration of sugars.

Sugar	Hydration		$\dfrac{36\,000\ V_x - \log_{10} J}{1.9}$
	Munton	Juszkiewicz	
Sucrose	8	7	7.4
Maltose	7	—	—
Lactose	3	8	—
Glucose	5	5	5.1
Mannose	—	5	—
Galactose	3	—	—
Fructose	3	—	—
Rhamnose	—	—	4.1
Arabinose	—	4	4.2
Xylose	3.5	4	—

sugars from partition coefficients reported by Collander [228,229]. For the polyols, 1,2-ethanediol, 1,2,3-propanetriol (glycerol) and 1,2,3,4-butanetetrol, $\underline{n}$ is close to the number of oxygen atoms in the molecules. The fully acetylated derivatives have almost the same values of $\underline{n}$ as the polyols themselves.

Siek, Albin, Sather and Lindsay [430] have suggested that taste intensity depends on molecular size and stereochemistry. Greenberg [431] has correlated the taste thresholds for compounds in some homologous series with partition coefficients between 1-octanol and water. Equation (101), which relates partition coefficients between biophase and water to characteristic volumes, has been given for the estimation of (physically) toxic concentrations C_t (see Chapter 6, (c))

$$-\log_{10} C_t = -\log_{10} C_B + kV_x - E \qquad (101)$$

This equation can be used to predict the effects of substitutions. On the formation of a glycoside, V_x is increased by 1.0303×10^{-4} m^3 mol^{-1} and $\underline{n}$ seems to increase by 3 (the difference between $\underline{n}$ for sucrose and glucose) so that the value of $\log_{10} C_t$ would be expected to increase by $36\,000\ V_x \times 1.0303 \times 10^{-4} - 3 \times 1.2 = 0.11$ since k for partition between water and the biophase seems to be about $36\,000$ mol m^{-3}. The formation of a glycoside might be expected to have little effect on biological activity. The formation of an acetate increases V_x by 2.975×10^{-5} m^3 mol^{-1} and that of a benzoate increases V_x by 7.644×10^{-5} m^3 mol^{-1}. Since neither of these changes seems to alter $\underline{n}$, each acetylation would make a compound about ten times more biologically active and each benzoylation over 500 times more biologically active. Increased biological activity can also be achieved by substitutions which reduce the number $\underline{n}$ of interactions. Replacement of a hydroxyl group by chlorine

Table 52. Number (n) of interactions for compounds related to sugars.

Compound	Formula (number of bonds)	V_x (calc.) (m^3 mol^{-1})	Partition coefficient (J)	$\dfrac{36\,000\,V_x - \log_{10}x}{1.9}$
1,2-Ethanediol	$C_2H_6O_2$ (9)	5.078×10^{-5}	5.3×10^{-3}	2.2
1,2-Ethanediol diacetate	$C_6H_{10}O_4$ (19)	1.1028×10^{-4}	2.0	2.2
1,2,3-Propanetriol	$C_3H_8O_3$ (13)	7.074×10^{-5}	6.6×10^{-4}	3.0
1,2,3-Propanetriol monoacetate	$C_5H_{10}O_4$ (18)	1.0049×10^{-4}	4.1×10^{-2}	2.6
1,2,3-Propanetriol diacetate	$C_7H_{12}O_5$ (23)	1.3024×10^{-4}	2.2×10^{-1}	2.8
1,2,3-Propanetriol triacetate	$C_9H_{14}O_6$ (28)	1.5999×10^{-4}	1.4	3.0
1-Ethoxy-2,3-propanediol	$C_5H_{12}O_3$ (19)	9.892×10^{-5}	2.6×10^{-2}	2.7
1,3-Diethoxy-2-propanol	$C_7H_{16}O_3$ (25)	1.2710×10^{-4}	8.4×10^{-1}	2.4
1,2,3,4-Butanetetrol	$C_4H_{10}O_4$ (17)	9.070×10^{-5}	1.1×10^{-4}	3.8
2,2-Bishydroxymethyl-1,3-propanediol	$C_5H_{12}O_4$ (20)	1.0479×10^{-4}	3.0×10^{-4}	3.6
2,2-Bishydroxymethyl-1,3-propanediol tetra-acetate	$C_{13}H_{20}O_8$ (40)	2.2379×10^{-4}	9.3	3.7
Glucose 2,3,4,5,6-penta-acetate	$C_{16}H_{22}O_{11}$ (49)	2.6066×10^{-4}	16	4.3
Methyl-α-D-glucopyranoside	$C_7H_{14}O_6$ (27)	1.3385×10^{-4}	5×10^{-5}	4.8

increases V_X by only 6.37×10^{-6} m^3 mol^{-1}. However, chlorine, unlike hydroxyl, can give no interaction and so the substitution can reduce E by 1.2. The net effect is to increase $\log_{10} C_t$ by $6.37 \times 10^{-6} \times 36\,000 + 1.2 = 1.429$: C_t is increased 27 times. It is of interest therefore that the substitution of the hydroxyl at either the $1'$ or $6'$ position in sucrose by chlorine increases the sweetness [432] by a factor of about 20 and that partition between water and some organic phase has been suggested as a factor, among others, which determines sweetness [432, 433].

(h) PROPERTIES OF BIOPHASE

It was noted earlier that for partitions of esters, alcohols and ketones between ether and water, $E = 1.9$ which roughly equals

$$\log_{10} \frac{[\text{water in ether-rich layer}]}{[\text{water in water-rich layer}]}.$$

The value of E for compounds containing one of these groups and partitioning between the biophase and water has been found [26, 38] to be -1.2. If it is assumed that one phase is pure water and the interactions in the biophase are caused solely by dissolved water, then

$$\log_{10} \frac{55344}{[\text{water in biophase}]} = 1.2$$

giving a concentration of water in biophase equal to 3492 mol m^{-3}. This value has been compared with the solubilities of water in some organic liquids in Table 53 and will be seen to be fairly high.

Since the biophase is an associated liquid, the equation (71) (see Chapter 5) will apply so that the solubility C_{SB} of a non-interacting compound in the biophase is given by (110)

$$\log_{10}(C_{SB}/C_L) = -k_B V_x + E \tag{110}$$

where C_L is the concentration of the (liquid) compound in its own pure liquid phase and k_B is the value of k for the biophase. McGowan [38, 424] has given a value of 4000 mol m^{-3} for k_B and this can be used for most examples of physical toxicity. However, cases are known (see Chapter 8, section (b)) where a higher value of k_B is required. The difference between the water concentrations of the two phases multiplied by 0.65, i.e. $0.65 [55\,344 - 3492] = 33\,700$ mol m^{-3} will give k for partitions between the biophase and water (see equation (78)) if all the association arises from the water in the biophase. This value is somewhat higher than the difference, 32\,000 mol m^{-3} between 36\,000 (see Chapter 5, section (b)), the figure suggested for solubilities of unassociated compounds in water and the k_B value of 4000.

There are four factors which determine the physical toxicities of compounds but it is not always necessary to consider all of them in any particular case.

Table 53. Solubilities in water in organic solvents at 298 K.

Solvent	Water concentration $(mol\ m^{-3})$	Reference
Cyclohexane	3.01	[434]
Carbon tetrachloride	8.87	[434]
o-Dichlorobenzene	24.0	[337]
Chlorobenzene	24.4	[337]
1-Chlorobutane	31.3	[337]
Benzene	35.2	[434]
1,1-Dichloroethane	56.7	[337]
1,1,1-Trichloroethane	74.2	[337]
1,2-Dichlorethane	128	[337]
Dichloromethane	145	[337]
Nitrobenzene	168	[337]
Diethyl ether	588	[233]
Ethyl acetate	1594	[435]
n-Octanol	2300	[237]
n-Heptanol	2453	[436, 437]
Biophase	3500	This work
n-Hexanol	3681	[436, 437]
n-Pentanol	5620	[436, 437]
n-Butanol	9152	[436, 437]

(I)   Allowance has to be made for *phase changes* and this involves the heat of the change and the temperature at which it occurs. The most important phase change is that involved in the solution of a solid compound.

(II) Allowance has to be made for the difference in isothermal *compressibility* of the solvent and the liquid solute. So far, it has been shown how to calculate the work for the change of solute to the compressibility of the solvent and so this will only apply to dilute solutions. What is really required is the work to bring both the solute and the solvent to the compressibility of the solution. The compressibility of the biophase is not known. However, something like 1000 K might be a reasonable value for its characteristic temperature. In order to allow for compressibility, the characteristic temperature and characteristic volume of the solute are required as well as the characteristic temperature of the solvent. The characteristic temperatures of water and of the biophase are probably not very different and so the allowance required for compressibility in the estimation of the toxicity of aqueous solutions may well be small.

(III) Allowance has to be made for the *association of the solvent* and this is often the major factor. It is estimated from the characteristic volume of the solute and a constant which measures the strength of the association of the solvent (at the temperature of the experiments).

(IV) Allowance has to be made for *interactions* between the solute and solvent. The hydroxyl content of the solvents frequently seem to be largely responsible for these interactions. Differences between the interactions of solvents can then be estimated from the concentrations of hydroxyl groups in the solvents and a number $\underline{n}$.

(i) THE 'CUT-OFF'

As the molecular volume of physically toxic compounds increase, their toxicities, measured as the reciprocals of the concentrations required to give a certain biological effect, also increase. This follows from equation (101). However, compounds which are solids or have large molecules are often biologically inactive and there is a fairly sharp 'cut-off' in the toxicity. The reason is that the solubilities of the compounds have fallen below the concentrations required for toxicity.

In Table 2, experimental values of Hutchinson, Hellebust, Tam, MacKay, Mascarenhas and Shiu [28] were given for concentrations of compounds required to halve the photosynthetic activities of algae. These workers noted that a number of the compounds were not sufficiently soluble in water to give 50% reduction in photosynthetic activity. These compounds did, however, reduce the photosynthetic activity and from the concentrations which gave reductions of less than 50%, concentrations were estimated for the 50% reduction. None of the compounds tested would be expected to give interactions and so from equation (101)

$$\log_{10} C_t = \log_{10} C_B - k V_x$$

The experimental values from Table 2 give, for C_t, the concentrations required to halve the photosynthetic activity of *Chlamydomonas angulosa*

$$\log_{10} C_t = 2.870 - 35\,580\, V_x \ (n = 30; r = 0.893)$$

The corresponding relationship for *Chlorella vulgaris* is

$$\log_{10} C_t = 2.889 - 35\,000\, V_x \ (n = 30; r = 0.906)$$

These correlations are not as good as many similar correlations but they are reasonable when it is considered how difficult it is to experiment with the extremely dilute solutions involved.

The relationships given above suggest that $\log_{10} C_B$ is about 2.88 so that C_B, the concentration in the biophase required to halve the photosynthetic activity of the algae, is about 760 mol m^{-3}. It has been suggested that the biophase is a somewhat associated liquid and a value of $k = 4000$ mol m^{-3} has been given [38, 424] (see Chapter 6, section (h)). This value of k is small and it would seem that the main factor which determines the 'cut-off' for liquid compounds is the low compressibility of the biophase. The compressibility of the biophase appears to be near that of water because it has not been found necessary to make any appreciable corrections for compressibilities when toxic concentrations in water are estimated with equation (101). The biophase seems to be a polymer and polymers have low compressibilities, that is, high characteristic temperatures T_X. The following values have been suggested [23, 85] for T_X:

polyolefines	about	800 K
polystyrene		1100 K
poly(methyl-methylacrylate)		1150 K

If T_X for water is calculated from the isothermal compressibility at 298.2 K according to the program given in Appendix II, T_X comes to 914 K. However, T_X obtained in this way is not a constant: as the temperature rises, T_X rises right up to the boiling point, 373 K, when it is 1081 K. The structure of water is probaly altered as pressure is applied in the measurement of compressibility. When equation (4) is used at 298 K a value of 1317 K is obtained for T_X from the density. Those compounds from Table 2 for which it has been possible to attribute reasonable values of T_X are listed in Table 54. Values of C_{calc} (mol m^{-3}) at 298 K have been calculated with the equation (67) and use of the program given in Appendix II with the T_X value of the compound from Appendix III and T_X for water equal to 1317 K. The program in Appendix II is for use with unassociated liquids but it does seem to be of value for estimation of solubilities of unassociated liquids in water (and probably in other associated liquids) provided the solubilities are low. Allowance is made in the calculation of C_{calc} for the lower solubility of solids compared with liquids. Values of 4000 V_X are used for association of the biophase and figures are given for $\log_{10} C_{calc} - 4000 V_X$, which are estimates of the logarithm of the solubility of the compound in the biophase.

It is interesting that all those compounds giving values of $\log_{10} C_{calc} - 4000 V_X$ greater than 2.88 have been found to halve the photosynthetic activity of the algae whilst all the those liquids giving values of $\log_{10} C_{calc} - 4000 V_X$ less than 2.88 will not give this 50% inhibition. The values of $\log_{10} C_{calc} - 4000 V_X$ for the solids naphthalene and phenanthrene are below 2.88 and this would suggest that these compounds should not be capable of halving the photosynthetic activity but in fact they were found to do this. It is not clear why this is so. It is possible that there are compounds in the biological systems which lower the melting points of the solids and increase the solubilities.

The 'cut-off' for inhibition of the growth of the fungus *Fomes annosus* has been mentioned earlier in this chapter (section (a)). In Table 47, $\log_{10} C_B$ for complete inhibition of growth was given as 2.8. Bateman [353] found that acenaphthene, diphenyl and 1,2,4,5-tetramethylbenzene did not give complete inhibition of growth: the inhibitions were 82.6, 84.0 and 95.6% respectively. The values of $[\log_{10} C_{calc} - 4000 V_X]$ are 2.61, 2.75 and 2.50 respectively. All are below 2.8 although they are not in the order of biological activity given by Bateman. If the compounds acted independently, it would be expected that C_B

for mixtures would equal the sum of the C_B values of the components so that if the antilogarithms of the $[\log_{10} C_{calc} - 4000\ V_x]$ values are added, the logarithm of the result would be $[\log_{10} C_{calc} - 4000\ V_x]$ for the mixture. Bateman gave 96.6% for the inhibition for a solution saturated with acenaphthene and diphenyl. When calculated as just described, $[\log_{10} C_{calc} - 4000\ V_x]$ is 2.99 and so the mixture might have been expected to give 100% inhibition. The value of $\log_{10} C_{calc} - 4000\ V_x$ for a solution saturated with all three compounds is 3.11 and this did give 100% inhibition.

In Table 54, values of $\log_{10} C_s$ (where C_s are the solubilities in water given in Table 2) are compared with $(\log_{10} C_{calc} - 37\,000\ V_x)$. It will be seen from the table in Appendix III, which lists properties required for calculation of C_{calc}, that the values of T_x for many of the more common organic solvents are around 500 K so that C_{calc} will be much the same for all of them. Moreover, T_x tends to rise with V_x and allowance can be made for this when k is chosen so that the simple equations (71) and (101) are often adequate for the estimation of partition coefficients, solubilities and physical toxicities. It is not possible at present to estimate the effects of pressure on interactions and associations. The equation (67) can only be used for the work of compression of unassociated liquids, and predictions of the 'cut-off' are limited to these. An example of the 'cut-off' for associated liquids which interact with water and probably with the biophase is given in Table 55. These results for the anaesthetic potency of normal alcohols agree with those obtained more recently by Pringle, Brown and Miller [438].

Gibbs [439] studied the effects of n-alcohols on the growth of roots of seedlings. He used *Pisum sativum*, *Cucurbita pepo*, *Helianthus annuus* and *Lupinus polyphyllus*. He expressed his results as the growth in the presence of the alcohols as a percentage of that in their absence. He found that this percentage fell as the size of the alcohol molecules increased up to 1-undecanol. The alcohols with larger molecules than this were almost without effect because they were insufficiently soluble in water.

(j) 1-OCTANOL/WATER PARTITIONS

An equation [14, 440] relating the changes in toxicity brought about by substitutions to changes in the partition coefficients between 1-octanol and water at 300 K resulting from the same substitution has been much used [13–17, 440–442]. If the biological effect is the toxic dose for a given effect (C_t) then

$$-\log C_t = k_H \pi^2 + k_H' \pi + \rho\sigma + k_H'' \tag{111}$$

Here, π is the logarithm of the ratio of the partition coefficient of a substituted (J^s) and unsubstituted compound (J^H).

σ is Hammett's sigma factor and k_H, k_H', k_H'' and ρ are constants. It has been pointed out [48, 49] that since π is derived from partition coefficients, it is given by

Table 54. Estimation of solubilities in the biophase and in water at 298 K.

Compound	$V_x \times 10^5$ (m³ mol⁻¹)	T_x	C_{calc} (mol m⁻³)	$\text{Log}_{10} C_{calc}$ $-4000 V_x$	$\text{Log}_{10} C_s$ (observed [28])	$\text{Log}_{10} C_{calc}$ $-37\,000 V_x$
Dichloromethane	4.944	505	7575	3.68	2.36	2.05
Benzene	7.164	570	5810	3.48	1.36	0.93
Trichloromethane	6.168	503	5010	3.45	1.82	1.42
Chlorobenzene	8.388	617	5583	3.41	0.62	0.65
Toluene	8.573	572	4319	3.29	0.75	0.46
1,4-Dimethylbenzene	9.982	581	3462	3.14	0.24	−0.14
1,3,5-Trimethylbenzene	11.392	606	3160	3.04	—	—
Naphthalene ($T_m = 353.4$ K $\Delta H_m = 18\,800$ J mol⁻¹)	10.854	740	1728	2.80	−0.61	−0.77
Diphenyl ($T_m = 341.5$ K $\Delta H_m = 18\,600$ J mol⁻¹)	13.242	800	1921	2.75	—	—
1-Methyl-4(2-propyl)benzene	12.801	559	1762	2.73	—	—
Hexane	9.541	454	972	2.61	−0.96	−0.60
Acenaphthene	12.586	811	1142	2.55	—	—

Table 54. (continued)

Compound	$V_x \times 10^5$ (m³ mol⁻¹)	T_x	C_{calc} (mol m⁻³)	$Log_{10} C_{calc}$ −4000 V_x	$Log_{10} C_s$ (observed [28])	$Log_{10} C_{calc}$ −37 000 V_x
Phenanthrene ($T_m = 369.5$ K $\Delta H_m = 18\,630$ J mol⁻¹)	14.543	970	1314	2.54	−2.14	−2.19
1,2,4,5-Tetramethylbenzene ($T_m = 352.5$ K $\Delta H_m = 21\,000$ J mol⁻¹)	12.801	688	1034	2.50	−	−
Octane	12.360	491	840	2.43	−2.24	−1.62
Nonane	13.769	506	771	2.34	−	−
Decane	15.178	520	714	2.25	−3.44	−2.76
Dodecane	17.996	543	604	2.06	−4.65	−3.87
Heptadecane	25.042	583	396	1.60	−	−
Anthracene ($T_m = 489.7$ K $\Delta H_m = 28\,500$ J mol⁻¹)	14.543	910	59	1.19	−3.64	−3.61

Table 55. Concentrations (mol m^{-3}) in water required for narcosis of tadpoles [6].

Alcohol	Concn for narcosis (mol m^{-3})
Ethanol	330
n-Propanol	110
n-Butanol	30
n-Pentanol	7
n-Heptanol	0.38
n-Octanol	0.13
n-Nonanol	0.025
n-Decanol	0.01
n-Undecanol	0.005
n-Dodecanol	0.0075
n-Tetradecanol	Inactive

$$\pi = \log_{10} J^S - \log_{10} J^H = k(V_x^S - V_x^H) + E_A^S - E_A^H \tag{112}$$

and it would be expected that

$$-\log_{10} C_t = k V_x^H + \pi + \text{ the algebraic sum of interaction terms.}$$

This equation, unlike equation (111), contains no π^2 term and the inclusion of this term seems difficult to justify. The π^2 term converts the linear curve into a parabola. Hyde [403] has pointed out that there are often few experimental points on the down-turn beyond the maximum value of $-\log_{10} C_t$ and for this, and other reasons, the curve here is usually ill-defined. He has suggested that instead of a parabola the points fall on two straight lines which is what would be expected [50] for a system where concentrations were measured in a liquid containing a non-aqueous as well as an aqueous phase. Other points may be low because the cut-off point is being neared and the toxic concentrations observed are high and somewhat uncertain. Partition coefficients of many compounds between 1-octanol (and other solvents) and water have been collected [237], and k seems to be somewhat below 36 000. Briggs [443] has applied equation (71) to partition coefficients J_{ow} between 1-octanol and water. He gives a relationship which when the parachor is replaced by $V_x \times 2.385 \times 10^6$ becomes

$$\log_{10} J_{ow} = 34\,000\, V_x - 1.2\,\Sigma n \tag{113}$$

Briggs used the following values of n to make up the sum Σn:

$n = 1$ for each oxygen not bonded or conjugated to an aromatic ring (but including ether oxygen in aryl alkyl ethers)

$n = 1$ for each nitrogen atom provided it is linked to other atoms by single bonds

$n = 1$ for each heterocyclic aromatic ring however many hetero atoms
                  it contains

$n = -0.25$ for each halogen atom attached to a saturated carbon atom.

Briggs measured the partition coefficients of a number of compounds between 1-octanol and water. He found for 26 compounds, most of which are used in agriculture,

$$\log_{10} J_{ow} + 1.2\Sigma n = 31\,200\, V_x \quad (r = 0.95) \tag{114}$$

When different factors are involved in producing some effect, under most conditions one factor is likely to be more important than others and only over a narrow range of conditions will two or more factors be of critical importance. It has been suggested [48] that k_H in equation (111) should be zero and, provided the compound involved does not associate or dissociate, k_H' should be unity. If the $\rho\sigma$ term of the equation is important, either the biological activity involves some chemical reaction or the interaction terms are proportional to σ.

(k) VARIATIONS IN PROPERTIES OF THE BIOPHASE

Brink and Posternak [20] have suggested that the biophase can vary somewhat for different types of physical toxicity. They estimated the concentrations of narcotics which produce 50% reduction in the number of responding cells involved in transmission of nerve impulses over synaptic and non-synaptic pathways for the cat and pointed out the difference between the two sets of values. The narcotic concentrations for both pathways are equal for n-butanol, the concentrations are higher for the synaptic pathways than for the non-synaptic pathways for the alcohols of molecular weight lower than n-butanol, and for alcohols with higher molecular weights, the reverse is true. In Fig. 21, the results are shown for eight alcohols. The results for the synaptic pathways give

$$\log_{10} C_t = -41\,680\, V_x + 4.71 \quad (r = 0.995)$$

and for the non-synaptic pathways

$$\log_{10} C_t = -29\,900\, V_x + 3.87 \quad (r = 0.989)$$

Lines corresponding to these relationships have been drawn in Fig. 21. It would seem that the biophases involved in the non-synaptic nerve transmission of cats is more associated than the biophases involved in the synaptic nerve transmission.

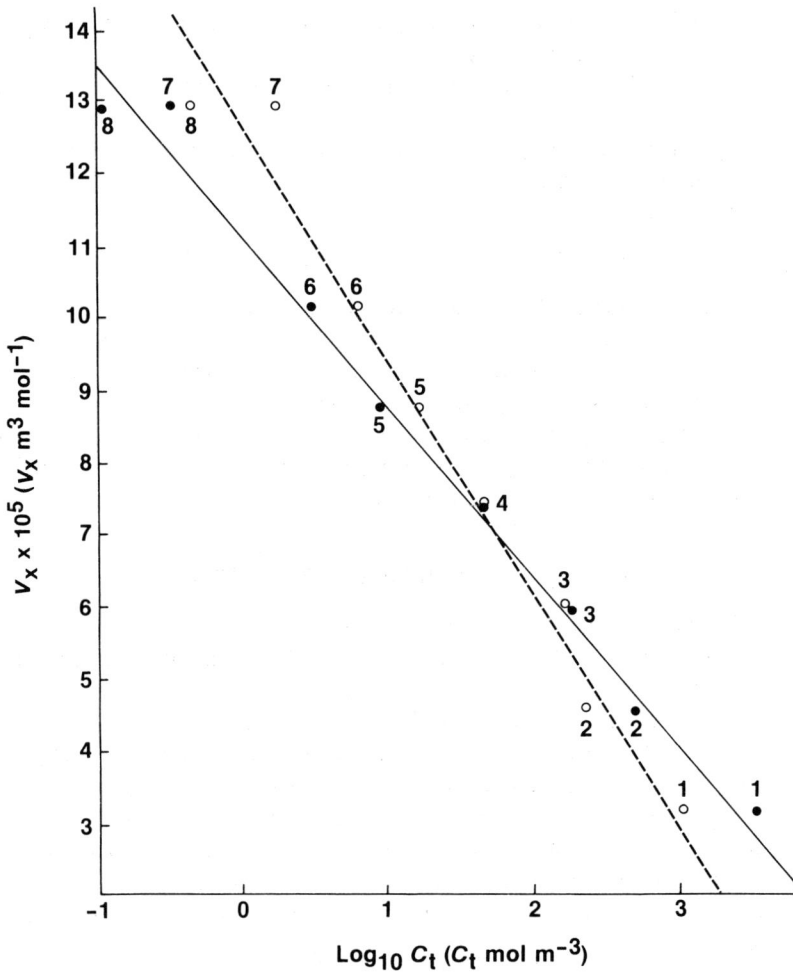

Fig. 21. Reversible suppression of transmission of nerve impulses [20]. ● ——— Synaptic pathways; ○ - - - - - - non-synaptic pathways. (1) Methanol; (2) ethanol; (3) propanol; (4) butanol; (5) Pentanol; (6) 2-hexanol; (7) 2-octanol; (8) octanol.

The Site of Action of Physically Toxic Substances

(a) ARE PROTEINS THE TARGETS OF ANAESTHETICS?

The success of the Meyer–Overton hypothesis for anaesthetic action [11, 12], at predicting the potency of many anaesthetics, has led to the assumption that the primary site of anaesthetic action is in a lipid region of nerve cells. Since anaesthesia is one aspect of physical toxicity, it has been assumed that all physical toxicity involves the solution of the toxic compound in a biophase which is composed of lipid. However from the evidence presented in the previous chapter it appears that the biophase cannot be composed solely of lipid.

Seifriz [444] reviewed early work on the effects of anaesthetics on protoplasm, and noted that in 1875 Bernard [445, 446] had suggested that anaesthesia involved the reversible coagulation of the cytoplasm of sensory nerves by the anaesthetic. Later work by Eyring and coworkers on the enzyme luciferase has led to more direct evidence that proteins may be the site of action of anaesthetics [447]. It has long been known that alcohols and other metabolic inhibitors suppress the luminescence of luminous bacteria [448]. It was shown that high pressures, 150–300 atmospheres, could reverse the inhibition by narcotics of light output in these organisms [449]. This finding led to the suggestion that high pressures might reverse the effects of anaesthetics on higher organisms.

This prediction was later verified by using high pressures to overcome anaesthesia in tadpoles [450] and in newts [451]. Another important consequence of the inhibition of bacterial luminescence by narcotics was the theory that anaesthesia may be caused by altered protein conformation [447].

As restated by Eyring [452], it is proposed that anaesthetic action is analogous to reversible heat-denaturation of proteins. The reversible unfolding of the native protein by heat or by anaesthetic would result in an increase in volume, and thus could be reversed by high pressures.

Later studies on a cell-free luciferase preparation from fireflies showed that only protein and anaesthetic were necessary for inhibition of the light production, and that 50% inhibition was given at anaesthetic concentrations of volatile halogenated hydrocarbons [453]. Bacterial luciferase is similarly inhibited by anaesthetics [454]. The enzyme is a dimer of molar mass 79 000, composed of α- and β-subunits [454]. The binding site for the substrates are on the α-subunits; one of the substrates is a long-chain fatty aldehyde and the active site contains a hydrophobic region, presumably the site of binding of the aldehyde [455]. The kinetics of inhibition by anaesthetics of bacterial luciferase give apparent competitive inhibition, in that high concentrations of the long-chain aldehyde substrate overcome the inhibition [456]. Similar apparent competitive inhibition was noted for the inhibition of bacterial luminescence by urethanes [447]. However the dependence of this inhibition on temperature led to the suggestion that anaesthetics promote thermal inactivation of the enzyme [451]. (Type II inhibition in the nomenclature of Eyring [452].) This inhibition is distinct from true competitive, or type I, inhibition, which is independent of thermal inactivation. Classical competitive inhibition of enzymes (type I) arises from close structural similarities between the inhibitors and the substrate, and it is unlikely that the inhibition of enzymes by anaesthetics, ranging in size from inert gases to large hydrocarbons, occurs by competitive binding of the anaesthetic to the substrate binding site of the enzyme. What then is the likely cause of reversal of enzyme inhibition by high concentrations of substrate? It is possible that the high concentrations of substrate stabilise the active conformation of the protein molecule and prevent reversible conformational changes by the anaesthetic. Substrates are frequently added to enzyme solutions to prevent thermal denaturation of the protein during storage [457].

Direct evidence for the binding of anaesthetics to proteins is sparse. Myoglobin forms a clathrate with xenon and with cyclopropane, but the specificity for binding appears to be much greater than that shown for anaesthetic action [458].

(b) INHIBITION OF ENZYMES BY PHYSICALLY TOXIC SUBSTANCES

Much indirect evidence for the binding of anaesthetics to enzymes has been obtained from enzyme inhibition studies on enzymes other than luciferase. Glutamate dehydrogenase (EC 1.4.1.2) from beef liver is a complex quaternary structure in which protein subunits associate through hydrophobic interactions. The active complex can be inhibited by a variety of hydrocarbons, which appear to dissociate the protein subunits. Inhibitors include steroids [459], tranquilisers [460] and anaesthetics [461, 462]. Similar non-specific inhibition of enzyme activity has been reported for β-glucuronidase (EC 3.2.1.31) [463].

As briefly mentioned in Chapter 6, physically toxic substances have long been known to inhibit enzymes in intact organisms, including micro-organisms, plants and animals. In Chapter 6 the relationship between partition coefficient and molecular volume was extended to equation (101), which relates the toxic concentration of physically toxic compounds (C_t) for a given biological effect to the characteristic volumes, V_X in m^3 mol^{-1}

$$-\log_{10} C_t = -\log_{10} C_B + kV_X - E \qquad (101)$$

C_B is the concentration in the biophase required to give the biological effect, E is the interaction term, which may be zero, and k is approximately 36 000 mol m^{-3}, the value for partitioning of compounds between diethyl ether and water.

An example of the use of equation (101) is given in Fig. 20: this refers to the inhibition of succinic acid oxidation catalysed by ox diaphragm tissue. Although the points in this figure do lie fairly near the line of slope -1, such a line is not the one which would have been drawn given the values of $\log_{10} C_t$ and 36 000 $V_X - E$. Most of the compounds are normal primary alcohols and α-methylketones and for these compounds with interactions all equal, a linear correlation gives $\log_{10} C_t = -27\,800\, V_X + 4.47$ ($n = 9$; $r = 0.982$). Measurements were also made at the same time by Batelli and Stern [404] on the oxidation of succinic acid catalysed by sheep liver homogenates. The corresponding correlation gives $\log_{10} C_t = -26\,900\, V_X + 4.39$ ($n = 9$; $r = 0.989$).

In marked contrast to Fig. 20, based on the figures of Batelli and Stern for the inhibition of the enzymic oxidation of succinate, are the results of Mattson, Volpenhein and Benjamin [464] for the inhibition by n-alkanols of the hydrolysis of methyl oleate by pancreatic lipase. These are used in Fig. 22 (with $E = 1.2$ for the hydroxyl group). The line is drawn with a slope of -1 and the points fall on a line with a steeper (negative) slope. Also, the line bends over to become approximately horizontal. For the first six alcohols tested, $\log_{10} I_{50}$ (concentration to give 50% inhibition) $= -43\,500\, V_X + 5.49$ ($n = 6$; $r = 0.997$). If all the alcohol, corresponding to the horizontal line in Fig. 22, were dissolved in the methyl oleate lipid phase taken initially, the concentration would be about 180 mol m^{-3} ($\log_{10} 180 = 2.3$) and this seems to be rather low. From the intercept (36 000 $V_X - E = 0$), however, a figure for $\log_{10} C_B = 3.5$ is given. This is high compared with the values given in Table 56 but a value between 2.3 and 3.5 would be expected. Mattson, Volpenhein and Benjamin observed that about 6000 mol m^{-3} of hexane, heptane and dodecane were required to give 50% inhibition of the lipase (calculated on the assumption that it is dissolved in the methyl oleate). This may mean that these hydrocarbons are insufficiently soluble in the biophase to give 50% inhibition and that the observed inhibition arises from the considerable dilution of the substrate by the hydrocarbons. Liu, Beppu and Arima [465] studied the inhibition of the hydrolysis of olive oil catalysed by *Humicola* lipase. They added a volume of inhibitor equal to one-tenth the volume of the olive oil and found that n-hydrocarbons did not inhibit the hydrolysis. This is considerably less hydrocarbon than was listed by Mattson, Volpenhein and Benjamin. Alcohols in these amounts did retard the hydrolysis.

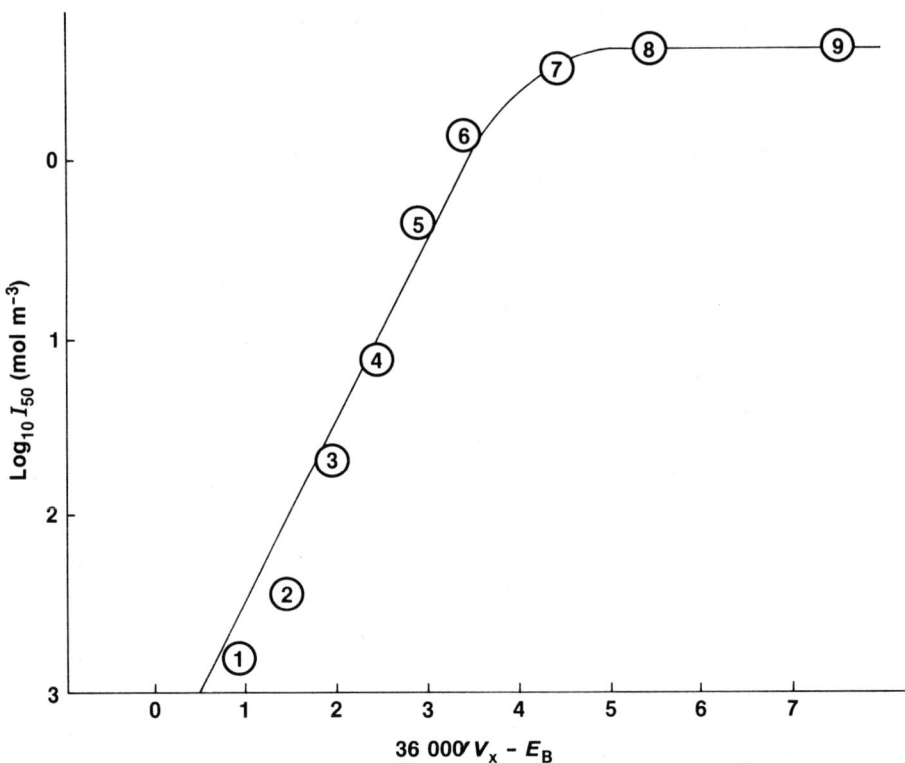

Fig. 22. The inhibition of hydrolysis of methyl oleate catalysed by pancreatic lipase [464]. The concentration of nine alcohols required for 50% inhibition of the hydrolysis was measured ($\log_{10} I_{50}$) and is plotted against 36 000 $V_x - E_B$. The compounds are: (1) n-propanol; (2) n-butanol; (3) n-pentanol; (4) n-hexanol; (5) n-heptanol, (6) n-octanol; (7) n-decanol; (8) n-dodecanol; (9) n-hexadecanol.

The inhibition caused by n-decanol was reduced by the addition of more olive oil but not by the addition of more enzyme. This would be expected since the extra olive oil would dilute the decanol and lower the concentration partitioning into the biophase. Mates [466] studied the hydrolyses of three triglycerides catalysed by lipase from *Staphylococcus aureus*. From the (approximate) results given of the 50% inhibitory concentrations of n-propanol, n-butanol, n-pentanol, n-hexanol and n-heptanol.

Trimyristin	$\log C_t = 6.64 - 39\,690\,V_x$
Tripalmitin	$\log C_t = 5.78 - 26\,650\,V_x$
Triolein	$\log C_t = 5.72 - 25\,630\,V_x$

The k values for tripalmitin and triolein are exceptionally low. The C_t values for alcohols with ten or more carbon atoms seemed to be constant.

Table 56. Effects of normal primary alcohols on enzymatic and other biological activities.

Biological activity	k	Intercept	Number of C atoms in alcohols used for correlation	r
Inhibition of action of (pig) pepsin on haemoglobin or N-carbobenzoxy-L-glutamyl-L-tyrosine [471]	28 560	3.64	1,2,3,4,5	0.999
Loss of potential pepsin activity of pepsinogen [472]	29 420	4.40	1,2,3,4,5,6	0.998
Inhibition of (Na$^+$ + K$^+$)−ATPase (EC 3.6.1.3) from plasma membranes of guinea pig kidney [473]	30 730	4.41	1,2,3,4,5,6,7	0.999
Inhibition of germination of *Bacillus subtilis* spores under influence of L-alanine [368]	34 120	3.90	1,2,3,4,5,6,7,8	0.996
Inhibition of adenosine 5′-phosphatase in tissue from spleen lymphocytes of mice [397] (see Fig. 18)	34 180	4.30	4,6,8,9,10	0.995
Action on frog's heart (see Table 1) [10]	36 850	4.73	1,2,3,4,7	0.9999
Narcosis of tadpoles (see Table 55) [6]	42 130	4.50	2,3,4,5,7,8,9	0.999
Reduction of osmotic haemolysis (see Fig. 19) [401]	42 180	4.77	4,5,6,7,8,9	0.994
Inhibition of hydrolysis of methyl oleate by pancreatic lipase (EC 3.1.1.3) [464]	43 550	5.49	3,4,5,6,7,8	0.997

Hansch and Dunn [467], and Smith, Hansch and Poindexter [468, 469] have given a table showing effects of inhibitors on enzymes and have allocated constants to fit the figures to equation (111). The work of Baker and colleagues on the inhibitory activities of over 1000 compounds on 14 enzymes has been reviewed [17, 470]. Molar volume correlations are difficult to apply in these studies since the data are presented as per cent inhibitions and not as concentrations required to produce the same inhibitions. Primary n-alcohols have been used in many experiments involving physical toxicity and in Table 56, results of the linear correlations of $\log_{10}$ (concentration required for a certain definite biological effect) with characteristic volume of the alcohol are given. These correlations are very good but the slopes (k) are sometimes below and sometimes above 36 000, which was taken as an average value. Alcohols are associated liquids and give interactions with many solvents: these properties make the interpretation of results more difficult.

It will be seen from Table 56 that the k value (from the experiments of Tang [471] for the inhibition by alcohols of the hydrolysis by hog pepsin of haemoglobin, or N-carbobenzoxy-L-glutamyl-L-tyrosine, is about as low as k from Batelli and Stern's experiments described above. Pepsin is formed from pepsinogen by treatment with acid, and Neumann and Shinitzky [472] found that alcohols cause a loss of potential activity of pepsinogen (see Table 56). The effect was reversible. Tang reported that chymotrypsin is similarly inhibited by alcohols but that trypsin is not inhibited by alcohols. Risley, Buffington and Arnow [474] found that bovine serum was digested by trypsin even in 60% ethanol.

Mitjavila, Lacombe and Carrera [475] studied the inhibition of enzymes in the brush border of enterocytes. Their results for the half-maximal inhibitory concentrations (C_t) of the first eight primary alcohols on $(Na^+ + K^+)$—APTase at 310 K gave $\log C_t = 4.02 - 30\,450\,V_x$ ($n = 8$; $r = 0.999$). This is very similar to the results of Hegyvary [473] (see Table 56). Mitjavila, Lacombe and Carrera [475] noted that V_x had a greater effect on the inhibition of Mg^{2+}–ATPase in the same system and for the same alcohols $\log C_t = 4.73 - 36\,650\,V_x$ ($n = 8$; $r = 0.999$).

Trypsin is anomalous in that it can be activated by high concentrations of alcohols. Schwert and Eisenberg [476] studied catalysis by trypsin of the hydrolyses of benzoyl-L-arginine esters. They found that the rate of hydrolysis of benzoyl-L-arginine methyl ester increased with the addition of ethanol up to 32 volume per cent when the rate was about 50% higher than that in water. As the ethanol concentration was increased further, the rate dropped and at 54 volume per cent ethanol, it was the same as that in water. The increases (per cent) of rates of hydrolysis of benzoyl-L-arginine methyl and ethyl esters were compared for four alcohols, all at 16 volume per cent. The results were: methanol 15%; ethanol 35%; n-propanol and t-butanol about 40%. Further studies of the hydrolysis of benzoyl-L-arginine methyl ester catalysed by trypsin were made by Inagami and Sturtevant [477] at pH 8; they found that the rate increased with addition of dioxane up to about 50% and then decreased. However, the maximum rate of hydrolysis did not vary greatly and even in 88 volume per cent dioxane, the rate was 68% of that in water itself at the same pH. Dimethyl sulphoxide showed similar effects with maximum rate of hydrolysis again at about 50 volume per cent. Kallen-Trummer, Hofmann and Rottenberg [478] confirmed that addition of t-butanol can accelerate reactions catalysed by trypsin. It is of interest that acidic solutions of purified crystalline trypsin can be heated to boiling for a short time without permanent loss of activity [479]. It has also been found [480, 481] that low concentrations (5%), of methanol, ethanol, n-propanol and isopropanol increase the rate of reaction of the enzyme β-D-galactosidase (from *Escherichia coli*) on o-nitrophenyl-β-D-galactopyrano-side. It was found earlier by Laidler and Ethier [482] that the hydrolysis of adenosine triphosphate catalysed by myosin was 20% higher in 40 volume per cent methanol than in water. They also used mixtures of dioxane and water and found the rate increased with addition of dioxane up to 20 volume per cent when it was about double the rate in water.

It therefore appears that methanol, ethanol, n-propanol, t-butanol, dioxane and dimethyl sulphoxide can increase the activity of trypsin and similar effects have been found with some other enzymes. These compounds are all completely miscible with water but they do not seem to share any chemical property which could explain the increase in biological activity. It seems possible that the explanation is to be found in the physical properties. It was suggested above that the normal action of physically toxic compounds which inhibit the action of enzymes might be to favour the formation of a phase rich in protein and relatively poor in water at the expense of a phase containing much water and little protein. The compounds which increase the activity of enzymes may be giving the reverse effect, i.e. giving increased amounts of the particular enzyme (and perhaps the substrate as well) in the largely aqueous phase. It was noted above that up to a certain limit, ethanol and dioxane do increase the solubility of tryptophan in water.

George, McMahan, Bowler and Elliott [483] believe that the apparent activation of some enzymes by organic compounds is really an inhibition of deactivation. They used pig heart malate dehydrogenase (EC 1.1.1.37) and found conditions for a 50% decrease in activity when the enzyme was acting on its own. Quantities of organic solvents were then introduced and the percentage loss of enzyme activity was measured again under the same conditions. Some of the results are given in Table 57. It will be seen that acetone and glycerol are particularly good inhibitors for the activation of the enzyme. When it comes to the interpretation of the effects of organic compounds on reactions with enzymes, it is obviously a complication if the compounds slow the spontaneous deactivation of the enzymes as well as acting as inhibitors of the physically toxic type.

Experiments with higher plants show their behaviour towards alkanols is similar to that of micro-organisms and enzymes. Sather and Thimann [484] studied the ability of oat seedlings (*Avena sativa*) to maintain chlorophyll in the dark and found the concentrations of the primary alcohols required for 50%

Table 57. Percentage of original activity of pig heart malate dehydrogenase (EC1.1.1.37) in the presence of organic solvents [483].

Solvent	Solvent concentration (v/v %)										
	0	1.5	2.5	5	10	20	30	40	50	60	70
Ethanol	50	–	–	75	72	87	87	76	79	68	62
1-Propanol	50	–	–	74	78	77	31	11	–	–	–
2-Propanol	50	–	–	85	–	99	105	–	–	–	–
1-Butanol	50	84	67	–	–	–	–	–	–	–	–
1-Propanol, 2-methyl-	50	79	88	–	–	–	–	–	–	–	–
Acetone	50	–	–	76	77	95	99	109	101	81	–
1,4-Dioxane	50	–	–	86	94	77	77	–	–	–	–
Dimethylsulphoxide	50	–	–	50	32	42	48	–	–	–	–
Glycerol	50	–	–	59	57	82	96	109	94	107	109
Tetrahydrofuran	50	–	–	59	63	73	78	21	–	–	–

maintenance of chlorophyll after 3 days dropped by 2.9 times (i.e. $k = 33\,000$ mol m^{-3}) for each additional CH_2 group at 303 K. Reynolds [485] found that the germination of lettuce seeds (*Lactuca sativa*) was inhibited by alcohols, aldehydes and ketones. The inhibitory activity increased with increasing length of the carbon chain, and k for the concentrations of 1-alkanols required to reduce the percentage germination to 50% at 303 K was $36\,000$ mol m^{-3}. The effects of alcohols on the growth of the roots of seedlings [439] have already been mentioned.

While on the subject of the physical toxicities of the normal primary alcohols, the work of Rang [486] should be mentioned. He used the eight alchohols from methanol to 1-octanol in the following four different biological experiments. He gives the concentrations required to give

(A) 50% immobilization of *Paramecium*
(B) 50% depression of the maximum contraction of guinea pig ileum (gut muscle) elicited by acetyl choline
(C) 50% reduction in the rate of uptake of oxygen by guine pig lung tissue (Warburg's method)
(D) 50% reduction of anaphylactic histamine release (method of Mongar and Schild [487])

It is of interest to compare Table 58 based on Rang's results with Table 56. Rang noticed that the slopes of plots of the logarithms of the toxic concentrations against the number of carbon atoms varied for different tests. This might be connected with the rather short times (about 15 min) taken for the tests. In tests C and D, 1-heptanol seemed to be marginally active. In test C, 1-octanol showed no significant activity at all and in test D, although 1-octanol

Table 58. Toxicities [486] of normal primary alcohols.

Biological activity	K	Intercept	Chain length of alcohol	r
(D) Anaphylactic histamine release	26 000	3.24	1,2,3,4,5,6	0.996
(A) Immobilization of *Paramecium*	34 070	4.36	1,2,3,4,5,6,7,8	0.998
(C) Reduction in oxygen uptake	34 120	4.53	1,2,3,4,5,6	0.997
(B) Depression of gut contractibility	37 870	4.26	1,2,3,4,5,6,7,8	0.997

showed some activity, it failed to give 50% inhibition. No 'cut-off' was observed in tests A and B. Ferguson [21, 22] had suggested that compounds with rather high toxicity were chemically toxic but Rang believes this is not necessarily so; some such compounds might owe their high biological activity to specific interactions leading to specially high solubility in the biophase. Rang suggested that as a solvent, the biophase had properties somewhere between those of ethanol and those of butanol.

It is usually assumed that an enzyme E combines with the substrate S to give a complex ES. This complex breaks down to give free enzyme and the product P.

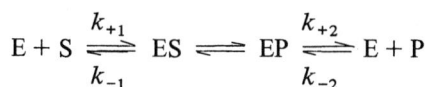

$$E + S \underset{k_{-1}}{\overset{k_{+1}}{\rightleftharpoons}} ES \rightleftharpoons EP \underset{k_{-2}}{\overset{k_{+2}}{\rightleftharpoons}} E + P$$

The reactions are assumed to be reversible and if [ES] attains a steady state

$$k_{+1}([E_T] - [ES])[S] = k_{-1}[ES] + k_{+2}[ES]$$

[ET] = the total enzyme concentration. From the above

$$\frac{[S]([E_T] - [ES])}{[ES]} = \frac{k_{-1} + k_{+2}}{k_{+1}} = K_m \tag{115}$$

K_m is called the Michaelis–Menten constant.

When the concentration of substrate is sufficiently high, the rate of the reaction reaches a constant value V_{max}: then the enzyme is considered to be saturated with the substrate so that $[ES] = [E_T]$ and

$$V_{max} = k_{+2}[ET_T] \tag{116}$$

The rate can be written as

$$v = k_{+2}[ES] = k_{+2}\frac{[E_7][S]}{K_m + [S]} \tag{117}$$

Miles, Robinson and Canady [488] studied the hydrolysis of hippurates ($C_6H_5CONHCH_2COOR$) catalysed by α-chymotrypsin. They found that there was little difference in the behaviour of methyl, ethyl, propyl and isopropyl hippurates. The Michaelis–Menten constants decrease in the presence of salts such as potassium chloride: K_m is approximately three times lower when the ionic strength is increased from 0.004 to 1.885. Salts had little effect on the dissociation of the enzyme–substrate complex, i.e. on k_{+2}. The authors studied the inhibition of the reaction by aromatic compounds. They expressed their results as constants K_i

$$\frac{v_0}{v} = 1 + \frac{K_i C_t}{1 + [S]/K_m}$$

where v_0 is the rate of the reaction in the absence of inhibitor and v is the rate when the inhibitor concentration is C_t. From the above expression the concentrations of inhibitors required to halve rates of hydrolyses were calculated with 2 mol m^{-3} substrate in 100 mol m^{-3} aqueous potassium chloride: i.e. with $K_m = 2.46$ mol m^{-3}. The results are given in Table 59. The additional hydrocarbons, pentane, cyclohexane and indene were studied by Hymes, Robinson and Canady [489] and figures for these are included in the table. For the 11 compounds

$$\log_{10} C_t = -43\,407\ V_x + 4.2944$$

with $r = 0.9216$. The values of k and the intercept fall within the range of the examples shown in Table 56. The authors related the degree of inhibition to the size of the molecules. They assumed that the molecules were spherical and calculated surface areas from the molecular refractions.

Table 59. Concentrations (mol m^{-3}) of inhibitors required to halve the rate of hydrolysis of methyl hippurate catalysed by α-chymotrypsin at 298.2 K in aqueous potassium chloride [488, 489].

Compound	V_x (m^3 mol^{-1})	Concentration of inhibitor (mol m^{-3})
Benzene	7.164×10^{-5}	21.7
Cyclohexene	8.025×10^{-5}	8.71
Pentane	8.132×10^{-5}	5.75
Chlorobenzene	8.388×10^{-5}	2.14
Toluene	8.573×10^{-5}	7.49
Nitrobenzene	8.871×10^{-5}	2.52
Indene	9.875×10^{-5}	0.22
Ethylbenzene	9.982×10^{-5}	4.76
Azulene	10.854×10^{-5}	0.16
Naphthalene	10.854×10^{-5}	0.31
Anthracene	14.543×10^{-5}	0.015

Wallace, Kurtz and Niemann [490] examined the inhibition by 136 compounds of the hydrolysis of acetyl-1-valine methyl ester catalysed by α-chymotrypsin at 298.2 K in aqueous sodium chloride (100 mol m^{-3}). Some of the compounds were too insoluble to show measurable inhibition and many would be expected to give interactions. Among the compounds were benzene and toluene. From the results (calculated for a substrate concentration of 2 mol m^{-3}), the concentrations required to halve the rates of hydrolyses were 30.6 and 15.9 mol m^{-3} respectively for benzene and toluene. These figures are close to those found by Miles, Robinson and Canady [488] (see Table 59). On the assumption that alcohols are competitive inhibitors of α-chymotrypsin, Berezin, Lerashov and Martinek [491] worked out binding constants for the alcohols with the enzyme and found that these constants when plotted against the logarithms of the partition coefficients between 1-octanol and water (equivalent to plotting against characteristic volumes [49], see Chapter 6), gave points close to a straight line up to the C$_5$ alcohol, with some falling away for alcohols with more carbon atoms. A review of the inhibition of α-chymotrypsin by organic compounds has been written by Hansch and Coats [492].

Backes and Canady [493] compared the effects of aromatic hydrocarbons on the following three enzyme reactions:

(1)   the hydrolysis of methyl hippurate catalysed by α-chymotrypsin [488]
(2)   the action of yeast alcohol dehydrogenase [494]
(3)   the action of human Cl-esterase of the complement cascade on N-acetyl-L-tyrosine ethyl ester [495]

The free energies of transfer from water to enzyme 'solvent' of the hydrocarbons were calculated from kinetic measurements on the inhibition of the enzyme actions. They found that in all three cases a plot of the free energy of transfer against the number of carbon atoms in the hydrocarbon gave straight lines and all had the same slope: 3 kJ mol^{-1} per carbon atom. This value of the slope corresponds to k = 36 500 mol m^{-3} at 298 K in equations (70) and (71) and this is almost identical to the value used for partitioning between organic solvents and water. In fact, Backes and Canady noted that the plot of the free energies of transfer for aromatic hydrocarbons from water to 1-octanol against number of carbon atoms also gave a slope of 3 kJ mol^{-1} per carbon atom. They suggested that the enzyme could act as a non-aqueous phase and 'extract' compounds from the aqueous medium. They state that 'the larger the hydrocarbon the greater its ability to leave water and to bind with the enzyme or transfer to a non-aqueous phase'. Also, according to them, the organic compound-induced spectral changes could arise from a new phase.

The increase in activity, mentioned above, of α-chymotrypsin in the presence of potassium chloride has been investigated further [496–498]. Torchilin, Martinek and coworkers [497, 498] have found that α-chymotrypsin becomes more thermally stable in the presence of salts and the rate constant of inactivation can be decreased by 100-fold. The best salt for inhibition of de-activation was sodium sulphate. Sodium chloride and potassium chloride were less effective but better than potassium trichloroacetate. The order of these salts follows that of the molecular volumes. However, trimethylammonium bromide was about as active as potassium chloride. The substrate for these experiments carried out by the Russian workers was N-acetyl-1-tyrosine ethyl ester.

(c) OTHER PROTEINS AS TARGETS OF ANAESTHETICS AND PHYSICALLY TOXIC SUBSTANCES

Enzymes have been widely studied as models for the actions of anaesthetics on proteins largely because the loss of biological activity in enzymes is relatively easy to measure. However for many enzymes the concentrations of drugs needed to alter biological activity greatly exceed concentrations needed for anaesthesia [499]. Other proteins have been suggested as potential sites of anaesthetic action, including the cytoskeletal proteins of microtubules and microfilaments.

Allison *et al.* [500, 501] studied the action of anaesthetics on microtubules, structures which are a major part of the mitotic spindle of dividing cells and important cytoskeletal elements of many living cells. These polymeric thread-like structures can be readily broken down into dimers, which can be further dissociated into monomers with a molecular weight of about 60 000 as determined by sedimentation. Allison *et al.* found that microtubules depolymerise in the presence of anaesthetics. At concentrations two to four times the minimum alveolar concentration required for anaesthesia in man, the anaesthetics brought about reversible collapse of the axopods of the heliozoon, *Actinosphoerium nucleofilum* and the axopods reappeared in a few minutes after withdrawal of the anaesthetic. Diethyl ether was, however, comparatively ineffective. It was also noted that exposure to a concentration of halothane (2-bromo-2-chloro-1,1,1-trifluorethane) sufficient to block impulse transmission led to disappearance of microtubules in the axons of the rat, as seen in the electron microscope. Allison *et al.* suggest that depolymerisation of microtubules in nerve cells is actually responsible for narcosis.

Evidence against the involvement of microtubules in anaesthesia has been presented, for example, pentobarbital and halothane fail to depolymerise mouse optic nerve axonal microtubules [502]. It has been shown that low concentrations of halothane increase the number of rabbit vagus nerve microtubules while axonal conduction is blocked, and that colchicine decreases the microtubule count without affecting electrical conduction [503].

Membrane proteins have been shown by electron spin resonance studies to require the presence of a layer of tightly bound lipids at the protein—liquid bilayer boundary [504]. The liquid crystalline fluidity of this boundary layer appears to modify the biological activity of the membrane protein [505]. It has been proposed that the effect of anaesthetics on the activity of the sodium channel proteins of nerve axons is to increase the fluidity of the boundary layer lipids surrounding the proteins, with a resultant reversible loss of protein structure and function [506]. Independent evidence that the site of action of anaesthetics might be a membrane protein or a boundary region between membrane protein and lipid comes from X-ray and neutron diffraction studies on model systems [507]. From these it appears that the site of action has both polar and non-polar characteristics, typical of protein or protein–lipid interfaces.

(d) PARTITIONING OF PROTEINS

In view of the evidence that anaesthesia and other manifestations of physical toxicity involve partition between an aqueous phase and a phase rich in protein, other phenomena which have been thought to involve the 'hydrophobicity' may depend upon partition between these phases. A subject in which there has been considerable interest recently, is the distribution of proteins and peptides between aqueous phases and membranes. This has been discussed by McGowan and Mellors [508].

An equation analogous to Henry's law [188] for vapour pressures of solutions, can be given for the lowering of the solubility of one liquid in another when a solute is present in one of the liquids. Lewis [193] considers a mixture of water and ether to illustrate this. The lower layer of this system is a solution of ether (concentration S_0) in water. This solubility will be reduced (concentration S) if a substance soluble in ether and not in water is dissolved in the upper layer. The ratio S_0/S is given by (118)

$$\log S_0/S = \frac{CM}{\rho_l} \tag{118}$$

where C is the concentration of the solute, M is the molecular mass of the solvent (ether) and ρ_l is its density. If in place of the ether, a protein were substituted, M would be very high and a low concentration C of solute would give quite a large change in $\log S_0/S$, which would mean a very large change in S_0/S. In equation (118), S_0 refers to a saturated solution but a higher concentration of solute than that required for a saturated solution could cause separation of the protein even if its aqueous phase was less than fully saturated.

$$\log_{10} J = kV_x - E \tag{71}$$

The equation (71) has been used to estimate partition coefficients between water and non-aqueous phases (see Chapter 5, section (b)). Interaction terms for partition between water and ether are given in Table 32. The term for compounds containing one alcoholic hydroxyl or one ester group was 1.9. The figures in the table suggest that the interaction E for amides is about twice 1.9. Amino acids are very insoluble in ether. However, Collander does give approximate partition coefficients for alanine, leucine and aminobutyric acid and these correspond to E values of 8.39, 8.98 and 8.63 respectively; these are somewhat higher than four times 1.9.

Amino acids are much more soluble in the phases given by a mixture of alkoxyethanols and water than in ether and partition coefficients have been

measured between such phases [509]. The k value for the mixture used was
13 500 mol m^{-3} and equation (71) was used with this value to give the interaction terms E listed in Table 60. The interactions for serine and threonine give
$E = 0.38$ for the addition of a hydroxyl group to unsubstituted amino acids,
which have E values about four times this. These and other results suggest that
if $E(1)$ is the interaction for the alcohol, ether, ester and ketone groups between
two phases then $E = nE(1)$ for other groups and the number n is the same for
many pairs of phases.

Table 60. Interactions from partition coefficients
between phases given by a mixture of potassium
phosphate buffer at pH 7.0, 2-methoxyethanol
and 2-butoxyethanol (3:1:1 by volume respectively) at 293 K.

Compound	Interaction E	$n = E/0.38$
Glycine	1.53	4.0
Alanine	1.51	4.0
Proline	1.60	4.2
Valine	1.55	4.1
Leucine	1.52	4.0
Isoleucine	1.61	4.2
Methionine	1.68	4.4
Phenylalanine	1.43	3.8
Tryptophan	1.33	3.5
Tyrosine	1.75	4.6
Serine	1.95	5.1
Threonine	1.90	5.0
Aspartic acid	1.92	5.1
Glutamic acid	1.91	5.0
Histidine	2.21	5.8
Ornithine	2.47	6.5
Lysine	2.70	7.1
Arginine	2.86	7.5

The interaction of chemical groups with water weakens as the temperature
rises and some compounds which are soluble in cold water separate out when
the solutions are warmed. This is most marked in the case of some polymers,
e.g. mixed polymers of ethanediol and propanediol, methyl cellulose [510], and
some poly(N-alkylacrylamides) [511–514]. Poly(N-isopropylacrylamide) is
isomeric with the peptides poly(leucyl) and poly(isoleucyl) and, as shown, all
these substances have very similar structures. Poly(N-isopropylacrylamide)
[511–513] is completely soluble in acetic acid, ethanol, acetone and butanol

$$
\left[\begin{array}{c} -CH_2-CH- \\ \quad | \\ \quad CO \\ \quad | \\ \quad NH \\ \quad | \\ \quad CH \\ \quad / \ \backslash \\ CH_3 \ \ CH_3 \end{array}\right]_n
\quad
\left[\begin{array}{c} -CHNHCO- \\ \quad | \\ \quad CH_2 \\ \quad | \\ \quad CH \\ \quad / \ \backslash \\ CH_3 \ \ CH_3 \end{array}\right]_n
\quad
\left[\begin{array}{c} -CHNHCO- \\ \quad | \\ CH-CH_3 \\ \quad | \\ \quad CH_2 \\ \quad | \\ \quad CH_3 \end{array}\right]_n
$$

Poly(N-isopropyl   Poly(leucyl)   Poly(isoleucyl)
acrylamide)

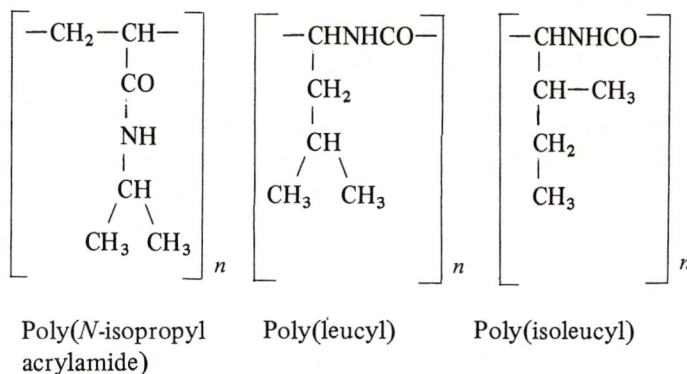

but it does not dissolve in hydrocarbons [512]. It is readily soluble in cold water but separates when the solution is warmed. It separates from a 5% solution at about 306 K. Copolymers of acrylamide and N-isopropylacrylamide containing 50 mol per cent or more acrylamide are soluble in hot and cold water [513]. Taylor and Cerankowski [514] have prepared many polymers which show temperature-inverse solubility in water. They give the following general solubility rule. 'As a polymer which is soluble in water at all temperatures is made increasing hydrophobic (i.e. substituents are introduced which increase the characteristic volume of the unit without the introduction of groups which interact with water), a range of compositions will be found which show temperature-inverse solubility and the more hydrophobic (i.e. the larger) the increment, the lower the cloud-point (often called 'the lower critical solution temperature')'.

Poly(L-proline) separates when its solutions in water are warmed. The phase which separates redissolves when cooled to 273.2 K. The separation on heating and solution on cooling may be carried out repeatedly [515]. These facts suggest that the kV_x and E terms in equation (71) for poly(proline) are almost equal at about room temperature. Values of k are high for the solubilities of compounds in water (see Chapter 5, section (b)) [38] and with k equal to 36 000 and V_x values for proline units calculated from the factors given in Table 4

$$\log_{10} J = 36\,000(7.113 \times 10^{-5}n + 1.674 \times 10^{-5})$$

$$- 2nE(1) - 2E(1) = \approx 0$$

where n is the number of amino acid units. The equation is corrected for the extra water molecule of the end group. With n at infinity, $E(1)$ is 1.28. The value of $E(1)$ falls somewhat as n decreases (at $n = 10$, it is 1.245) so $E(1)$ is close to the value of 1.2 (see Chapter 6, section (c)). The biophase thus resembles the protein-rich phase which separates when solutions of some polypeptides and related compounds are warmed. The equation (71) can be written in the form (119)

$$\log_{10} J = 36\,000 \, V_x - 1.2n \tag{119}$$

This equation was used [508] to interpret studies of the distribution of proteins and peptides between aqueous solutions and membranes. It is convenient to calculate $\log_{10} J$ for peptides and proteins from those of the separate units. For example, $\log_{10} J$ for leucine (also isoleucine and poly(isopropylacrylamide) for which the formulae are given above is.

6 carbons give $V_x \times 10^5$		9.810
11 hydrogens give $V_x \times 10^5$		9.581
1 nitrogen gives $V_x \times 10^5$		1.439
1 oxygen gives $V_x \times 10^5$		1.243
19 bonds	Sum	22.073
	Less	12.464
	V_x	9.609×10^{-5}

The values for E, the interactions found from partition coefficients, have been divided by 0.38 to give values of n (see Table 60). Whole numbers have been used for n except for the value for tyrosine: this amino acid contains a phenolic group for which n has been found to be 0.5 (see Chapter 6, section (c)). A value of n equal to 4.5 has been used for tyrosine. For asparagine and glutamine, n was taken as 4 and for arginine, it was taken as 5. Amide units have n values two less than the corresponding amino acids. There is one amide group in leucine for which $n = 2$ and so from equation (119) for this amino acid

$$\log_{10} J = 36\,000 \times 9.609 \times 10^{-5} - 2 \times 1.2 = 1.059$$

Values of $\log_{10} J$ for units in proteins and peptides are given in Table 61.

Davis and Model [516] have studied a protein from a virus (bacteriophage) which infects the bacterium *Escherichia coli*. This protein becomes fixed in the membrane of the bacterial cell. If, however, 23 amino acids are removed from near the carboxyl terminal end of the molecule, the protein passes out through the membrane and is secreted into the periplasm. Davis and Model used techniques of genetic engineering to alter the carboxyl terminal end of the viral protein from the virus. They introduced the unit Leu—Ala—Leu—Val from one to six times near the carboxyl terminal end of the protein from the virus. The $\log_{10} J$ value for Leu—Ala—Leu—Val is 2.24. When tested in order to see which proteins became fixed in the cell membrane, the proteins with no added unit and with addition of one unit were found in the supernatant liquid. The proteins containing three or more of the units were located in the membrane. Although much of the protein with two added units was found in the membrane, some was also present in the supernatant liquid. Units of Thr—Ser—Ala—Ser were also introduced near the carboxyl terminal end of the protein. The $\log_{10} J$ value for this group is -4.28 and none of the proteins containing this group were fixed in the membrane. Davis and Model inserted units Leu—Ala—Leu—Val into the protein at different places in addition to near the end and obtained similar results. They concluded that what was required was water repellency and not any feature of the structure or the sequence of the units. The water repellency appeared to be the sum of those values for the individual units and was related to the hydrophobicities suggested by von Heijne [517]. Some modifications were made earlier [518] to the end of the same protein and with one exception, the distributions of these follow the $\log_{10} J$ values [508].

Gething and Sambrook [519] carried out experiments with a haemagglutinin protein from an influenza virus. This protein was located in the plasma membrane but when 38 amino acids having $\log_{10} J = +1.59$ at the C-terminus were replaced with 11 amino acids having $\log_{10} J = -8.21$, the protein was present with the cell extract and medium. The virus protein is made up of 562 amino acids [520] and $\log_{10} J$ for the whole protein is -227.8. The protein would be expected to be largely in the aqueous phase and Gething and Sambrook seem to be correct in their view that regions with a positive $\log_{10} J$ can 'anchor' the protein into the membrane. There are no specific amino acid sequences which cause proteins to be located in membranes, as proposed by Blobel [521].

Table 61. Values of $\log_{10} J$ for units in peptides and proteins.

Peptide/protein	$\log_{10} J$ for unit
Lys	−2.18
Asn	−1.94
Arg	−1.62
Ser	−1.45
Gln	−1.43
His	−1.32
Gly	−0.97
Thr	−0.9
Asp	−0.89
Ala	−0.43
Glu	−0.29
Cystine/2	−0.14
Cys	0.13
Pro	0.16
Val	0.55
Leu	1.06
Ile	1.06
Met	1.14
Tyr	1.33
Phe	1.73
Trp	2.55

8

Physical Toxicities of Vapours

(a) TOXICITIES OF VAPOURS

Most of the discussion has so far been concerned with aqueous solutions. The toxicities of vapours are also important: anaesthetics are often administered as vapours, there is concern about human exposure to solvent vapours, and vapours are much used for fumigation of grain in stores. The distribution law and its application to vapours in Henry's law have been discussed in Chapter 4. According to the law

$$\frac{\text{concentration in vapour phase}}{\text{concentration in liquid phase (solution)}} = \text{a constant} \tag{120}$$

so that if vapour pressures are assumed to be proportional to vapour concentrations, application of (120) to the toxic concentrations and saturated solutions gives (121)

$$\log (p_t/p_s) = \log (C_B/C_{SB}) \tag{121}$$

where p_t is the toxic vapour pressure of the liquid with saturated vapour pressure p_s; C_B is the toxic concentration and C_{SB} the saturated concentration in the biophase. The biophase appears to be somewhat associated and in order to allow for this McGowan [38, 424] used (122)

$$\log_{10} C_{SB} = \log_{10} C_L - 4000\, V_x + E \tag{122}$$

The toxicities of vapours are often expressed as parts per million (ppm) by volume in air at atmospheric pressure ($101\,325\ \mathrm{N\,m^{-2}}$) so that C_t (ppm) corresponds to $p_t \times 101\,325 \times 10^{-6}$ ($\log_{10} 0.101325 = -0.99$) and

$$\log_{10} C_t(\text{ppm}) = \log_{10} p_s + \log C_B + 0.99$$
$$- \log_{10} C_L + 4000\, V_x - E \qquad (123)$$

In Chapter 6, it was suggested that the biophase has a low compressibility and it is important that corrections should be made for this. In equations (122) and (123) C_L, the concentration of the liquid in its own pure liquid state, should be replaced by the smaller C_{calc}, which is the solubility estimated for the compound by equation (67) with $T_x = 1317$ K.

A number of sets of values for the toxic concentrations of vapours to insects have been given. Ferguson and Pirie [30] measured toxicities to grain weevils (*Calandra granaria*). The observed toxicities were compared with the values estimated with equation (123). The vapour pressures given by Stull [522] were used and it was assumed that $\log_{10} C_B$ equalled 3.30 for the median lethal dose of vapours to grain weevils at 298.2 K. This same value for $\log_{10} C_B$ served for the median lethal doses of vapours [4] towards wireworms (larvae of *Agriotes* species) but $\log_{10} C_B$ equal to 3.60 was used for the concentrations of vapour [523, 524] required to kill 100% weevils (*Sitophilus oryzae*) in 24 hours. The replacement of $\log_{10} C_L$ in equation (123) by the smaller $\log_{10} C_{calc}$ reduces the value of $\log_{10} C_B$ required by about 0.5.

Ferguson [22] also measured directly the ratio of the toxic vapour pressure to the saturated vapour pressure p_t/p_s for the toxicities of the vapours of many organic compounds to grain weevils. In these experiments, air was saturated with the vapour and then mixed in definite proportions with air containing no vapour. These mixtures were passed through chambers holding 50 grain weevils. The behaviour of the insects under the influence of the air containing the vapour was observed at half-hourly intervals for a period of 5 hours. Narcosis was noted at two stages, 'threshold' narcosis and 'complete' narcosis. The experiments were all carried out at 298.2 K. If equations (121) and (122) are combined and C_L is replaced by C_{calc}, the equation (124) is obtained

$$\log_{10}(p_t/p_s) = \log_{10} C_B - \log_{10} C_{calc} + 4000\, V_x - E \qquad (124)$$

This equation was applied to the results of Ferguson and gave $\log_{10} C_B$ for threshold narcosis of grain weevils $= 2.2 \log_{10} C_B$; for complete narcosis of grain weevils $= 2.5$ and it is suggested that $\log_{10} C_B$ for death (median lethal dose) of grain weevils or wireworms $= 2.8$.

In Chapter 6 the 'cut-off' point for physical toxicity was discussed. The 'cut-off' occurs when the solubility in the biophase, C_{SB}, is lower than C_B, the concentration in the biophase required to give the toxicity [21, 26, 525]. The value given above of $\log_{10} C_B$ for the toxicity of vapours to wireworms was 2.8 and the 'cut-off' will not depend on what saturated phase is used to apply the toxic compound. Tattersfield and Roberts [4] found that the saturated vapours of phenanthrene (2.54) and anthracene (1.19) were non-toxic to wireworms. The values of $\log_{10} C_{calc} - 4000\, V_x$ ($= \log_{10} C_{SB}$) from Table 54 are given in

brackets and these are well below 2.8. Some compounds were listed as
marginally toxic; among these were naphthalene (2.8), 1-methyl-4(2-propyl)-
benzene (2.73) and 1,3,5-trimethylbenzene (3.04). The values of $\log_{10} C_{calc}$ —
4000 V_x for these compounds are near although it might have been expected
from the figures that 1,3,5-trimethylbenzene would have shown more than
marginal toxicity.

Tattersfield and Roberts [4] suggested that factors could be used to relate
the effects of some substitutions on the toxicities of vapours to wireworms.
They list ratios (toxic concentration of substituted compound)/(toxic concen-
traction of unsubstituted compound). The logarithms of these ratios give the
following factors for changes in $\log_{10} C_t$:

addition of $-CH_2-$	-0.34
replacement of C—H by C—Cl	-0.6
replacement of C—H by C—OH	-1.8

These ratios can be used for other cases of physical toxicity of vapours and a
more extensive list of factors has been given [424]. These factors are listed in
Table 62. They are intended to be used with C_B values based on C_L. If they are
to be used with C_B based on C_{calc}, which is about 0.5 smaller on the average,
the C_B value, or the estimated C_t, will have to be reduced by 0.5.

Table 62. Factors for calculation of
the toxicities of vapours by means of
equation (124).

Ethane	3.02
Cyclohexane	1.48
Benzene	1.14
Naphthalene	-0.84
Substitution of:	
C=C by CH—CH	-0.1
C—C by C—O—C	-0.3
C—H by C—CH$_3$	-0.34
C—C by C—CH$_2$—C	-0.34
C—H by C—Cl	-0.74
C—H by N	-0.75
C—C by C—S—C	-1.17
C—H by C—Br	-1.23
C—H by C—OH	-1.4
C—C by C—O—C—C	-1.42
$\quad\quad\quad\quad\quad \overset{\|}{O}$	
C—H by C—I	-1.67

Table 62. (continued)

Substitution of:	
C—H by C—CH=O	−1.75
C—C by C—C—C $\overset{\|}{\underset{O}{}}$	−1.75
C—H by C—CN	−2.15
C—H by C—NO$_2$	−2.4
C—H by C—C$_6$H$_5$	−2.56

(b) PHYSICAL TOXICITIES OF VAPOURS AND BOILING POINTS

The ratio of the toxic vapour pressure p_t to the saturated vapour pressure p_s is given by equations (121) and (122). Since experimental values for p_s at normal temperatures are not always available, methods for the prediction of p_s are of interest. One value of p_s is usually known and that is at the boiling point T_B where p_s is 101 325 N m^{-2} (i.e. 1 atmosphere). An equation of Littlewood [201] can be combined with equation (123) to relate C_t (ppm) to the boiling point T_B as follows:

$$\log_{10} C_t = \log_{10} C_B - 4.8\, T_B/T - 10.8 - \log_{10} C_{calc}$$
$$+ 4000\, V_x - E \tag{125}$$

McGowan [526] has suggested (126) as an alternative:

$$\log_{10} p_s = 7.70 - 2.7\, (T_B/T)^{1.7} \tag{126}$$

Examples used by Littlewood [201] to illustrate the use of his equation (125) for the estimation of vapour pressures of unassociated liquids are given in Table 63 with the values estimated from equation (126) for comparison. A combination of (123) and (126) gives (127)

$$\log_{10} C_t = \log_{10} C_B - 2.7\, (T_B/T)^{1.7} + 8.7$$
$$- \log_{10} C_L + 4000\, V_x - E \tag{127}$$

Examples of the use of this equation have been given [5].

Relationships between boiling points of liquids and the toxicities of their vapours to insects have been noted in the past. Holt [1] found that the toxicities of the vapours of liquids to cockroaches increased with the boiling point up to a certain value above which there was little, if any toxicity. Moore [2, 3] studied the toxicities of vapours to house flies (*Musca domestica*) at about 294 K and found that the higher the boiling point of the liquid, the more toxic the vapour except that compounds boiling above 520 K were usually so slightly volatile that not enough would evaporate to given an effect. Tattersfield and Roberts [4] in their work with wireworms (*Agriotes* species) at about 288 K got results similar

Table 63. Estimation of vapour pressures of unassociated liquids.

| Compound | Boiling point (K) | Vapour pressure (N m^{-2}) at 323.2 K | | |
| | | Observed | Calculated | |
			from (125)	from (126)
n-Hexane	341.5	5.33×10^4	5.43×10	5.43×10^4
n-Heptane	371.6	1.93×10^4	1.92×10^4	1.89×10^4
2,2,4-Trimethylpentane	372.6	1.87×10^4	1.84×10^4	1.84×10^4
n-Decane	447.3	0.10×10^4	0.14×10^4	0.10×10^4
Benzene	353.3	3.60×10^4	3.59×10^4	3.63×10^4
p-Xylene	411.5	0.44×10^4	0.49×10^4	0.42×10^4
n-Butylbenzene	456.3	0.07×10^4	0.11×10^4	0.07×10^4
Ethyl acetate	350.3	3.76×10^4	3.93×10^4	4.02×10^4
Diethyl carbonate	399.0	0.52×10^4	0.73×10^4	0.69×10^4
Methyl benzoate	472.7	0.03×10^4	0.06×10^4	0.035×10^4

to those of Moore. They found that the inert compounds (such as hydrocarbons) boiling above 440 K were uncertain in their action on wireworms and compounds boiling about 510 K had too low a volatility to produce any effect on the wireworms.

(c) PHYSICAL TOXICITY AND HUMAN EXPOSURE

Smith *et al.* and others [527–531] have investigated the teratogenic effects of anaesthetics on chick embryos, and similar effects have been noted for rats [532]. There is a significant increase in the risk of spontaneous abortion among women working in operating rooms [533, 534] and an increased risk of congenital abnormality for the live-born children of anaesthetists (both men and women) [535]. It is of interest that Sice [536] has found that some n-alkanes and n-alkanols promote papilloma growth in the skin of mice which had been treated with a non-carcinogenic dose of 7,12-dimethylbenz[a] anthracene. The effect was related to chain length and each alkane was approximately equipotent with the alkanol containing two fewer carbon atoms. 1-Dodecanol, dodecane and tetradecane were the most potent of the compounds tested. 1-Hexanol, hexane and octane were inactive. The cocarcinogenic activity of decane and tetradecane has been confirmed by van Duuren [537].

Further investigation may show these long-term effects of hydrocarbons to be of great importance but there is currently much interest too in the short-term aspects. The addiction of persons to physically toxic compounds of all kinds is of increasing social concern.

In Europe and North America glue-sniffing has become a significant form of drug abuse, especially among juveniles. The inhalation of solvents of many kinds has resulted in death and physical impairment and has led to calls for legislative controls on the sale and manufacture of solvent-based products [538, 539]. The number of deaths from glue-sniffing recovered in the United Kingdom were 22 in 1980, 39 in 1981 and 66 in 1982 [540].

The medical aspects of glue-sniffing have been reviewed [541]. The cases of 19 children admitted to the Royal Hospital for Sick Children, Glasgow between 1974 and 1980 with acute encephalopathy caused by glue-sniffing are described. Toluene, which is the main solvent used in Britain for contact adhesives, was determined in the blood of the children by gas chromatography. The values ranged from 0.8 to 8 ppm. Higher concentrations of toluene in the blood, up to 40 ppm, were found for some fatal cases of glue-sniffing and the concentrations in brain tissue were higher than in the blood.

In order to overcome the problems associated with 'glue-sniffing', it has been suggested [542] that some unpleasant substance might be added to the solvents. Perhaps allyl isothiocyanate (the main constituent of mustard oil) or one of the more volatile nitroethylenes would be suitable additives. These compounds would be harmful themselves at high concentrations but merely disagreeable at very low concentrations. The most satisfactory method of solving the problems, however, would be to use solvents sufficiently insoluble in the biophase to bring them above the 'cut-off' and so make them non-toxic. As the biological effect becomes less severe, the concentration in the biophase C_B required to produce it falls. As shown in Chapter 8, section (a), $\log_{10} C_B$ is 2.8 for death, 2.5 for complete narcosis and 2.2 for threshold narcosis of grain weevils. To be safe as a solvent, C_B might have to be about four times lower than that giving the threshold narcosis, i.e. $\log_{10} C_B = 1.6$. In Table 54, some values estimated for $\log_{10} C_B$ ($= \log_{10} C_{calc} - 4000\, V_x$) are given and for heptadecane the value is 1.6. This compound and others such as olive oil would be expected to be harmless. Unfortunately, these solvents have low volatility and would be useless when evaporation of the solvent was required.

For guidance in industry, toxic limits of compounds are laid down. The choice of a value of C_B for the maximum atmospheric concentrations of physically toxic vapours, to which people may safely be exposed, has been discussed [424]. The equation (123) with the term $\log_{10} C_L$ was used and a value of 1.06 for $\log_{10} C_B$ was suggested since p_t depends on $\log_{10} C_B - \log_{10} C_{calc}$ (see equation (124)); the estimated values of p_t will be largely unchanged when C_L is replaced by C_{calc} because C_B will have to be lowered also.

(d) PHYSICAL TOXICITY AND INDUSTRIAL HYGIENE

The equations discussed above are useful not only for the prediction of concentrations which will cause the death of various organisms, but also for the prediction of the concentrations that will give rise to milder toxic symptoms. At certain places of work individuals may be exposed for long periods to comparatively low concentrations of vapours and in order to protect these individuals, safe working limits have been proposed. It might be expected that a value could be given to C_B so that the equations (123) and (124) could be used as a guide to the maximum average atmospheric concentrations of physically toxic vapours to which men may be safely exposed and a figure of $\log_{10} C_B = 1.6$ has been suggested [424]. This can be used with the calculated or the observed values of $\log_{10} C_t - \log_{10} C_B$ in Table 64 to suggest a limiting concentration (ppm) above which a person should not be exposed for a long period.

With $\log_{10} C_B$ equal to 1.6 equation (124) becomes (128)

$$\log_{10} C_t = \Sigma f + 1.6 \tag{128}$$

and equation (125) becomes (129)

$$\log_{10} C_t = \log_{10} p_s + 2.6 - \log_{10} C_L + 4000 \, V_x - E \tag{129}$$

Table 64. A comparison of threshold limits with figures calculated from equations (128) and (129).

Compound	Toxic concentration (ppm)		
	Suggested value	Calculated from equation:	
		(128)	(129)
(a) *Hydrocarbons and their halogen derivatives*			
Benzene	10	550	590
Benzene, chloro-	75	100	100
Benzene, 1,2-dichloro-	50	18	14
Benzene, dimethyl-	100	110	100
Benzene, ethyl	100	110	110
Benzene, 2-methylpropyl- 4-methyl-	10	11	
Benzene, 2-propyl-	50	52	
Benzene, 1,3,5-trimethyl-	25	52	52
Cyclohexane	300	1 150	960
Cyclohexane, methyl-	400	550	600
Cyclohexene	300	1 500	–
Ethane, 1,2-dichloro- 1,1,2,2-tetrafluoro-	1 000	–	16 000
Ethan, 1,1,1-trichloro-	350	250	1 070
Ethane, 1,2-dichloro-	200	5 000	1 450
Ethene, tetrachloro-	100	60	170
Ethene, trichloro-	100	320	560
Heptane	400	590	830
Hexane	100	1 820	2 000
Methane, dichloro-	200	2 900	1 780
Methane, dichlorofluoro-	1 000	–	7 200
Methane, tetrachloro-	10	100	890
Methane, trichloro-	10	550	1 180

Table 64. (continued)

Compound	Suggested value	Toxic concentration (ppm) Calculated from equation: (128)	(129)
Methane, trichlorofluoro-	1 000	—	5 900
Octane	300	380	280
Pentane	600	4 000	5 400
Toluene	100	250	270
Toluene, 2-chloro-	50	46	
(b) *Alcohols and phenols*			
1-Butanol	50	320	
1-Butanol, 1,3-dimethyl-	25	48	
Cyclohexanol	50	50	
Cyclohexanol, methyl-	50	25	
Ethanol	1 000	1 600	
Methanol	200	4 000	
Phenol	5	20	
Phenol, methyl-	5	10	
2-Propanol	400	790	
(c) *Ketones*			
Acetone (2-propanone)	1 000	740	1 100
2-Butanone	200	340	710
Cyclohexanone	50	50	40
Cyclohexanone, methyl-	50	20	—
2-Hexanone	25	71	
2-Cyclohexen-1-one, 3,5,5-trimethyl-	5	6	8
2-Pentanone	200	150	140
2-Pentanone, 4-methyl-	100	70	80
(d) *Miscellaneous*			
Acetic acid, butyl ester	150	151	
Acetic acid, ethyl ester	400	720	510
Acetic acid, methyl ester	200	1 600	1 200
Acetic acid, 3-methylbutyl ester	100	69	83
Acetic acid, 1-methylpentyl ester	50	32	
Acetic acid, 2-methylpropyl ester	150	151	263
Acetic acid, propyl ester	200	330	350

Table 64. (continued)

Compound	Toxic concentration (ppm)		
	Suggested values	Calculated from equation: (128)	(129)
Aniline	2	40	3
Aniline, *N,N*-dimethyl-	5	10	10
Benzamine, methyl-	5	20	2
Benzene, nitro-	1	2	2
1,4-Dioxane	50	1 600	260
Ethane, nitro-	100	160	96
Ethanol, 2-butoxy-	50	40	—
Ethanol, 2-methoxy-	25	400	—
Ethanol, 2-methoxy-, acetate	25	160	—
Methane, dimethoxy-	1 000	5 000	—
Methane, nitro-	100	400	115
Propane, 1-chloro-1-nitro	20	14	—
Propane, 2-nitro-	25	80	115
Propane, 2,2'-oxybis-	250	1 000	2 500
Toluene, nitro- (benzene, methyl-nitro-)	5	1	2.5

In Table 64, some of the threshold limits proposed [543] for the maximum average concentrations of vapours to which workers may be exposed for an 8-hour working day without injury to health are compared with figures for C_t calculated from equations (128) and (129). The agreement between the suggested limits and those calculated, whilst not good, is nevertheless encouraging. The suggested limits are subject to review as more information becomes available.

Some of the suggested limits are chosen because it is known that toxic symptoms will be produced if the threshold given is much exceeded and in such cases the equations would be expected to give reasonable agreement when the compound is physically toxic. Other suggested limits are based on concentrations which are known to be safe although higher concentrations might well not be toxic: in these cases the equations could not be expected to agree with the suggested limits.

In Table 64, an effort has been made to exclude groups of chemically toxic compounds. Some compounds containing the groupings $CH_2 = C<$ and $XCH_2 CH< (X = halogen)$ seem to be chemically toxic towards rats [24] and compounds containing these groupings have been omitted from the table. Ferguson and Pirie [30] considered that ammonia, carbon disulphide, aliphatic amines and compounds containing the $-CHO$ group were chemically toxic towards grain weevils and none of these compounds have been included in Table

64. In section (a) of Table 64, hydrocarbons and their halogen derivatives are listed and E is taken as zero for equation (129). It has already been mentioned (Chapter 2) that carbon tetrachloride causes damage to the liver [74, 75]. Benzene is also not purely physically toxic: a characteristic feature of chronic benzene poisoning is injury to the bone marrow. The suggested threshold limits for benzene and carbon tetrachloride are therefore, as expected, much lower than the calculated figures from (128) and (129). In section (b) of Table 64, figures are given for alcohols and phenols. Since it is at present difficult to allot values for the interactions, equation (129) has not been used for these compounds. The agreement between the suggested threshold limits and the figures calculated from the factors in Table 62 and equation (128) is satisfactory except for methanol, exposure to which can lead to blindness. Table 64 gives figures for ketones (section (c)) and for miscellaneous compounds (section (d)). On the whole, the results are quite encouraging. Equations (128) and (129) may prove of value in the interpretation of toxicity data and also when the toxic limit of some physically toxic chemical has to be fixed for the first time or when the revision of a limit is under consideration. Sato and Nakajima [544] found a correlation between the threshold limit values recommended by the American Conference of Governmental Industrial Hygienists and the partition coefficients between blood and air. Exceptions were carbon tetrachloride, which is chemically toxic, and o-dichlorobenzene, which seemed to.be less toxic than the threshold limit suggested. The authors suggest that the threshold limit for this compound should be re-evaluated.

9

Chemical and Physical Toxicity

(a) CHEMICAL REACTIVITY AND TOXICITY

When the observed toxicity of a compound is considerably greater than that estimated for physical toxicity, 'chemical toxicity' is to be suspected. Ferguson and Pirie [30] considered that among the compounds which they tested for toxicity to grain weevils, iodides, most bromides, formates, aliphatic amines, aldehydes, methyl chloride, ethylene dibromide and carbon disulphide were chemically toxic because the p_t/p_s values for these were so low.

The effects of substituents can often be used to distinguish compounds showing chemical toxicity from physically toxic compounds. Physical toxicities (measured by the concentration in water or air to produce a given biological effect up to a 'cut-off') will increase with molecular volume: for example in a homologous series physical toxicity increases with the addition of each carbon atom. Chemical reactivity does not depend upon molecular volume unless there is at the same time a steric or electronic change at the reaction site. In a homologous series, the chemical toxicity usually remains nearly constant after perhaps the first one or two members. An example of this is the toxicities [545] of alkyl thiocyanoacetates $ROCOCH_2SCN$ to micro-organisms (see Table 65). Here toxicities are high and within experimental error are in independent of the group R. The compounds become inactive (i.e. there is a 'cut-off') when they become so insoluble that toxic doses cannot be attained. This 'cut-off' is earlier for *Salmonella typhosa* than for *Fusarium caeruleum*. The former organism requires about ten times as much thiocyanoacetate to kill it as the latter. In these examples, there is no sign of physical toxicity right up to the 'cut-off'. In some

Table 65. Toxic concentrations (mol m^{-3}) of alkyl thiocyano-acetates towards *Fusarium caeruleum* and *Salmonella typhosa* [54].

Group R in ROCOCH$_2$ SCN	Toxic concentration (mol m^{-3}) towards.	
	Fusarium caeruleum	*Salmonella typhosa*
CH$_3$	0.1	2.0
C$_2$H$_5$	0.2	2.0
n—C$_4$H$_9$	0.3	0.7
n—C$_6$H$_{13}$	0.1	1.0
n—C$_8$H$_{17}$	0.4	Inactive
n—C$_{10}$H$_{21}$	0.2	Inactive
n—C$_{12}$H$_{25}$	Inactive	Inactive

cases [545], however, lower members of a homologous series may be chemically toxic and the higher members are physically toxic.

Ferguson and Pirie [30] considered that, with the exception of methyl chloride, alkyl chlorides are physically toxic to grain weevils. (The work of Hassall [546] suggests that t-butyl and t-amyl chlorides are chemically toxic.) They point out that methyl halides are more reactive than the corresponding ethyl halides. There was some uncertainty about the type of toxicity shown by the higher members of the series of alkyl bromides but all the alkyl iodides seemed to be chemically toxic. Chemical reactions are known in which iodides are much more reactive than bromides, and bromides are in turn more reactive than chlorides.

Many examples can be found in which biological activities are related to chemical reactivities. The chemical reactivities of substituted aromatic compounds can frequently be related to the sigma factor of Hammett [547, 548] and good correlations have been found [16, 549] between log (toxic concentration) for certain biological effects and Hammett's sigma factor or the effective charge [550]. The relationship between fungistatic activity and ease of formation of positive iodine [78] has been given earlier (Chapter 2, Table 6) as an example of the influence of atomic volumes on the reactivities of compounds through steric effects.

In 1936, McGowan [551] put forward the following rule: 'Substitution in the phenyl derivative C$_6$H$_5$A by electrophilic reagents will give largely *ortho* and *para* derivatives if the dissociation constant

$$K_a = \frac{[AO^-][H^+]}{[AOH]}$$

of the compound AOH (measured in dilute aqueous solution at room temperature) is smaller than 10^{-4} mol m^{-3} and will give largely the *meta* derivative if K_a is greater than 10^{-2} mol m^{-3}'. The ionisation constant K_a of the compound was later used as a convenient rough measure of the attraction of the group A for electrons and has related to the fungicidal activities of ethylenic derivatives

$$\overset{\backslash}{\underset{/}{C}}=\overset{/}{\underset{\backslash}{C}}\overset{}{\underset{A}{}}$$

[552, 553]. The concentrations of some ethylenic compounds required to inhibit the germination of *Botrytis allii* spores under standard conditions have been used for Table 66. It will be seen from the table that all the compounds containing the $-C=CNO_2$ grouping are powerful fungicides. If β-nitrostyrene were acting as a physically toxic compound, the introduction of methylene groups would increase the biological activity. Bosquet, Kirby and Searle [554] tested some β-alkyl-β-nitrostyrenes and some of their results are shown in Table 67. It will be seen that the introduction of methylene groups does not increase the toxicity to the fungus.

Table 66. Concentrations C_t (mol m^{-3}) required to inhibit germination of *Botrytis allii* spores under standard conditions [552].

Compound	Formula	$Log_{10} C_t$
β-Nitrostyrene	$C_6H_5CH=CHNO_2$	-1.4
4-Chloro-β-nitrostyrene	$4\text{-}ClC_6H_4CH=CHNO_2$	-1.4
4-Methoxy-β-nitrostyrene	$4\text{-}CH_3OC_6H_4CH=CHNO_2$	-1.4
Diethenyl sulphone	$(CH_2=CH)_2SO_2$	-0.9
Methyl ethenyl sulphone	$CH_2=CHSO_2CH_3$	-0.2
n-Butyl ethenyl sulphone	$CH_2=CHSO_2C_4H_9$	$+0.2$
Benzalacetophenone	$C_6H_5CH=CHCOC_6H_5$	-0.6
Dehydracetic acid		-0.5

$$\begin{array}{c} CH_3 \\ | \\ O \overset{C=CH}{\underset{C-CH}{<}} \hspace{-6pt} > C=O \\ \underset{O \quad COCH_3}{\overset{\|\ \ |}{}} \end{array}$$

Sorbic acid	$CH_3CH=CH-CH=CHCOOH$	-0.3
Cinnamic aldehyde	$C_6H_5CH=CH-CHO$	0
Cinnamic acid	$C_6H_5CH=CH-COOH$	$+0.2$
Methyl fumarate	$CH_3OOCCH=CHCOOCH_3$	$+0.2$
Ethyl fumarate	$C_2H_5OOCCH=CHCOOC_2H_5$	$+0.5$
Benzal acetone	$C_6H_5CH=CHCOCH_3$	$+0.5$
Croton aldehyde	$CH_3CH=CHCHO$	$+0.9$

Table 67. Toxic Concentrations C_t (mol m^{-3}) of β-substituted-β-nitrostyrenes

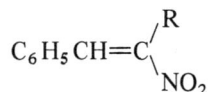

$$C_6H_5 CH = C \overset{\displaystyle R}{\underset{\displaystyle NO_2}{\big<}}$$

towards *Aspergillus niger* at pH 5.7 [554].

R	$Log_{10} C_t$
H-	-1.0
CH$_3$	-0.7
C$_2$H$_5$-	-0.4
n-C$_3$H$_7$-	-0.5

The alkyl sulphonic acids are fairly strong acids but not as strong as nitric acid; vinyl sulphones, which contain the $CH_2 = CHSO_2 R$ grouping, are fungicides but are rather less active than nitroethylenes. Again chemical toxicity is indicated for these compounds since methyl ethenyl sulphone has, if anything, greater toxicity than the more bulky n-butyl ethenyl sulphone (Table 65). Compounds having a group of the type -COOR, -COR, -COOH or -CHO attached to the ethylenic bond show in general less activity than the vinyl sulphones. Some may be physically toxic but there is evidence that some at least can be combined with groupings in proteins [555–557]. Geiger and Conn [555] found that a number of α, β-unsaturated ketones reacted very readily with certain compounds containing sulphydryl groups. The products of the reactions were much less bactericidal than the original α, β-unsaturated ketones. Also in a medium containing cysteine, or some other compound containing an -SH grouping, the α, β-unsaturated ketones often showed reduced bactericidal activity. It has been found that ethylenes with electron-attracting substituents react with cysteine and with p-aminobenzoic acid [558–562]. The bacteriostatic activities of a large number of β-benzoylacrylic acids towards *Staphylococcus aureus* and *Salmonella typhosa* have been measured and it was found that related compounds without the double bond (i.e. β-benzoylpropionic acids) were practically biologically inactive [561].

Dixon and Needham [563] found that lachrymators, including those which contained reactive ethylenic bonds, irreversibly inhibited enzymes, the activity of which depended on sulphydryl groups. Among those enzymes were succinic dehydrogenase, triosephosphate dehydrogenase, yeast alcohol dehydrogenase, hexokinase, the pyruvate dehydrogenase system, papain and urease. The vesicants seemed to owe their activity to reaction with hexokinase.

In the course of the work described above, McGowan, Brian and Hemming [552] discovered that sorbic acid (2,4-hexadienoic acid) and dehydracetic acid (3-acetyl-6-methyl-2,4-pyrandione) had quite high fungistatic activity but they did not consider this of special significance. However, later when it was realised that these compounds have low toxicity to humans, they became commercially important. Sorbic acid is particularly useful for the preservation of foods because it does not impart an adverse flavour and dehydracetic acid has proved to be of value for the pre-harvest treatment of fruit. A large amount of study has been devoted to these two fungicides and this has been reviewed [564].

(b) ACTIONS OF PHYSICALLY TOXIC COMPOUNDS

The equation (101) reproduced below has already been given for the estimation of the toxic concentrations for physically toxic compounds

$$-\log_{10} C_t = -\log_{10} C_B + kV_x - E \qquad (101)$$

The concentrations in the biophase, C_B, vary and increase as the intensities of the biological effects increase but for any one compound kV_x and E will usually be constant and $\log_{10} C_t$ will vary linearly with $\log_{10} C_B$. This will hold for other physically toxic compounds and, in general, physically toxic compounds all give the same sequence of symptoms of toxicity. Frequently, when presented with a toxic compound, a higher organism shows signs of excitation. Respiration may increase as the organism reacts against the compound and, if it is mobile, it may attempt to move away. However, with physically toxic compounds at a high enough concentration narcosis occurs and this is reversible unless it is too deep or too prolonged. Quite different symptoms are often found with compounds which are chemically toxic. Irritant compounds are usually chemically toxic [4] but chemically toxic compounds need not be irritants.

As well as being dependent on the intensity of the biological effect, C_B varies from one species to another for what appears to be the same biological effect, e.g. death under a given set of conditions. Thus the toxicities of various physically toxic compounds will appear in the same order towards different species. A different order will in general be found with chemically toxic compounds [421]. Busvine [565] studied toxic doses for seven insect species. He found (Table 68) the same order of toxicities for benzene, toluene, trichloroethylene, tetrachloroethylene, carbon tetrachloride and chloroform. The toxicities of other compounds (methyl acetate, ethyl acetate, ammonia, hydrogen cyanide and sulphur dioxide) were in a different order and compounds in this last set might be expected to be chemically toxic. Ratios of toxicities in different tests may also be used to distinguish between chemical and physical toxicity. The ratios of the toxic concentrations found by Ferguson and Pirie [30] for grain weevils to the concentrations required to produce narcosis in mice of ethyl chloride, dichloroethylene and chloroform are 8.4, 9.4 and 10.1 respectively. Ferguson and Pirie considered this was further evidence for their view that these compounds are physically toxic. On the other hand, they believe that methyl chloride, ethyl bromide and carbon disulphide were chemically toxic towards grain weevils and the corresponding ratios for these compounds were much lower: 1.2, 2.4 and 0.9 respectively. Ratios of toxicities to different bacteria had been noted earlier by Cooper and Forstner [421]. They found that

Table 68. Relative resistance of insects to vapours and gases [565].

Species (stage)	Median lethal dose (mol m^{-3}) for 5 h at 293 K									1 hr at 298 K		1 h at 293 K
	Benzene	Toluene	Trichloro-ethylene	Tetrachloro-ethylene	Carbon tetra-chloride	Chloro-form	Methyl acetate	Ethyl acetate	Ammonia	Hydrogen cyanide	Ethylene oxide	Sulphur dioxide
Flour moth (*Ephestia kuehniella*) – pupa	3.11	>Sat	2.28	>Sat	>Sat	3.24	–	–	–	0.06	0.84	–
Grain weevil (*Calandra granaris*) – adult	2.73	0.98	1.91	0.61	3.84	3.01	0.94	1.12	0.52	0.81	0.39	0.16
Rice weevil (*Calandra oryzae*) – adult	2.34	0.82	1.67	0.54	3.08	2.13	0.51	0.41	0.43	0.89	0.27	0.48
Flour moth (*Ephestia kuehniella*) – larva	1.95	0.67	1.55	0.55	2.91	2.14	0.59	0.57	0.45	0.01	0.59	0.25
Clothes moth (*Tineola bisselliella*) – larva	1.75	0.60	1.34	0.52	2.29	1.80	–	0.78	–	0.24	0.41	0.37
Flour beetle (*Tribolium castaneum*) – adult	0.82	0.36	0.78	0.30	0.89	1.52	0.88	0.77	0.35	0.02	0.93	0.27
Bed bug (*Cimex lectularis*) – adult	0.79	0.27	0.51	0.25	0.73	0.89	0.22	0.28	0.70	0.005	0.59	0.10

Pseudomonas aeruginosa was more sensitive than *E. coli* to compounds of what they called the 'physicochemical' type and gave the following figures for the ratio (toxic dose for *E. coli*)/(toxic does for *P. aeruginosa*), for 48 hours of exposure at 310 K: methanol (1.6); ethanol (2.0); n-propanol (1.6); isopropanol (1.4); benzyl alcohol (1.5); phenol (1.6). *P. aeruginosa* is also more susceptible to heat than *E. coli*. However, towards many chemically toxic compounds *E. coli* is more susceptible than *P. aeruginosa*. For example, ratios corresponding to those above are: *p*-nitrophenol (0.01); *p*-nitrosoaniline (0.3); benzoquinone (0.6).

There is evidence that k in equation (101) can vary somewhat and, because of this, plots of $\log C_t$ against V_x for different biological activities can sometimes intersect. An example of this is the effect of alcohols on the transmission of nerve impulses by the synaptic and non-synaptic pathways (see Fig. 21). The toxic concentrations for both pathways are equal for n-butanol. For the primary alcohols of lower molecular weight than n-butanol, higher toxic concentrations are required for the synaptic pathways than for the non-synaptic pathways; for the alcohols with higher molecular weights, the reverse is the case. From the figures for biological activities given in Table 56, it would be expected that the concentrations of 1-heptanol and lower primary alcohols required to inhibit the hydrolysis of methyl oleate by pancreatic lipase would be higher than those concentrations required for the inhibition of pepsin in the hydrolysis of haemo-globin or *N*-carbobenzoxy-1-glutamyl-1-tyrosine. However, the concentrations of 1-octanol and higher alcohols required to inhibit the lipase would, up to the cut-off, be lower than those required to inhibit pepsin. The number of exceptions of this kind to the generalisations given above are likely to be very few.

(c) SPECIFIC INTERACTIONS AND CHEMICAL TOXICITY

It seems probable that the biophase, like some enzymes which are affected by physically toxic compounds, is a protein. Proteins interact with water and indeed, if this were not so they would not form aqueous solutions. Physical toxicity seems to occur when the toxic compound brings about the separation of a phase containing much protein and relatively little water. The examples of chemical toxicity given above involve chemical reactions which are practically irreversible and impair something essential for the proper functioning of the living organism. It is relatively easy to distinguish between what might be called 'pure physical toxicity' and this 'pure chemical toxicity'. However, there are cases where it is not so easy to make the distinction.

The term E in equation (101) was originally introduced to account for increases of solubilities brought about by specific interactions. Water in the largely non-aqueous phase can also give interactions and it has been found (Chapter 5) that the terms E for partitions between water and organic com-pounds can often be related to the solubilities of water in these compounds. The biophase appears to be somewhat associated. This means that it interacts with itself and it will therefore interact with some other compounds also. If the specific interactions are weak and reversible, the bulk of the biophase would remain largely unchanged and some increase in toxicity beyond that predicted by equation (101) may be found. Examples of this which have been suggested already are the toxicities of ketones towards grain weevils [5] and the narcotic effects of ethers on the same insects (Chapter 8). If, however, the specific interaction of a compound with the biophase were strong, whether reversible or not, the biological activity could hardly be classed as 'physical toxicity'. There should be a graduation between 'pure physical toxicity' and 'pure chemical toxicity' and the action of a compound with a strong interaction might indistinguishable from the effect of an anti-metabolite on an enzyme.

Equations (128) and (129) can be applied to the specific interaction between a compound C and biophase B. These equations resemble those which were used (Chapter 5, section (b)) for the interaction of a compound with water and other solvents

$$nC + mB \rightleftharpoons C_n B_m \tag{130}$$

$$k_{BC} = \frac{[C_n B_m]}{[C]^n [B]^m} \tag{131}$$

The equations (130) and (131) are identical with those used for the combination of an enzyme with a substrate, metabolite antagonist or coenzyme. For example, the combination of haemoglobin (Hb) with oxygen to give oxyhaemoglobin (HbO_2) is described by equation (130) with $n = m = 1$. It is interesting that oxygen, although essential for life of the higher animals, is chemically toxic under pressure [32, 566, 567]. Poisoning by carbon monoxide is the result of the reversible combination of the gas with haemoglobin. This was first stated by Bernard [445]. Linas and Limousin [568] used pure oxygen in the treatment of carbon monoxide poisoning. Douglas, Haldane and Haldane [569] applied the equations (130) to reaction of oxygen and of carbon monoxide with haemoglobin. The results were combined to give the relationship (132)

$$\frac{[HbCO]}{[HbO_2]} = K_{co} \frac{[CO]}{[O_2]} \tag{132}$$

where K_{co} is the relative affinity constant, which was found [570] to be 210 for man. There are many reviews (for example those of Woolley [571–574] on anti-metabolites and it is not proposed to discuss the subject further.

(d) CONCLUSION

Much of modern toxicological research is devoted to compounds which are chemically toxic, that is which show specific chemical interactions with the molecular components of living cells. The theme of the preceding chapters has been toxicity, an area which, though it is frequently encountered and used in anaesthesia, narcosis and chemical sterilization, has received little attention from toxicologists in recent years. Physical toxicity is also encountered frequently by life science researchers in the course of their studies, when living cells or cellular molecules are affected by chemicals or solvents in a non-specific manner. The purpose of this book has been to illustrate the connection between physical toxicity and the molecular volume of the chemical. There is an awareness in the scientific community that partition coefficients greatly influence biological activities of molecules. However it is often not clear from such studies whether the partitioning of the molecule between the aqueous and biophase regions of the cell results in chemical or physical toxicity effects. The preceding chapters give means of recognising physically toxic effects of chemicals through use of molecular volumes. It has been shown that toxicity arises when a compound reaches a certain concentration in some biophase within a living cell. The partition coefficients between water and this biophase depend on characteristic volumes which can be used for the estimation of relative concentrations of compounds in water required for a given manifestation of physical toxicity. Compounds which are useful to the living organism, even some essential for its life, may give physical toxicity. However, solubilities in the biophase decrease somewhat as the characteristic volumes increase and compounds with large enough volumes are not sufficiently soluble in the biophase to show toxicity. It has been shown that the dose required for a given biological effect of compounds on living cells will vary with the proportion of lipid material in that cell, higher concentrations of drug being needed for cells rich in lipids. In higher animals the proportion of body weight which is adipose tissue will have a strong influence on the anaesthetic potency or physical toxicity of lipophilic chemicals. Further, compounds which are too insoluble in the biophase to be harmful by themselves may nevertheless contribute to a toxic concentration of a mixture. Normal metabolites and nutrients may at sufficiently high concentrations be physically toxic to an organism. The fat-soluble vitamins A and D for example show considerable toxicity at high concentration, while being essential for human nutrition in lower doses. The theme of this work has been the correlation between physical toxicity and molecular volumes and to the well-known remark of Paracelsus that 'everything is harmful; everything is safe; it all depends on the dose', one might add 'and the dose may depend on the molecular volume'.

Appendix I.

Instructions and examples for computer programs dealing with molecular volumes in chemistry and biology.

First a list of the more common elements is shown and for each compound a request is made for the symbol for an atom contained in it followed by a comma and then the number of these atoms in the compound. The instruction is:

ENTER DETAILS OF COMPOUND

H	C	N	O
F	Cl	Br	I
Si	P	S	As

ENTER SYMBOL FOR ATOM, COMMA, NUMBER OF THESE ATOMS

Next the number of double bonds after the symbol D and the number of triple bonds after the symbol T has to be given, if such bonds are present. To count these bonds, formulae have to be written so that the atoms have the electronic structure of the inert gas with the next higher atomic number. For example:

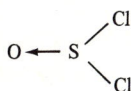

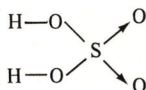

$$O \leftarrow S \overset{Cl}{\underset{Cl}{<}} \qquad \underset{H-O}{\overset{H-O}{>}} S \overset{O}{\underset{O}{<}} \qquad \text{No double bonds}$$

H — O — N = O   Formulae with one double bond

O = C = O   Two double bonds

O ⧤ C   H — C ≡ N   H — N ⧤ C   One triple bond

          Three double and one triple bond

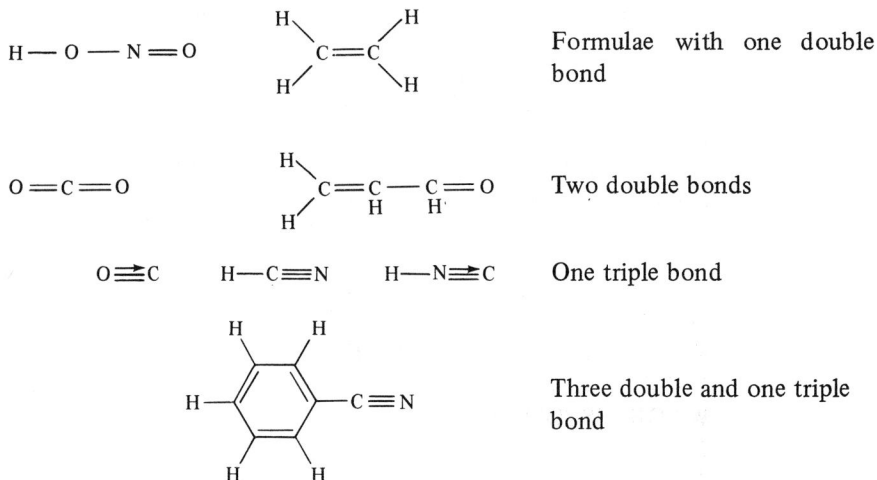

After these details z,999 is entered and the characteristic volume of the compound will be calculated: so the program proceeds:

ENTER D FOR DOUBLE AND T FOR TRIPLE BOND, COMMA, NUMBER FINALLY ENTER z, 999

?

(1) PROPERTIES OF LIQUIDS

This program calculates first the characteristic volume and the mass per mol of the compounds, details of which are entered as described above. The display then shows:

MASS OF ONE MOL EQUALS (Value) KILOGRAMS
CHARACTERISTIC VOLUME OF ONE MOL EQUALS (Value) CUBIC METRES

For characteristic volumes of other compounds, the program can be re-run to this point.

When any key is now pressed, the program is ready either (option a) to receive, or (option b) to estimate the characteristic temperature for the compound from some property of the liquid state. The most convenient property is often the density of the liquid minus the density of the vapour at the same temperature. The density of the vapour may be so low that it can be neglected and if it is somewhat higher, it can be calculated from the gas laws and the vapour pressure. Other properties are the isothermal compressibility, the surface tension and viscosity. The viscosity should not be used [51] if the characteristic volume of the compound is greater than 2×10^{-4} m^3 mol^{-1}. The temperature at which the property was measured has to be entered and, on request, the value of the property in SI units. The estimated characteristic temperature will be displayed and the program runs:

PRESS ANY KEY TO CONTINUE
OPTION (a) ENTER CHARACTERISTIC TEMPERATURE OR OPTION
(b) ESTIMATE IT FROM A PROPERTY:

      ? a or b

ENTER LETTER TO SELECT PROPERTY
D FOR DENSITY
K FOR ISOTHERMAL COMPRESSIBILITY
G FOR SURFACE TENSION
W FOR VISCOSITY
?
TEMPERATURE FOR PROPERTY ?
THE CHARACTERISTIC TEMPERATURE IS (Value)

The characteristic temperature should be based if possible on some value of the property which the program is now ready to estimate. The code letters for those properties which can be estimated are those given above with one other.

PROPERTY TO BE ESTIMATED
TYPE INDICATED LETTER TO SELECT PROPERTY
H FOR LATENT HEAT OF EVAPORATION
?
TEMPERATURE FOR PROPERTY?

The estimate for the property at the temperature selected will be printed. Options will be given as follows for the next action:

CHOOSE OPTION
1 – ANOTHER PROPERTY FOR SAME COMPOUND AND CHARAC-
    TERISTIC TEMPERATURE
2 – ANOTHER PROPERTY FOR SAME COMPOUND
3 – ANOTHER COMPOUND
4 – END
         WHAT NEXT?

Example: chlorobenzene

    Enter   C,6
                H,5
                Cl,1
                D,3
                z,999

The display shows:

Mass of one mol equals 0.112559 kilograms
Characteristic volume of one mol equals 8.3880×10^{-5} cubic metres

Enter a

617   (characteristic temperature from Appendix III)
D
298.2

The display shows

Density (kg per cubic metre) = 1100.7;

Enter   1
         K
         298.2

The display shows:;

Isothermal compressibility (square metres per Newton) 7.36×10^{-10}

Enter   2
         b
         D
         298.2
         1101.0

The display shows:

Characteristic temperature is 617.48

Enter   K
         298.2

The display shows:

Isothermal compressibility (square metres per Newton) 7.35×10^{-10}

The density of chlorobenzene has been given [177] as 1101.0 kg per cubic metre and the isothermal compressibility as [575] 7.51×10^{-10} square metres per Newton.

Example: polypropylene

The program can be used to estimate densities, surface tensions and isothermal compressibilities of polymers. Although volumes for the mass and the characteristic volume per mol are not known, the ratio of these quantities can be calculated from the values of the repeating unit.

Enter   C,3
           H,6 (for repeating unit)
           z,999

See Table A1 for values [217] for the densities and surface tensions of liquid polypropylene. The characteristic temperature is calculated from these and the properties are estimated from the characteristic temperatures 750 K and 800 K which cover the range found from the experiments.

(2) SOLUBILITIES

In order to calculate the characteristic volumes of solute and solvent, the symbols and numbers of the atoms are entered as already described. Then the characteristic temperatures are calculated from experimental values of the density of the liquid minus the density of the saturated vapour at the same temperature. The melting point and the latent heat of fusion of the solute are requested if the solute is a solid. The program runs:

     ENTER DETAILS OF SOLUTE
     (These are entered as described above)
     IS THE SOLUTE A SOLID?
     (MELTING POINT?)
     (HEAT OF FUSION?)
     ENTER A VALUE FOR THE DENSITY OF THE LIQUID STATE
     TEMPERATURE FOR THIS DENSITY
     ENTER DETAILS OF THE SOLVENT
     (These are entered as for solute)

The solubility as a volume fraction will now be estimated. After the result has been printed three options are offered.

     ON 1 CHANGE THE TEMPERATURE
     ON 2 CHANGE THE SOLVENT
     ON 3 END

Example: The estimation of the solubilities of anthracene in hexane at 298.2 K and in carbon disulphide at 298.2 K and 313.2 K

Enter   C,14
           H,10
           D,7
           z,999

Y
489.0   Melting point and latent heat of fusion (J mol^{-1})
29 400   [576]
945.7   Density (kg m^{-3}) at
527.7   Temperature [577]
C,6
H,14
z,999
654.9   Temperature and density for hexane at
298.2   temperature [68]
298.2

The display shows: VOL FRACTION = 1.327×10^{-3}

2
C,1
S,2
D,2
z,999
1255.9   Density of carbon disulphide at
298.2   temperature [68]
298.2

The display shows: VOL FRACTION = 5.863×10^{-3}

1
313.2

The display now shows: VOL FRACTION = 9.96×10^{-3}

3
READY

The volume fractions given above are for anthracene in the liquid state. If it is assumed that the densities of anthracene in the liquid state at around room temperature can be estimated by the preceding program, from the value for the characteristic temperature of 912.2 K, derived above from the figures Marti [577]; and that there would be no volume change on solution, values for the volume fraction can be suggested. J. Mahieu [219] gives the solubility of anthracene in hexane at 298.2 K as 3.1×10^{-3} kg per kg solvent corresponding to a volume fraction equal to

$$\frac{3.1 \times 10^{-3} \times 654.9}{1.0031 \times 1088.2} = 1.86 \times 10^{-3}$$

Mahieu also gives solubilities in carbon disulphide at 298.2 K, 2.03×10^{-2} kg per kg solvent, from which the volume fraction is

$$\frac{2.03 \times 10^{-2} \times 1255.9}{1.0203 \times 1088.2} = 2.30 \times 10^{-2}$$

and at 3.13 K, 3.14×10^{-2} from which the volume fraction is

$$\frac{3.14 \times 10^{-2} \times 1232.3}{1.0314 \times 1080.2} = 3.47 \times 10^{-2}$$

Estimated solubilities depend upon small differences between much larger figures and this may, at least in part, account for the rather poor agreement between the two sets of volume fractions.

(3) BIOLOGICAL ACTIVITIES (IN SOLUTION)

This program will either calculate biological activity of a compound from a given equation $\log_{10} C - E = F V_x + D$ or create the equation by correlation of concentrations for a given biological effect with characteristic volumes. The display shows:

> CHOOSE OPTION (a) ESTIMATE BIOLOGICAL ACTIVITY FROM EQUATION LOG(10) C − E = FV + D OR (b) CORRELATE CONCENTRATIONS FOR A GIVEN BIOLOGICAL EFFECT WITH CHARACTERISTIC VOLUMES a or b?

If a is selected, volumes are requested for F and D. The value of F will normally be negative and the negative sign has to be entered. The display shows.

> F − USUALLY A NEGATIVE NUMBER?
> D ?

Then details of the compound are required as usual

> H   C   N   O
> F   Cl   Br   I
> Si   P   S   As
> ENTER SYMBOL FOR ATOM, COMMA THEN NUMBER OF THESE ATOMS
> ENTER D FOR DOUBLE, T FOR TRIPLE BOND, COMMA, NUMBER
> WHEN COMPLETE ENTER z,999
> ?
> ESTER, ALCOHOL, ALDEHYDE, KETONE AND ETHER GROUPS
> GIVE INTERACTIONS,
> ENTER NUMBER OF SUCH GROUPS
> ?

Other groups such as urethanes (H_2NCOOR) also give a similar interaction.

The estimation of the concentration for the biological effect will then be printed.

After this, options are offered.

---- CONTINUATION OPTIONS ----
1 – ESTIMATE CONCENTRATION FOR BIOLOGICAL EFFECT OF A
    COMPOUND
2 – PUT RESULTS IN CORRELATION
3 – PLOT POINTS AND CORRELATION

4 – END PROGRAM
WHAT NEXT?

If b was chosen originally instead of a, details of the compound for the correlation have to be entered as described above plus the concentration for the biological effect. The same details and the concentrations have to be entered for the other compounds and then finally z,999 is entered. The number of compounds, the correlation coefficient, and the equation which relates $\log_{10} C$ to characteristic volumes are displayed. The options 1, 2, 3 and 4 given above are then offered. Under option 2, further compounds can be included in the correlation.

Examples: Vernon [578] studied the narcosis of tadpoles by a variety of compounds under different conditions. The concentrations of some compounds required to produce narcosis in 60 min of tadpoles about 20 days old have been used as examples. The option b is chosen and then figures from the columns in Table A2 are entered. For the eight primary alcohols the correlation is given as:

NUMBER OF PAIRS 8
CORRELATION COEFFICIENT 0.997
LOG(10) C+E = −42471 ∗ V + 3.2285

This can then be used to estimate the concentration of 1-butanol for the biological effect. Proceed as follows:

    1
    C,4
    H,10
    O,1
    z,999
    1

The result given is:

CONCENTRATION FOR BIOLOGICAL EFFECT 20.37

This can be compared with the value of 21.5 given by Vernon for 1-butanol and 32 for the isomeric 1,1'-oxybis-ethane (diethyl ether). Vernon gave the concentrations for four esters and five urethanes. The interactions for these seem to be the same as for alcohols and the entries for them can be included in the correlation with option 2. All the results from Table A2 give:

NUMBER OF PAIRS 17
CORRELATION COEFFICIENT 0.980
LOG(10) C+E = −40068 * V + 3.1931

This can be used to estimate the concentration of 1-butanol (or of 1,1'-oxybis-ethane) for the biological effect.

1
C,4
H,10
O,1
z,999
1

The result given is:

CONCENTRATION FOR BIOLOGICAL EFFECT 28.2

This is not as close as the estimate of 20.37 from the correlation based on results for alcohols alone for 1-butanol (experimental 21.5) but is closer for diethyl ether (experimental 32).

Hegyvary [473] studied the inhibition of $(Na^+ + K^+)$−ATPase (EC 3.6.1.3) of the plasma membranes of guinea pig kidney. The entries required for correlation of characteristic volumes and his results with primary alcohols are given in Table A3. Option b is used. The result is:

NUMBER OF PAIRS 7
CORRELATION COEFFICIENT 0.9986
LOG(10) C+E = −30447 * V + 3.2006

In order to use this to estimate the biological activities of the isomeric butanols and 1,1-oxybis-ethane, option 1 is chosen and then the following entries are made:

1
C,4
H,10
O,1
z,999
1

CONCENTRATION FOR BIOLOGICAL EFFECT 146.0

The experimental values of Hegyvary are:

    1-Butanol 160
    2-Methylpropanol 200
    1,1'-Oxybis-ethane 290

Hegyvary also gives the value 23 mol m^{-3} for chloroform.
  The program gives from the entries:

    1
    C,1
    H,1
    Cl,3
    z,999
    0
    20.9 mol m^{-3}

Table A1. Densities and surface tensions of liquid polypropylene [217].

Property at temperature		Experimental value	T_X from property	Estimate of property with: $T_X = 750$ K	$T_X = 800$ K
Density					
(kg m^{-3})	438.2 K	775	774	765	785
	461.2 K	761	780	748	769
	472.2 K	755	784	739	762
	495.2 K	741	791	720	745
Surface tension					
(N m^{-1})	438.2	0.0225	749	0.0225	0.0249
	461.2	0.0215	768	0.0206	0.0230
	472.2	0.0211	779	0.0196	0.0221
	495.2	0.0202	798	0.0177	0.0203

Table A2. Entries for the concentration of compounds required to produce narcosis of tadpoles [578].

(a) *Alcohols*

C,1	C,2	C,3	C,4	C,5	C,6	C,7	C,8	z,999
H,4	H,6	H,8	H,10	H,12	H,14	H,16	H,18	
0,1	0,1	0,1	0,1	0,1	0,1	0,1	0,1	
z,999	z,999	z,999	z,999	z,999	z,999	z,999	z,999	

Table A2. (continued)

(The concentrations in the following line are in mol m^{-3})							
980	460	100	21.5	4.2	0.95	0.28	0.107
1	1	1	1	1	1	1	1

(b) *Esters*

C,4	C,5	C,6	C,7
H,8	H,10	H,12	H,14
0,2	0,2	0,2	0,2
D,1	D,1	D,1	D,1
z,999	z,999	z,999	z,999
30	7.7	2.8	1.3
1	1	1	1

(c) *Urethanes*

C,2	C,3	C,4	C,5	C,6	z,999
H,5	H,7	H,9	H,11	H,13	
0,2	0,2	0,2	0,2	0,2	
N,1	N,1	N,1	N,1	N,1	
D,1	D,1	D,1	D,1	D,1	
z,999	z,999	z,999	z,999	z,999	
300	35	6.6	3.2	1.18	
1	1	1	1	1	

Table A3. Entries for concentrations (mol m^{-3}) of primary alcohols required to halve the activity of $(Na^+ + K^+)-ATPase$ [473].

C,1	C,2	C,3	C,4	C,5	C,6	C,7	z,999
H,4	H,6	H,8	H,10	H,12	H,14	H,16	
0,1	0,1	0,1	0,1	0,1	0,1	0,1	
z,999	z,999	z,999	z,999	z,999	z,999	z,999	
2520	1170	390	160	62	17	7.3	
1	1	1	1	1	1	1	

Appendix II.

Computer programs, written in BASIC, for the estimation of characteristic temperature, density, isothermal compressibility, surface tension, viscosity and solubility of liquids, and for the estimation of concentration required for physical toxicity.

```
1000 PRINT"    ***********************"
1010 PRINT"    *                     *"
1020 PRINT"    *   LIQUID PROPERTY    *"
1030 PRINT"    *                     *"
1040 PRINT"    *   This Program       *"
1050 PRINT"    *                     *"
1060 PRINT"    *   (1) Calculates the*"
1070 PRINT"    *   characteristic     *"
1080 PRINT"    *   volume of a        *"
1090 PRINT"    *   compound from its *"
1100 PRINT"    *   chemical formula   *"
1110 PRINT"    *                     *"
1120 PRINT"    *   (2) Calculates a   *"
1130 PRINT"    *   characteristic     *"
1140 PRINT"    *   temperature from   *"
1150 PRINT"    *   a property of the *"
1160 PRINT"    *   compound           *"
1170 PRINT"    *                     *"
1180 PRINT"    *   (3) Estimates some*"
1190 PRINT"    *   properties of      *"
1200 PRINT"    * unassociated liquids*"
1210 PRINT"    *                     *"
1220 PRINT"    ***********************"
```

```
1230 PRINT"PRESS ANY KEY TO CONTINUE"
1240 A$=INKEY$: IF A$="" GOTO 1240
1250 CLS
1260 DIM a$(15),v(15),m(15)
1270 FOR n=1 TO 15
1280 READ a$(n):NEXT n
1290 FOR n=1 TO 15
1300 READ v(n):NEXT n
1310 FOR n=1 TO 15
1320 READ m(n):NEXT n
1330 P1=4.455E+09
1340 REM FIND CHARACTERISTIC VOLUME
1350 REM FROM THE CHEMICAL FORMULA
1360 GOSUB 2550
1370 PRINT"Choose Option"
1380 PRINT"(a) Enter characteristic"
1390 PRINT"temperature or"
1400 PRINT"(b) Estimate Characteristic"
1410 PRINT"temperature from a property"
1420 PRINT"enter (a) or (b)"
1430 INPUT j$
1440 IF j$="a" GOTO 1870
1450 GOSUB 2830
1460 INPUT A$
1470 PRINT"Enter Temperature"
1480 PRINT "of Property"
1490 INPUT T
1500 IF A$="D" THEN 1570
1510 IF A$="K" THEN 1640
1520 IF A$="G" THEN 1710
1530 IF A$="W" THEN 1770
1540 PRINT:PRINT"Invalid Option!"
1550 PRINT "Try Again"
1560 GOTO 1450
1570 PRINT"Enter Density"
1580 PRINT "In Kgm per Cubic Metre"
1590 INPUT D
1600 B=V*D/(M*1000)
1610 P=B^(10/3)
1620 F=T/(1-P)
1630 GOTO 1840
1640 PRINT"Enter Compressibility"
1650 PRINT"In Square Metres per Newton"
1660 INPUT K
1670 B=P1*K
```

```
1680 P=B^(5/9)
1690 F=T*P/(P-1)
1700 GOTO 1840
1710 PRINT"ENTER SURFACE TENSION"
1720 PRINT"(Newtons per Square Metre)"
1730 INPUT G
1740 B=(G/0.0646)^(5/6)
1750 F=T/(1-B)
1760 GOTO 1840
1770 PRINT"Viscosity (Newton Seconds"
1780 PRINT"per Square Metre)?"
1790 INPUT W
1800 B=LOG10(W)
1810 P=(B+3.88)*T*0.12878
1820 R=(P/V)^(2/3)
1830 F=T/(1-R)
1840 PRINT:PRINT"The Characteristic"
1850 PRINT"Temperature is ";INT(F)
1860 GOTO 1900
1870 PRINT "The Characteristic "
1880 PRINT "Temperature is ?"
1890 INPUT F
1900 PRINT"Property to be estimated"
1910 GOSUB 2830
1920 PRINT"      H for Latent Heat of"
1930 PRINT"      Evaporation"
1940 INPUT B$
1950 PRINT"Temperature at which ";
1960 PRINT "property is required"
1970 INPUT T
1980 B=1-(T/F)
1990 C=B^0.3
2000 IF B$="D" THEN 2050
2010 IF B$="K" THEN 2100
2020 IF B$="G" THEN 2160
2030 IF B$="W" THEN 2220
2040 IF B$="H" THEN 2280
2050 D=M*(10000)*C/V
2060 PRINT"Density ";
2070 PRINT"(Kgms per cubic metre) ";
2080 PRINT"equals    ";(INT(D))/10
2090 GOTO 2310
2100 PRINT"Isothermal Compressibility (
2110 PRINT"Square metres per newton)"
2120 K=1/(P1*C^6)
```

```
2130 K=(INT(K*1E+12))/1E+12
2140 PRINT K
2150 GOTO 2310
2160 PRINT"Surface Tension ";
2170 PRINT"(Newtons per metre) equals "
2180 S=0.0646*(C^4)
2190 S=(INT(S*100000))/100000
2200 PRINT S
2210 GOTO 2310
2220 PRINT"Viscosity (Newton Seconds "
2230 PRINT"per square metre) equals"
2240 S=17.88*(C^5)*v/T-8.934
2250 X=INT(EXP(S)*1000000)/1000000
2260 PRINT X
2270 GOTO 2310
2280 PRINT"Latent Heat of Evaporation"
2290 PRINT"(Joules per mol) equals"
2300 PRINT INT(8.314*T+P1*v*C/9000000)
2310 PRINT"PRESS ANY KEY TO CONTINUE"
2320 A$=INKEY$:IF A$="" GOTO 2320
2330 CLS
2340 PRINT:PRINT:PRINT"Choose Option"
2350 PRINT
2360 PRINT:PRINT"1-Another Property"
2370 PRINT"for same compound and"
2380 PRINT"characteristic temperature"
2390 PRINT
2400 PRINT:PRINT"2-Another property"
2410 PRINT"for same compound"
2420 PRINT
2430 PRINT:PRINT"3-Another Compound"
2440 PRINT
2450 PRINT:PRINT"4-End"
2460 PRINT
2470 PRINT
2480 PRINT:PRINT"WHAT NEXT?"
2490 INPUT Q
2500 IF Q=4 THEN END
2510 IF Q=1 THEN 1900
2520 IF Q=2 THEN 1370
2530 IF Q=3 THEN 1360
2540 REM ENTER FORMULA OF COMPOUND
2550 FOR n=1 TO 12:PRINT a$(n),
2560 NEXT n
2570 v=0:M=0
```

```
2580 PRINT"Enter symbol for atom,comma"
2590 PRINT"then number of these atoms"
2600 PRINT"enter D for double, T for"
2610 PRINT"triple bond,comma,number"
2620 PRINT"when complete enter z,999"
2630 INPUT b$,q
2640 IF b$="z" GOTO 2710
2650 FOR n=1 TO 14
2660 IF a$(n)=b$ THEN w=n
2670 NEXT n
2680 v=v+v(w)*q
2690 M=M+M(w)*q
2700 GOTO 2630
2710 CLS
2720 PRINT"MASS OF ONE MOL EQUALS";
2730 PRINT(INT(M*100))/(100000) ";
2740 PRINT"KILOGRAMS"
2750 PRINT:PRINT
2760 PRINT"CHARACTERISTIC VOLUME "
2770 PRINT "OF ONE MOL EQUALS ";
2780 PRINT (INT(v*100))/100000000
2790 PRINT
2800 PRINT"PRESS ANY KEY TO CONTINUE"
2810 A$=INKEY$: IF A$="" GOTO 2810
2820 RETURN
2830 PRINT"Type Letter to indicate ";
2840 PRINT" property"
2850 PRINT"     D for DENSITY"
2860 PRINT"     K for ISOTHERMAL ";
2870 PRINT"        COMPRESSIBILITY"
2880 PRINT"     G for SURFACE TENSION"
2890 PRINT"     W for VISCOSITY"
2900 RETURN
2910 END
2920 DATA H,C,N,O,F,Cl,Br
2930 DATA I,Si,P,S,As,Sn,D,T
2940 DATA 5.43,3.23,4.55,5.87,7.20
2950 DATA 17.67,22.93,31.25,13.71
2960 DATA 15.03,16.35,19.58
2970 DATA 26.23,6.56,13.12
2980 DATA 1.008,12.011,14.007,16,19
2990 DATA 35.453,79.91,126.9,28.086
3000 DATA 30.974,32.064,74.922,118.69
3010 DATA 0,0
```

```
1000 PRINT"    ***********************"
1010 PRINT"    *                     *"
1020 PRINT"    *     SOLUBILITY      *"
1030 PRINT"    *                     *"
1040 PRINT"    *    IN this program  *"
1050 PRINT"    *    solubilities are *"
1060 PRINT"    *    estimated as     *"
1070 PRINT"    *    volume fractions *"
1080 PRINT"    *    from the chemical*"
1090 PRINT"    *    formulae and the *"
1100 PRINT"    *    densities of the *"
1110 PRINT"    *    solvent and the  *"
1120 PRINT"    *    solute           *"
1130 PRINT"    *                     *"
1140 PRINT"    *    The melting point*"
1150 PRINT"    *     and the latent  *"
1160 PRINT"    *    heat of fusion are*"
1170 PRINT"    *    required for a    *"
1180 PRINT"    *    solid solute      *"
1190 PRINT"    *                     *"
1200 PRINT"    ***********************"
1210 PRINT:PRINT
1220 PRINT"Press any key to continue"
1230 A$=INKEY$: IF A$="" GOTO 1230
1240 CLS
1250 DIM a$(15),v(15),m(15)
1260 FOR n=1 TO 15
1270 READ a$(n):NEXT n
1280 FOR n=1 TO 15
1290 READ v(n):NEXT n
1300 FOR n=1 TO 15
1310 READ m(n):NEXT n
1320 PRINT"ENTER DETAILS OF SOLUTE"
1330 GOSUB 1990
1340 U1=v*0.000001
1350 W1=M*0.001
1360 PRINT
1370 PRINT"IS THE SOLUTE A SOLID?"
1380 PRINT"ANSWER Y OR N"
1390 INPUT E$
1400 IF E$="N" THEN H=0:P1=1:GOTO 1480
1410 PRINT "ENTER MELTING POINT"
1420 INPUT P1
1430 PRINT"ENTER HEAT OF FUSION"
1440 PRINT"Joules per Mol)"
```

```
1450  INPUT H
1460  REM FIND CHARACTERISTIC
1470  REM TEMPERATURE FOR SOLUTE
1480  GOSUB 1860
1490  F1=F
1500  PRINT:PRINT
1510  PRINT"ENTER DETAILS OF SOLVENT"
1520  GOSUB 1990
1530  U2=V*0.000001
1540  M2=M*0.001
1550  REM FIND CHARACTERISTIC
1560  REM TEMPERATURE FOR SOLVENT
1570  GOSUB 1860
1580  F2=F
1590  PRINT"TEMPERATURE AT WHICH"
1600  PRINT"SOLUBILITY IS REQUIRED"
1610  INPUT T
1620  B1=(1-T/F1)^(3/10)
1630  B2=(1-T/F2)^(3/10)
1640  Y=B1/B2
1650  K=(1/((Y^8)*72)+Y/9-0.125)
1660  L=53580000*U1*K*(B1^5)/T
1670  L=L+H*(1/T-1/F1)/8.314
1680  E=EXP(-L)
1690  PRINT"SOLUBILITY"
1700  PRINT"AS A VOLUME FRACTION"
1710  PRINT (INT(E*1000000))/1000000
1720  PRINT"PRESS ANY KEY TO CONTINUE"
1730  A$=INKEY$:IF A$="" GOTO 1730
1740  CLS
1750  PRINT:PRINT"ENTER ACTION"
1760  PRINT
1770  PRINT"ON 1,CHANGE THE TEMPERATURE"
1780  PRINT
1790  PRINT"ON 2,CHANGE THE SOLVENT"
1800  PRINT:PRINT"ON 3,END"
1810  PRINT"ACTION": INPUT B
1820  ON B GOTO 1590,1510,1830
1830  END
1840  REM CALCULATE THE
1850  REM CHARACTERISTIC TEMPERATURE
1860  PRINT:PRINT"ENTER A DENSITY FOR"
1870  PRINT"THE LIQUID STATE"
1880  INPUT D1
1890  PRINT"ENTER THE TEMPERATURE"
```

```
1900 PRINT"FOR THIS DESIITY"
1910 INPUT T1
1920 B=v*D1*(0.001)/M
1930 P=B^(10/3)
1940 F=T1/(1-P)
1950 RETURN
1960 REM CALCULATE CHARACTERISTIC"
1970 REM VOLUME AND MASS PER MOL
1980 REM OF THE COMPOUND
1990 FOR n=1 TO 12:PRINT a$(n),
2000 NEXT n
2010 v=0:M=0
2020 PRINT"Enter symbol for atom,comma"
2030 PRINT"then number of these atoms"
2040 PRINT"enter D for double, T for"
2050 PRINT"triple bond,comma,number"
2060 PRINT"when complete enter z,999"
2070 INPUT b$,q
2080 IF b$="z" GOTO 2150
2090 FOR n=1 TO 14
2100 IF a$(n)=b$ THEN w=n
2110 NEXT n
2120 v=v+v(w)*q
2130 M=M+M(w)*q
2140 GOTO 2070
2150 CLS
2160 PRINT
2170 PRINT"PRESS ANY KEY TO CONTINUE"
2180 A$=INKEY$: IF A$="" GOTO 2180
2190 RETURN
2200 END
2210 DATA H,C,N,O,F,Cl,Br
2220 DATA I,Si,P,S,As,Sn,D,T
2230 DATA 5.43,3.23,4.55,5.87,7.20
2240 DATA 17.67,22.93,31.25,13.71
2250 DATA 15.03,16.35,19.58
2260 DATA 26.23,6.56,13.12
2270 DATA 1.008,12.011,14.007,16,19
2280 DATA 35.453,79.91,126.9,28.086
2290 DATA 30.974,32.064,74.922,118.69
2300 DATA 0,0
```

```
1000 MEMORY &A9FF
1010 FOR i%=&AA00 TO &AA9E
1020 READ m$
1030 POKE i%,VAL("&"+m$)
1040 NEXT
1050 POKE &AA4F,0
1060 DATA CD,06,B9,3E,1B,CD,91,AA,3E
1070 DATA 41,CD,91,AA,3E,04,CD,91,AA
1080 DATA 21,8E,01,22,9B,AA,3E,09,CD
1090 DATA 91,AA,3E,1B,CD,91,AA,3E,4B
1100 DATA CD,91,AA,3E,40,CD,91,AA,3E
1110 DATA 01,CD,91,AA,21,00,00,22,99
1120 DATA AA,01,20,00,ED,43,9D,AA,48
1130 DATA 2A,9B,AA,A7,ED,42,ED,5B,99
1140 DATA AA,C5,CD,DF,BD,C1,FE,00,28
1150 DATA 08,2A,9D,AA,7D,84,32,9E,AA
1160 DATA 21,9D,AA,A7,CB,1E,0C,0C,79
1170 DATA FE,08,20,D8,3A,9E,AA,CD,91
1180 DATA AA,2A,99,AA,23,23,22,99,AA
1190 DATA 01,80,02,A7,ED,42,20,BA,3E
1200 DATA 0A,CD,91,AA,2A,9B,AA,01,08
1210 DATA 00,A7,ED,42,22,9B,AA,30,88
1220 DATA C9,47,CD,2B,BD,78,30,FA,C9
1230 DATA 00,00,00,00,00,00
```

```
1240 PRINT"    *************************"
1250 PRINT"    *                       *"
1260 PRINT"    *   BIOLOGICAL ACTIVITY*"
1270 PRINT"    *                       *"
1280 PRINT"    *   This program will   *"
1290 PRINT"    *   calculate from the  *"
1300 PRINT"    *   chemical formulae   *"
1310 PRINT"    *   characteristic      *"
1320 PRINT"    *   volumes and then    *"
1330 PRINT"    *   correlate these     *"
1340 PRINT"    *   with logarithms of  *"
1350 PRINT"    *   the concentrations  *"
1360 PRINT"    *   for a biological    *"
1370 PRINT"    *   effect              *"
1380 PRINT"    *                       *"
1390 PRINT"    *   Either the equation*"
1400 PRINT"    *   of the correlation  *"
1410 PRINT"    *   or one found in     *"
1420 PRINT"    *   other ways,can be   *"
1430 PRINT"    *   used to estimate    *"
1440 PRINT"    *   biological          *"
1450 PRINT"    *   activities          *"
1460 PRINT"    *                       *"
1470 PRINT"    *************************"
1480 PRINT" PRESS ANY KEY TO CONTINUE"
1490 A$=INKEY$: IF A$="" GOTO 1490
1500 CLS
1510 DIM a$(14),v(14),T(50),C(50)
1520 FOR n=1 TO 14
1530 READ a$(n):NEXT n
1540 FOR n=1 TO 14
1550 READ v(n):NEXT n
1560 PRINT"choose option - (a) estimate"
1570 PRINT"biological activity from"
1580 PRINT"equation log(10)c=f*v+d+e"
1590 PRINT"or - (b) correlate";
1600 PRINT"concentrations with"
1610 PRINT" characteristic volumes"
1620 PRINT"enter (a) or (b)"
1630 INPUT j$
1640 IF j$="b" GOTO 1700
1650 PRINT"Enter f - Usually a negative"
1660 PRINT"number ": INPUT f
1670 INPUT "d";d
1680 CLS: GOSUB 3040
```

```
1690 GOTO 1960
1700 N1=0:X1=0:Y1=0:X2=0:Y2=0:P=0
1710 GOSUB 2820
1720 IF v=0 GOTO 1870
1730 PRINT"enter concentration in water"
1740 PRINT"to give biological effect"
1750 INPUT c
1760 I2= LOG10(c)
1770 GOSUB 2980
1780 I2=I2-I3*1.2
1790 X1=X1+I1
1800 X2=X2+I1*I1
1810 P=P+I1*I2
1820 Y1=Y1+I2
1830 Y2=Y2+I2*I2
1840 N1=N1+1
1850 T(N1)=I2:C(N1)=I1
1860 GOTO 1710
1870 L=(N1*P-X1*Y1)/(N1*X2-X1*X1)
1880 R=L*SQR((N1*X2-X1*X1)/(N1*Y2-Y1*Y1))
1890 PRINT"NUMBER OF PAIRS ";N1
1900 R=(INT(R*10000))/10000
1910 PRINT"CORRELATION COEFFICIENT=";R
1920 D=(Y1-L*X1)*10000/N1
1930 D=(INT(D))/10000
1940 F=INT(L*1000000)
1950 PRINT "LOG(10)C+E= ";F;"*V+";D
1960 PRINT"PRESS ANY KEY TO CONTINUE"
1970 A$=INKEY$: IF A$="" GOTO 1970
1980 CLS
1990 PRINT
2000 PRINT"  CONTINUATION OPTIONS"
2010 PRINT
2020 PRINT"1-ESTIMATE CONCENTRATION FOR"
2030 PRINT"BIOLOGICAL EFFECT OF COMPOUND
2040 PRINT: PRINT"2-PUT FURTHER"
2050 PRINT"RESULTS IN CORRELATION"
2060 PRINT
2070 PRINT"3-PLOT POINTS AND CORRELATION"
2080 PRINT"Switch on printer"
2090 PRINT" Press key B to transfer"
2100 PRINT "plot to paper"
2110 PRINT"To continue"
2120 PRINT"Press any other key"
2130 PRINT: PRINT"4 - END PROGRAM"
```

```
2140 PRINT: PRINT"WHAT NEXT"
2150 INPUT J: IF J=4 THEN END
2160 IF J=1 THEN GOSUB 3040
2170 IF J=2 THEN GOTO 1710
2180 IF J=3 THEN GOTO 2200
2190 GOTO 1960
2200 CM=C(1)
2210 FOR J= 1 TO N1
2220 IF C(J)>CM THEN CM=C(J)
2230 NEXT J
2240 CL=C(1)
2250 FOR J= 1 TO N1
2260 IF C(J)<CL THEN CL=C(J)
2270 NEXT J
2280 TL=T(1)
2290 FOR J=1 TO N1
2300 IF T(J)<TL THEN TL=T(J)
2310 NEXT J
2320 TM=T(1)
2330 FOR J=1 TO N1
2340 IF T(J)>TM THEN TM=T(J)
2350 NEXT J
2360 XM=(CL+CM)/2
2370 YM=(TL+TM)/2
2380 TM=(INT(TM*1000)/1000)
2390 TL=(INT(TL*1000)/1000)
2400 YM=(INT(YM*1000)/1000)
2410 CLS
2420 PRINT:PRINT
2430 PRINT USING"££.£££";TM;
2440 PRINT" "; CHR$(159)
2450 FOR J=1 TO 9:PRINT TAB(8)CHR$(151)
2460 NEXT
2470 PRINT USING"££.£££";YM;
2480 PRINT" "; CHR$(159)
2490 FOR J=1 TO 9:PRINT TAB(8) CHR$(151)
2500 NEXT
2510 PRINT USING"££.£££";TL;
2520 PRINT" "; CHR$(159);
2530 FOR J= 1 TO 14:PRINT CHR$(158);
2540 NEXT
2550 PRINT CHR$(159);
2560 FOR J=1 TO 14:PRINT CHR$(158);
2570 NEXT
2580 PRINT CHR$(159)
```

```
2590 PRINT TAB(5) CL;SPACE$(8);
2600 PRINT XM;SPACE$(6);CM
2610 DC=(CM-CL)/30
2620 DT=(TM-TL)/20
2630 T=D+(F*CL/1000000)
2640 U=16*(T-TL)/DT
2650 UM=INT(U)+40
2660 T=D+(F*CM/1000000)
2670 U=16*(T-TL)/DT
2680 UL=INT(U)+40
2690 PLOT 128,UM
2700 DRAW 608,UL
2710 FOR I=1 TO N1
2720 C=C(I)
2730 X=(C-CL)/DC
2740 H=INT(X)+8
2750 T=T(I): U=(TM-T)/DT
2760 G=INT(U)+3
2770 LOCATE H,G
2780 PRINT CHR$(42): NEXT I
2790 A$=INKEY$:IF A$="" GOTO 2790
2800 IF A$="B" THEN CALL &AA00
2810 GOTO 2000
2820 FOR n=1 TO 12: PRINT a$(n),
2830 NEXT n
2840 v=0
2850 PRINT"enter symbol for atom,comma"
2860 PRINT"then number of these atoms"
2870 PRINT"enter d for double, t for "
2880 PRINT"triple bond,comma,number"
2890 PRINT"when complete enter z,999"
2900 INPUT b$,m
2910 IF b$="z" GOTO 2970
2920 FOR n=1 TO 14
2930 IF a$(n)=b$ THEN w=n
2940 NEXT n
2950 v=v+v(w)*m
2960 GOTO 2900
2970 I1=v:RETURN
2980 PRINT: PRINT"Ester,alcohol"
2990 PRINT"aldehyde,ketone and ester"
3000 PRINT"groups give interactions"
3010 PRINT"Enter number of such groups"
3020 INPUT I3
3030 RETURN
```

```
3040 GOSUB 2820
3050 GOSUB 2980
3060 L1=f*v/ 1000000+d+1.2*I3
3070 J=EXP(2.3026*L1)
3080 PRINT"CONCENTRATION FOR BIOLOGICAL"
3090 PRINT"EFFECT EQUALS "
3100 PRINT (INT(J*1000))/1000
3110 RETURN
3120 END
3130 PRINT"PRESS Y FOR ESTIMATION OF"
3140 PRINT"A BIOLOGICAL ACTIVITY"
3150 J$=INKEY$: IF J$="" GOTO 3150
3160 IF J$="Y" THEN GOSUB 1680
3170 END
3180 DATA H,C,N,O,F,Cl,Br
3190 DATA I,Si,P,S,As,D,T
3200 DATA 5.43,3.32,4.55,5.87,7.20
3210 DATA 17.67,22.93,31.25,13.71
3220 DATA 15.03,16.35,19.58,6.56,13.12
```

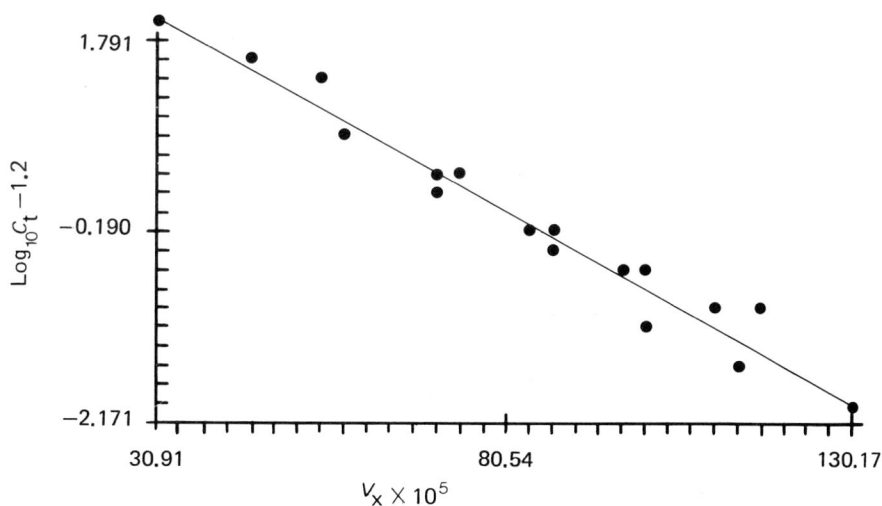

Fig. 23. Plot of results for concentrations of compounds required to produce narcosis of tadpoles ($E = 1.2$).

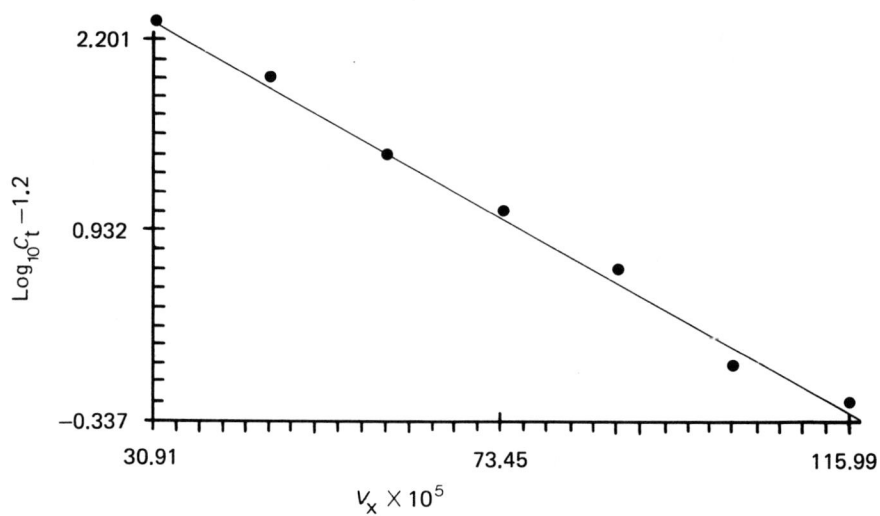

Fig. 24. Plot of results for enzyme inhibition by primary alcohols ($E = 1.2$).

Appendix III.

Data for estimation of solubilities

DATA FOR ESTIMATION OF SOLUBILITIES

Formula	Compound	M Molecular mass ($kg\ mol^{-1}$)	V_x Characteristic volume ($m^3\ mol^{-1}$)	T_M Melting point (K)	T_x Characteristic temperature (K)	ΔH_m Molecular heat of fusion ($J\ mol^{-1}$)
$CHCl_3$	Trichloromethane	1.1938×10^{-1}	6.168×10^{-5}	209.7	503	8 800
CH_2Cl_2	Dichloromethane	8.493×10^{-2}	4.944×10^{-5}	178.1	505	6 000
CH_3Br	Bromomethane	9.494×10^{-2}	4.245×10^{-5}	179.5	470	5 980
CH_4O	Methanol	3.204×10^{-2}	3.083×10^{-5}	175.4	492	3 180
CH_3NO_2	Nitromethane	6.104×10^{-2}	4.238×10^{-5}	252.7	534	9 700
CCl_4	Tetrachloromethane	1.5382×10^{-1}	7.392×10^{-5}	250.2	500	3 280
CO_2	Carbon dioxide	4.401×10^{-2}	2.810×10^{-5}	215.6	320	7 855
CS_2	Carbon disulphide	7.614×10^{-2}	4.905×10^{-5}	161.7	589	4 396
C_2HCl_3	Trichloroethene	1.3139×10^{-1}	7.146×10^{-5}	186.8	550	3 350
C_2H_4	Ethylene	2.805×10^{-2}	3.474×10^{-5}	104.0	281	10 840
$C_2H_4Br_2$	1,2-Dibromoethane	1.8787×10^{-1}	7.404×10^{-5}	283.1	734	8 709
$C_2H_4Cl_2$	1,2-Dichloroethane	9.896×10^{-2}	6.353×10^{-5}	237.9	566	11 540
$C_2H_4O_2$	Acetic acid	6.005×10^{-2}	4.649×10^{-5}	289.7	580	4 452
C_2H_5Cl	Chloroethane	6.452×10^{-2}	5.129×10^{-5}	138.6	422	4 938
C_2H_6O	Dimethyl ether	4.607×10^{-2}	4.492×10^{-5}	134.7	375	5 021
C_2H_6O	Ethanol	4.607×10^{-2}	4.492×10^{-5}	158.7	612	11 235
$C_2H_6O_2$	1,2-Ethanediol	6.207×10^{-2}	5.079×10^{-5}	261.7	1 090	–
C_2H_6SO	Sulphinylbismethane	7.813×10^{-2}	6.126×10^{-4}	291.6	746	6 396
$C_3H_6Cl_2$	1,2-Dichloropropane	1.1299×10^{-1}	7.762×10^{-5}	172.7	546	5 690
C_3H_6O	2-Propanone	5.805×10^{-2}	5.471×10^{-5}	177.9	469	

Formula	Compound	M Molecular mass (kg mol^{-1})	V_x Characteristic volume (m^3 mol^{-1})	T_M Melting Point (K)	T_x Characteristic temperature (K)	ΔH_m Molecular heat of fusion (J mol^{-1})
C$_3$H$_7$NO$_2$	Ethyl carbamate	8.909×10^{-2}	7.056×10^{-5}	322.7	735	15 200
C$_3$H$_8$O	1-Propanol	6.011×10^{-2}	5.901×10^{-5}	146.7	540	4 800
C$_3$H$_8$O$_3$	Glycerol	9.211×10^{-2}	7.075×10^{-5}	293.2	2 700	18 480
C$_4$H$_4$S	Thiophene	8.414×10^{-2}	6.411×10^{-5}	234.9	582	4 970
C$_4$H$_8$O	2-Butanone	7.212×10^{-2}	6.880×10^{-5}	186.8	501	8 490
C$_4$H$_8$O$_2$	Ethyl acetate	8.811×10^{-2}	7.466×10^{-5}	189.6	495	10 480
C$_4$H$_{10}$	n-Butane	5.813×10^{-2}	6.723×10^{-5}	134.8	380	4 670
C$_4$H$_{10}$O	1-Butanol	7.412×10^{-2}	7.310×10^{-5}	183.6	557	9 280
C$_4$H$_{10}$O	1,1'-Oxybis-ethane	7.412×10^{-2}	7.310×10^{-5}	156.9	427	7 273
C$_5$H$_{10}$O	3-Pentanone	8.614×10^{-2}	8.289×10^{-5}	233.4	527	—
C$_5$H$_{10}$O$_2$	Methyl butyrate	1.0213×10^{-1}	8.877×10^{-5}	188.4	523	—
C$_5$H$_{10}$O$_2$	Ethyl propionate	1.0213×10^{-1}	8.877×10^{-5}	199.3	511	—
C$_5$H$_{10}$O$_2$	n-Propyl acetate	1.0213×10^{-1}	8.877×10^{-5}	178	508	—
C$_5$H$_{11}$Cl	1-Chloropentane	1.0660×10^{-1}	9.356×10^{-5}	174.2	513	—
C$_5$H$_{12}$	Pentane	7.215×10^{-2}	8.132×10^{-5}	143.5	426	8 420
C$_5$H$_{12}$	2-Methylbutane	7.215×10^{-2}	8.132×10^{-5}	113.3	420	5 150
C$_5$H$_{12}$O	1-Pentanol	8.815×10^{-2}	8.720×10^{-5}	194.3	573	9 830
C$_6$H$_4$Cl$_2$	1,2-Dichlorobenzene	1.4701×10^{-1}	9.612×10^{-5}	256.2	720	12 930
C$_6$H$_4$Cl$_2$	1,4-Dichlorobenzene	1.4701×10^{-1}	9.612×10^{-5}	326.3	669	10 210
C$_6$H$_5$Br	Bromobenzene	1.5702×10^{-1}	8.914×10^{-5}	242.3	693	10 620
C$_6$H$_5$Cl	Chlorobenzene	1.1256×10^{-1}	8.388×10^{-5}	227.6	617	9 610
C$_6$H$_5$I	Iodobenzene	2.0401×10^{-1}	9.746×10^{-5}	241.9	808	9 760

Formula	Compound	M Molecular mass (kg mol^{-1})	V_x Characteristic volume (m^3 mol^{-1})	T_M Melting point (K)	T_x Characteristic temperature (K)	ΔH_m Molecular heat of fusion (J mol^{-1})
$C_6H_5NO_2$	Nitrobenzene	1.2311×10^{-1}	8.9065×10^{-5}	278.9	800	11 590
C_6H_6	Benzene	7.8114×10^{-2}	7.164×10^{-5}	278.7	570	9 840
C_6H_6O	Phenol	9.411×10^{-2}	7.751×10^{-5}	314.9	855	11 290
C_6H_7N	Aniline	9.313×10^{-2}	8.155×10^{-5}	266.9	939	10 560
C_6H_{12}	Cyclohexane	8.416×10^{-2}	8.455×10^{-5}	279.8	520	2 630
$C_6H_{12}O$	Cyclohexanol	1.0016×10^{-1}	9.042×10^{-5}	298.3	727	1 760
$C_6H_{12}O_3$	2,4,6-Trimethyl-1,3,5-trioxane	1.3216×10^{-1}	1.0217×10^{-4}	285.8	503	13 835
C_6H_{14}	Hexane	8.6178×10^{-2}	9.541×10^{-5}	177.9	454	13 078
$C_6H_{14}O$	Dipropyl ether	1.0218×10^{-1}	1.0129×10^{-4}	147.1	465	8 833
$C_6H_{14}O$	1-Hexanol	1.0218×10^{-1}	1.0129×10^{-4}	226.5	588	–
C_7H_8	Toluene	9.215×10^{-2}	8.573×10^{-5}	178.1	572	6 620
C_7H_8O	Benzyl alcohol	1.0815×10^{-1}	9.160×10^{-5}	257.9	872	8 970
C_7H_8O	o-Cresol	1.0815×10^{-1}	9.160×10^{-5}	304.1	873	–
C_7H_8O	m-Cresol	1.0815×10^{-1}	9.160×10^{-5}	284.7	815	–
C_7H_8O	p-Cresol	1.0815×10^{-1}	9.160×10^{-5}	308.0	805	11 890
C_7H_{14}	Methylcyclohexane	9.819×10^{-2}	9.864×10^{-5}	146.6	510	6 750
$C_7H_{15}Cl$	1-Chloroheptane	1.3465×10^{-1}	1.2175×10^{-4}	–	544	–
C_7H_{16}	Heptane	1.0021×10^{-1}	1.0951×10^{-4}	182.6	474	14 160
$C_7H_{16}O$	1-Heptanol	1.1621×10^{-1}	1.1537×10^{-4}	239.1	600	–
C_8H_{10}	1,2-Dimethylbenzene	1.0616×10^{-1}	9.982×10^{-5}	248.0	628	13 600
C_8H_{10}	1,3-Dimethylbenzene	1.0616×10^{-1}	9.982×10^{-5}	225.4	586	11 560
C_8H_{10}	1,4-Dimethylbenzene	1.0616×10^{-1}	9.982×10^{-5}	286.4	581	17 100

Formula	Compound	M Molecule mass (kg mol^{-1})	V_x Characteristic volume (m^3 mol^{-1})	T_M Melting point (K)	T_x Characteristic temperature (K)	ΔH_m Molecular heat of fusion (J mol^{-1})
$C_8H_{17}Cl$	1-Chloro-octane	1.4868×10^{-1}	1.3584×10^{-4}	–	640	–
C_8H_{18}	Octane	1.1423×10^{-1}	1.2360×10^{-4}	216.4	491	20 650
C_8H_{18}	2,2,4-Trimethylpentane	1.1423×10^{-1}	1.2360×10^{-4}	165.8	475	9 210
$C_8H_{18}O$	Dibutylether	1.3023×10^{-1}	1.2947×10^{-4}	177.9	496	–
$C_8H_{18}O$	1-Octanol	1.3023×10^{-1}	1.2947×10^{-4}	256.5	612	–
C_9H_{12}	1,3,5-Trimethylbenzene	1.2020×10^{-1}	1.1392×10^{-4}	228.5	606	9 500
C_9H_{12}	1,2,4-Trimethylbenzene	1.2020×10^{-1}	1.1392×10^{-4}	317.0	633	3 760
C_9H_{20}	Nonane	1.2826×10^{-1}	1.3769×10^{-4}	219.7	506	15 470
$C_9H_{20}O$	1-Nonanol	1.4426×10^{-1}	1.4358×10^{-4}	267.7	617	–
$C_{10}H_7Br$	1-Bromonaphthalene	2.0708×10^{-1}	1.2603×10^{-4}	279.4	1 010	–
$C_{10}H_7Cl$	1-Chloronaphthalene	1.6262×10^{-1}	1.2078×10^{-4}	270.9	888	–
$C_{10}H_8$	Naphthalene	1.2819×10^{-1}	1.0853×10^{-4}	353.4	740	18 800
$C_{10}H_{14}$	1,2,4,5-Tetramethylbenzene	1.3422×10^{-1}	1.2801×10^{-4}	352.5	688	21 000
$C_{10}H_{22}$	Decane	1.4229×10^{-1}	1.5178×10^{-4}	243.50	520	28 750
$C_{11}H_{24}$	Undecane	1.5632×10^{-1}	1.6587×10^{-4}	247.6	532	22 200
$C_{12}H_{10}$	Acenaphthene	1.5421×10^{-1}	1.2586×10^{-4}	366.4	811	20 710
$C_{12}H_{10}$	Diphenyl	1.5421×10^{-1}	1.3242×10^{-4}	341.5	800	18 600
$C_{14}H_{10}$	Anthracene	1.7823×10^{-1}	1.4543×10^{-4}	489.7	910	28 500
$C_{16}H_{33}Cl$	1-Chlorohexadecane	2.6090×10^{-1}	2.4857×10^{-4}	291.1	618	–
$C_{16}H_{34}$	Hexadecane	2.2645×10^{-1}	2.3633×10^{-4}	291.4	576	53 360
$C_{16}H_{34}O$	1-Hexadecanol	2.4245×10^{-1}	2.4221×10^{-4}	323.2	662	34 300
$C_{16}H_{34}O$	Dioctyl ether	2.4245×10^{-1}	2.4221×10^{-4}	–	580	–

Appendix III

Formula	Compound	M Molecular mass (kg mol^{-1})	V_x Characteristic volume (m^3 mol^{-1})	T_M Melting point (K)	T_x Characteristic temperature (K)	ΔH_m Molecular heat of fusion (J mol^{-1})
C$_{17}$H$_{34}$O	Heptadecan-9-one	2.5446×10^{-1}	2.5199×10^{-4}	326	627	–
C$_{17}$H$_{36}$	Heptadecane	2.4048×10^{-1}	2.5042×10^{-4}	295.1	583	40 480
C$_{18}$H$_{38}$	Octadecane	2.5450×10^{-1}	2.6451×10^{-4}	301.4	–	61 380
H$_2$O	Water	1.80153×10^{-2}	1.674×10^{-5}	273.2	1 317	6 009
I$_2$	Iodine	2.5381×10^{-1}	6.2504×10^{-5}	386.7	750	15 700
S$_8$	Sulphur	2.5651×10^{-1}	1.3079×10^{-4}	368.5	1 580	9 870
SiCl$_4$	Silicon(IV) chloride	1.6990×10^{-1}	8.439×10^{-5}	203	462	7 720
SnCl$_4$	Tin(IV) chloride	2.6050×10^{-1}	9.691×10^{-5}	240.2	630	9 160

References

[1]   Holt, J.J.H., *Lancet* 1916, **5**, 1136–1137.

[2]   Moore, W., *J. Agric. Res.* 1917, **9**, 371–381.

[3]   Moore, W. and Graham, S.A., *J. Agric. Res.* 1917, **10**, 365–371.

[4]   Tattersfield, F. and Roberts, A.W.R., *J. Agric. Sci. Camb.* 1920, **10**, 199–232.

[5]   McGowan, J.C., *J. Appl. Chem., London* 1966, **16**, 103–104.

[6]   Meyer, K.H. and Hemmi, H., *Biochem. Z.* 1935, **277**, 39–71.

[7]   Richet, C. *C.r. de la Soc. Biol. Paris* 1893, **45**, 775–776.

[8]   Bradbury, F.R., McCarthy, M.C. and Suckling, C.W., *Chem. and Ind.* 1972, 105.

[9]   Snow, J., *On Chloroform and Other Anaesthetics*. London, 1858, pp. 353–354 and 386.

[10]   Fühner, H., *Biochem. Z.* 1921, **120**, 143–162.

[11]   Overton, E., *Studien über Narkose*. Jena, G. Fischer, 1901.

[12]   Meyer, K.H., *Trans. Faraday Soc.* 1937, **33**, 1062–1064.

[13]   Hansch, C., Maloney, P.P., Fujita, T. and Muir, R.M., *Nature, Lond.* 1962, **194**, 178–180.

[14]   Hansch, C. and Fujita, T., *J. Am. Chem. Soc.* 1964, **86**, 5175–5180.

[15]   Iwasa, J., Fujita, T. and Hansch, C., *J. Med. Chem.* 1965, **8**, 150–153.

[16]   Hansch, C., *Acc. Chem. Res.* 1969, **2**, 232–239.

[17]   Silipo, C. and Hansch, C., *J. Med. Chem.* 1976, **19**, 62–71.

[18]   Miller, W. L., *J. Phys. Chem.* 1920, **24**, 562–569.

[19]   Fraser, C.G., *J. Phys. Chem.* 1921, **25**, 1–9.
[20]   Brink, F. & Posternak, J.M., *J. Cell Comp. Physiol.* 1948, **32**, 211–233.
[21]   Ferguson, J., *Proc. Roy. Soc. (B)* 1939, **127**, 387–403.
[22]   Ferguson, J., *'Mecanisme de la Narcose'*, Extract from the 26th Colloques Internationaux de Centre National de la Recherche Scientifique, 1951, pp. 25–39.
[23]   McGowan, J.C., *J. Appl. Chem. Biotechnol.* 1978, **28**, 599–607.
[24]   McGowan, J.C., *J. Appl. Chem. Lond.* 1951, **1**, S120–S126.
[25]   Mullins, L.J., *Chem. Rev.* 1954, **54**, 289–323.
[26]   McGowan, J.C., Society of Chemical Industry Monograph No. 29 on *'Physico-Chemical and Biophysical Factors Affecting the Activity of Pesticides'*, 1968, pp. 141–158.
[27]   Ferguson, J., *Chem. and Ind.* 1964, 818–824.
[28]   Hutchinson, T.C., Hellebust, J.A., Tam, D., Mackay, D., Mascarenhas, R.A. and Shiu, W.Y., *Hydrocarbons and Halogenated Hydrocarbons in the Aquatic Environment* (B.K. Afghan and D. Mackay, eds.). Plenum Press, New York, 1980, pp. 577–586.
[29]   Mackay, D. & Shiu, W.Y., *J. Chem. Eng. Data* 1977, **22**, 399–402.
[30]   Ferguson, J. and Pirie, H., *Ann. Appl. Biol.* 1948, **35**, 532–550.
[31]   Ferguson, J. and Hawkins, S.W., *Nature, Lond.* 1949, **164**, 963–964.
[32]   Ferguson, J., Hawkins, S.W. and Doxey, D., *Nature, Lond.* 1950, **165**, 1021–1022.
[33]   Smith, H.W., *J. Phys. Chem.* 1921, **25**, 204–263.
[34]   Smith, H.W., *J. Phys. Chem.* 1921, **25**, 605–615 and 616–627.
[35]   Smith, H.W., *J. Phys. Chem.* 1921, **25**, 721–734.
[36]   Smith, H.W., *J. Phys. Chem.* 1921, **26**, 256 and 349.
[37]   McGowan, J.C., *J. Appl. Chem., Lond.* 1952, **2**, 323–328.
[38]   McGowan, J.C., *J. Appl. Chem., Lond.* 1954, **4**, 41–47.
[39]   Flory, P.J., Orwoll, R.A. and Vrij, A., *J. Am. Chem. Soc.* 1964, **86**, 3507–3514 and 3515–3520.
[40]   Flory, P.J., *J. Am. Chem. Soc.* 1965, **87**, 1833–1838.
[41]   Abe, A. and Flory, P.J., *J. Am. Chem. Soc.* 1965, **87**, 1838–1846.
[42]   McGowan, J.C., In *Handbook of Chemistry and Physics*, 63rd edn (R.C. Weast and M.J. Astle, eds.). C.R.C. Press, Boca Raton, Florida, USA, 1982/1983, pp. F14–F18.
[43]   Biltz, W. *Raumchemie der festen Stoffe*. Leipzig, 1934.
[44]   Biltz, W., Fischer, W. and Wunnenberg, E., *Z. Physik. Chem.* 1930, **141**, 13–55.
[45]   McGowan, J.C., *Rec. Trav. Chim. Pays-Bas.* 1957, **76**, 155–164.
[46]   Reed, T.M. *Fluorine Chemistry*, Vol. 5 (J.H. Simons, ed.). Academic Press, 1964, p. 164.
[47]   McGowan, J.C., *J. Appl. Chem., Lond.* 1952, **2**, 651–658.
[48]   McGowan, J.C., Atkinson, P.N. and Ruddle, L.H., *J. Appl. Chem., Lond.* 1966, **16**, 99–102.
[49]   McGowan, J.C., *Nature, Lond.* 1963, **200**, 1317.

[50] Greenberg, J.H., Mellors, A. and McGowan, J.C., *J. Med. Chem.* 1978, **21**, 1208–1212.

[51] Cogswell, F.N. and McGowan, J.C., *Brit. Polymer. J.* 1972, **4**, 183–198.

[52] McGowan, J.C., *Rec. Trav. Chim. Pays. Bas.* 1956, **75**, 193–208.

[53] Partington, J.R., *An Advanced Treatise of Physical Chemistry*, Vol. II. Longmans Green and Co., London, 1951, pp. 17–20.

[54] Schroeder, H., *Chem. Ber.* 1880, **10**, 848–853.

[55] Schroeder, H., *Chem. Ber.* 1880, **10**, 1070–1076.

[56] Reid, R.C., Prausnitz, J.M. and Sherwood, T.K., *The Properties of Gases and Liquids*, 3rd edn. McGraw-Hill, New York, 1977, p. 57.

[57] Sugden, S., *J. Chem. Soc.* 1924, 1177–1189.

[58] Sugden, S., *The Parachor and Valency*. Routledge, London, 1929, p. 31.

[59] Sugden, S., *Thorpe's Dictionary of Applied Chemistry*, 4th edn, Vol. 9, pp. 225–300.

[60] Exner, O., *Coll. Czech. Chem. Commun.* 1967, **32**, 24–55.

[61] Quayle, O.R., *Chem. Rev.* 1953, **53**, 439–589.

[62] Vogel, A.I., Cresswell, T., Jeffrey, G.I. and Leicester, J., *J. Chem. Soc.* 1952, 514–519.

[63] Mumford, S.A. and Phillips, J.W.C., *J. Chem. Soc.* 1929, 2112–2133.

[64] Exner, O., *Coll. Czech. Chem. Commun.* 1966, **31**, 3222–3251.

[65] Benson, S.W. and Buss, J.H., *J. Chem. Phys.* 1958, **29**, 546–572.

[66] Copley, G.N., *Chem. and Ind.* 1940, **59**, 675–677.

[67] McGowan, J.C., *Chem. and Ind.* 1952, 495–496.

[68] Timmermanns, J., *Physico-Chemical Constants of Pure Organic Compounds*. Elsevier, New York, 1950, p. 224.

[69] Nisel'son, L.A. and Sokolova, T.D., *Zhur. neorg. Khim.* 1965, **10**, 18; *Russ. J. Inorg. Chem.* 1965, **10**, 9–11.

[70] Ewens, R.V.G. and Lister, M.W., *Trans. Farad. Soc.* 1938, **34**, 1358–1362.

[71] Sands, D.E. and Zalkin, A., *Acta Cryst.* 1959, **12**, 723–726.

[72] Robinson, W.T., Fergusson, J.E. and Penfold, B.R., *Chem. Commun.* 1963, 116.

[73] Fergusson, J.E., Penfold, B.R., Elder, M. and Robinson, B.H., *J. Chem. Soc.* 1965, 5500–5502.

[74] Recknagel, R.O., Glende, E.A. and Hruzkewycz, A.M., *Free Radicals in Biology*, Vol. 3 (W.A. Pryor, ed.). Academic Press, New York, 1977, pp. 97–122.

[75] Reynolds, E.S. and Moslen, M.T., *Free Radicals in Biology*, Vol. 4 (W.A. Pryor, ed.). Academic Press, New York, 1980, pp. 49–94.

[76] Poyer, J.L., Floyd, R.A., McCay, P.B., Janzen, E.G. and Davis, E.R., *Biochim. Biophys. Acta* 1978, **539**, 402–409.

[77] Atherton, F.R. and Todd, A.R., *J. Chem. Soc.* 1947, 674–678.

[78] Muirhead, I., *Annals of Applied Biology* 1949, **36**, 250–256.

[79] Shorter, J., *Chem. Soc. Quarterly Reviews* 1970, **24**, 433–453.

[80] Taft, R.W., *Steric Effects in Organic Chemistry* (M.S. Newman, ed.). Wiley, New York, 1956, Chapter 13.

[81] Hancock, C.R., Meyers, E.A. and Yeger, B.J., *J. Am. Chem. Soc.* 1961, **83**, 4211–4213.

[82] Hansch, C. *Farmaco* 1968, **23**, 293–320.

[83] Bondi, A. and Simkin, D.J., *Am. Inst. Chem. Eng. J.* 1960, **6**, 191–197.

[84] Bondi, A., *J. Phys. Chem.* 1964, **68**, 441–451.

[85] McGowan, J.C., *Polymer* 1969, **10**, 841–848.

[86] Traube, J., *Chem. Ber.* 1892, **25**, 2524–2533.

[87] Traube, J., *Chem. Ber.* 1894, **27**, 3173–3178.

[88] Traube, J., *Chem. Ber.* 1895, **28**, 2722–2728.

[89] Traube, J., *Annalen der Chemie* 1896, **90**, 43–122.

[90] Traube, J., *Chem. Ber.* 1909, **42**, 2185–2188.

[91] Traube, J., *J. Phys. Chem.* 1910, **14**, 452–470.

[92] Traube, J., *Chem. Ber.* 1909, **42**, 86–94.

[93] Cohn, E. and Edsall, J.T., *Proteins, Amino-Acids and Peptides*. Reinhold Publishing Corp., New York, 1943, p. 157, pp. 370–381.

[94] McDuffie, G.E., Forbes, J.W., Madigosky, W.M. and von Bretzel, J.J., *Journ. Chem. Engng. Data* 1969, **14**, 176–180.

[95] Whalley, E. and Heath, J.B.R., *Canad. J. Chem.* 1976, **54**, 2249–2251.

[96] McMeekin, T.L. and Marshall, K., *Science* 1952, **116**, 142–143.

[97] Traube, J., *Chem. Ber.* 1898, **31**, 130–137.

[98] Masson, D.O., *Phil. Mag. (7)* 1929, **8**, 218–235.

[99] Redlich, O. and Rosenfeld, P., *Z. Physik. Chem.* 1931, **A155**, 65–74.

[100] Redlich, O. and Rosenfeld, P., *Z. Elektrochem.* 1931, **37**, 705–711.

[101] Redlich, O.J., *Phys. Chem.* 1940, **44**, 619–629.

[102] Harned, H.S. and Owen, B.B., *The Physical Chemistry of Electrolytic Solutions*, 3rd edn. Rheinhold Publishing Corp., New York, 1958, p. 361.

[103] Couture, A.M. and Laidler, K.J., *Canad. J. Chem.* 1956, **34**, 1209–1216.

[104] Zana, R. and Yeager, E., *J. Phys. Chem.* 1967, **71**, 534–536.

[105] Roux, A., Mushally, M., Perron, G. Desnoyers, J.E., Singh, P.P., Woolley, E.M. and Hepler, L.G., *Canad. J. Chem.* 1978, **56**, 24–28.

[106] Redlich, O. and Bigeleisen, J., *Chem. Rev.* 1942, **30**, 171–179.

[107] Redlich, O. and Meyer, D.M., *Chem. Rev.* 1964, **64**, 221–227.

[108] Millero, F.J., *Chem. Rev.* 1971, **71**, 147–176.

[109] Millero, F.J., *Structure and Transport Processes in Water and Aqueous Solutions* (R.A. Horne, ed.). Wiley–Interscience, New Yori, 1971, Ch. 15.

[110] Hammick, D.L. and Andrew, L.W., *J. Chem. Soc.* 1929, 754–759.

[111] Bowden, S.T. and Butler, E.T., *J. Chem. Soc.* 1939, 79–83.

[112] Bhagwat, W.V., Shukla, R.P. and Gupta, M.M., *J. Indian Chem. Soc.* 1952, **29**, 701–705.

[113] Washburn, E.W. (ed.), *International Critical Tables*, Vol. 3, New York, 1928.
[114] Belton, J.W., *Trans. Faraday Soc.* 1935, **31**, 1413–1419.
[115] Goard, A.K., *J. Chem. Soc.* 1925, **127**, 2451–2458.
[116] Jones, G. and Ray, W.A., *J. Am. Chem. Soc.* 1937, **59**, 187–198.
[117] Herz, W. and Knaebel, E., *Z. Physik. Chem.* 1928, **131**, 389–404.
[118] Stocker, H., *Z. Physik. Chem.* 1920, **94**, 149–180.
[119] Whatmough, W.H., *Z. Physik. Chem.* 1902, **39**, 129–193.
[120] Gibson, R.E., *J. Am. Chem. Soc.* 1935, **57**, 284–293.
[121] Thomas. W.G., and Perman, E.P., *Proc. Roy. Soc. (A)* 1934, **146**, 640–650.
[122] Scott, A.F., Obenhaus, V.M., and Wilson, R.W., *J. Phys. Chem.* 1934, **38**, 931–940.
[123] McGowan, J.C., *Nature, Lond.* 1951, **168**, 601–602.
[124] McGowan, J.C., *Rec. Trav. Chim.* 1966, **85**, 777–790.
[125] Perman, E.P. and Urry, W.D., *Proc. Roy. Soc. (A)* 1929, **126**, 47–78.
[126] Cupples, H.L., *J. Am. Chem. Soc.* 1945, **67**, 987–990.
[127] Hawkins, W.D. and Gilbert, E.C., *J. Am. Chem. Soc.* 1926, **48**, 604–607.
[128] Jones, G. and Ray, W.A., *J. Am. Chem. Soc.* 1942, **64**, 2744–2745.
[129] Forch, C., *Ann. Physik [4]* 1905, **17**, 744–762.
[130] Pappenheimer, J.R., Lepie, M.P. and Wyman, J., *J. Am. Chem. Soc.* 1936, **58**, 1851–1855.
[131] Belton, J.W., *Trans Farad. Soc.* 1939, **35**, 1293–1298.
[132] Daniel, J. and Cohn, E.J., *J. Am. Chem. Soc.* 1936, **58**, 415–423.
[133] Browne, C.A. and Zerbon, F.W., *Physical and Chemical Methods of Sugar Analysis*. Wiley, New York, 1941, pp. 547–548.
[134] Weast, R.C. (ed.), *Handbook of Chemistry and Physics*, 56th edn. CRC Press, Cleveland, Ohio, 1975, pp. D229–230.
[135] Hildebrand, J.H. and Scott, R.L., *Regular Solutions*. Prentice-Hall, New Jersey, 1962.
[136] Hildebrand, J.H. and Scott, R.L., *The Solubility of Non-electrolytes*, 3rd edn. Reinhold, New York, 1950.
[137] Hildebrand, J.H., Prausnitz, J.M. and Scott, R.L., *Regular and Related Solutions*. Van Nostrand Reinhold Co., 1970.
[138] Waals, J.D. van der, *Z. Physik. Chem.* 1890, **5**, 133–176.
[139] Bakker, G., *Z. Physik. Chem.* 1892, **10**, 558–562.
[140] Bakker, G., *Z. Physik. Chem.* 1895, **18**, 519–520.
[141] Partington, J.R., *Z. Physik. Chem.* 1914, **88**, 297–306.
[142] Partington, J.R., *An Advanced Treatise on Physical Chemistry*, Vol. 2, *The Properties of Liquids*. Longmans Green, London, 1951, p. 316.
[143] Dupré, A., *Chim. Phys.* 1865, **6**, 274–290.
[144] Stefan, J., *Ann. Phys.* 1886, **29**, 655–665.
[145] Laar, J.J. Van and Lorenz, R., *Z. anorg. allgem. Chem.* 1925, **146**, 42–44.

[146]   Scatchard, G., *Chem. Rev.* 1931, **8**, 321–333.

[147]   Murnagham, F.D., *Proc. Natl. Acad. Sci. U.S.A.* 1944, **30**, 244–247.

[148]   Moelwyn-Hughes, E.A., *J. Phys. Chem.* 1951, **55**, 1246–1254.

[149]   Harrison, D. and Moelwyn-Hughes, E.A., *Proc. Roy. Soc. (A)* 1954, **239**, 230–246.

[150]   Gilvarry, J.J., *Phys. Rev.* 1956, **102**, 325–331.

[151]   Gilvarry, J.J., *J. Appl. Phys.* 1957, **28**, 1253–1261.

[152]   Macdonald, J.R. and Barlow, C.A., *J. Chem. Phys.* 1962, **36**, 3062–3080.

[153]   Macdonald, J.R., *Rev. Mod. Phys.* 1960, **38**, 669–679.

[154]   Macdonald, J.R., *J. Chem. Phys.* 1964, **40**, 1792–1804.

[155]   Ryabinin, Yu.N., *Zhur. Tekh. Fiz.* 1960, **30**, 739–741.

[156]   Cook, M.A. and Rogers, L.A., *J. Appl. Phys.* 1963, **34**, 2330–2336.

[157]   Anderson, O.L., *Physics Chem. Solids* 1966, **24**, 547–565.

[158]   Bridgeman, P.W., *International Critical Tables*, Vol. III (E.W. Washburn, ed.). McGraw-Hill, New York, 1928, p. 39.

[159]   Eduljee, H.E., Newitt, D.M. and Weale, K.E., *J. Chem. Soc.* 1951, 3086–3091.

[160]   Blagoi, Yu.P. and Sorkin, V.A., *Russian J. Phys. Chem.* 1970, **44**, 1563–1566.

[161]   McGowan, J.C., *Polymer* 1970, **11**, 436–439.

[162]   McGowan, J.C. and Weeks, J.C., *Nature Physical Science* 1971, **234**, 119–120.

[163]   McGowan, J.C., *Chem. Communications (J. Chem. Soc. D)* 1971, 514–515.

[164]   Aircart, E., Tardajos, G. and Diaz Pena, M., *J. Chem. Engrg. Data* 1980, **25**, 140–145.

[165]   Mathot, V. and Desmyter, J., *Chem. Phys.* 1953, **21**, 782–788.

[166]   Laar, J.J. van, *J. Chim. Phys.* 1916, **16**, 3–24.

[167]   Arkel, A.E. van and de Groot, W., *Physica* 1932, **12**, 211–217.

[168]   Liempt, J.A.M. van, *Rec. Trav. Chim.* 1933, **52**, 123–128.

[169]   McGowan, J.C., *J. Appl. Chem. Biotechnol.* 1984, **34A**, 38–42.

[170]   Watson, K.M., *Ind. Eng. Chem.* 1934, **35**, 398–406.

[171]   Einstein, A., *Ann. Phys. [4]* 1901, **4**, 513–523.

[172]   Einstein, A., *Ann. Phys. [A]* 1911, **34**, 1165–1169.

[173]   Scatchard, G., *Chem. Rev.* 1949, **44**, 7–35.

[174]   Small, P.A., *J. Appl. Chem., Lond.* 1953, **3**, 71–80.

[175]   Hoy, K.L., *J. Paint Technol.* 1970, **42**, 76–78.

[176]   Krevelen, D.W. van and Hoftyzer, P.J., *Properties of Polymers. Their Estimation and Correlation with Chemical Structure*, 2nd edn. Elsevier, Amsterdam, 1976, p. 13.

[177]   Timmermanns, J., *Physico-Chemical Constants of Pure Organic Compounds*, Vol. II. Elsevier, Amsterdam, 1965.

[178]   Bunn, A., Cudby, M.E.A. and McGowan, J.C., *Rec. Trav. Chim.* 1968, **87**, 599–608.

[179] Grosse, A.V. and Cady, G.H., *Ind. Eng. Chem.* 1947, **39**, 367–374.

[180] Fowler, R.D., Hamilton, J.M., Kasper, J.S., Weber, D.E., Burford, W.B. and Anderson, H.C., *Ind. Eng. Chem.* 1947, **39**, 375–378.

[181] Hazeldine, P.N. and Smith, F., *J. Chem. Soc.* 1951, 603–608.

[182] Rowlinson, J.S. and Thacker, R., *Trans. Faraday Soc.* 1957, **53**, 1–8.

[183] Counsell, J.F., Green, J.H.S., Hales, J.L. and Martin, J.F., *Trans. Faraday Soc.* 1965, **61**, 212–218.

[184] Hurd, C.B., *J. Am. Chem. Soc.* 1946, **68**, 364–370.

[185] Ross, M. and Hildebrand, J.H., *J. Phys. Chem.* 1963, **67**, 1301–1303.

[186] Hildebrand, J.H. and Scott, R.L., *Regular Solutions*. New Jersey, Prentice-Hall Inc, 1962, p. 155.

[187] Lewis, W.C. McC., *A System of Physical Chemistry*, Vol. I. Longmans Green & Co., London, 1929, p. 289.

[188] Henry, W., *Phil. Trans. Roy. Soc.* 1803, **93**, 29–42 and 274–276.

[189] Gerrard, W., *Chem. and Ind.* 1969, 1460 only.

[190] Berthelot, M. and Jungfleisch, E., *Ann. Chim. Phys.* 1872, **26** [4], 396–407.

[191] Nernst, W., *Z. Physik. Chem.* 1891, **8**, 110–139.

[192] Herz, W. and Fischer, H., *Chem. Ber.* 1905, **38**, 1138–1144.

[193] Lewis, W.C.McC., *A System of Physical Chemistry*, Vol. II, *Thermodynamics*. Longmans, Green and Co., London, 1920, p. 121.

[194] Gerrard, W., *Solubility of Gases and Liquids*. Plenum Press, New York, 1976, p. 260.

[195] Lindenberg, A.B. and Massin, M., *J. Chim. Phys.* 1964, **61**, 1120–1121.

[196] Rider, P.E. and Hammaker, R.M., *Spectrochimica Acta* 1973, **29A**, 501–509.

[197] Kuntz, I.D., Gasparro, E.P., Johnston, M.D. and Taylor, R.P., *J. Am. Chem. Soc.* 1968, **90**, 4778–4781.

[198] Ben-Naim, A., *J. Phys. Chem.* 1978, **82**, 792–803.

[199] Smith, E.B., Walkley, J. and Hildebrand, J.H., *J. Phys. Chem.* 1959, **63**, 703–704.

[200] Trouton, F.T., *Phil. Mag. [5]* 1884, **18**, 54–57.

[201] Littlewood, A.B., *Gas Chromatography*. Academic Press, New York and London, 1962.

[202] Hildebrand, J.H. and Jenks, C.A., *J. Am. Chem. Soc.* 1920, **42**, 2180–2189.

[203] Benesi, H.A. and Hildebrand, J.H., *J. Am. Chem. Soc.* 1948, **70**, 3978–3981.

[204] Hildebrand, J.H. and Scott, R.L., *The Solubility of Non-Electrolytes*, 3rd edn. Reinhold, New York, 1950, p. 280.

[205] Hildebrand, J.H. and Jenks, C.A., *J. Am. Chem. Soc.* 1921, **43**, 2172–2177.

[206] Smith, E.G. and Walkley, J., *Trans. Faraday Soc.* 1960, **56**, 220–224.

[207] Hildebrand, J.H. and Scott, R.L., *Regular Solutions*. Prentice-Hall, New Jersey, 1962, p. 11.

[208] Hildebrand, J.H., Fisher, B.B. and Benesi, H.A., *J. Am. Chem. Soc.* 1950, **72**, 4348–4351.

[209] Shinoda, K. and Hildebrand, J.H., *J. Phys. Chem.* 1957, **61**, 789–791.

[210] Lannung, A., *J. Am. Chem. Soc.* 1930, **52**, 68–80.

[211] Cleaver, H.L., Saylor, J.H. and Gross, P.M., *J. Phys. Chem.* 1958, **62**, 89–91.

[212] Saylor, J.H. and Battino, R., *J. Phys. Chem.* 1958, **62**, 1334–1337.

[213] Evans, F.D. and Battino, R., *J. Chem. Thermodynamics* 1971, **3**, 753–760.

[214] Wilcock, R.J., Battino, R., Danforth, W.F. and Wilhelm, E., *J. Chem. Thermodynamics* 1978, **10**, 817–822.

[215] Riess, J.G. and LeBlanc, M., *Angew. Chem. (Intern. ed.)* 1978, **17**, 621–700.

[216] Michaels, A.S. and Bixler, H.J., *J. Polymer Sci.* 1961, **50**, 393–412.

[217] Schonhorn, H. and Sharpe, L.H., *J. Polymer. Sci. A.* 1965, **3**, 569–573.

[218] Cogswell, F.N., *Plastics & Polymers* 1970, **38**, 391–394.

[219] Mahieu, J., *Bull. Soc. Chim. Belg.* 1936, **45**, 667–675.

[220] Apelblat, A., *J. Chem. Soc. Phys. Org.* 1970, **8B**, 1459–1461.

[221] Apelblat, A., *J. Chem. Soc. Phys. Org.* 1969, **7B**, 175–177.

[222] Rossini, F.D. Pitzer, K.S., Arnett, R.L., Braun, R.M. and Pimental, G.C., *Selected Values of Physical and Thermodynamic Properties of Hydrocarbons and Related Compounds*. Pittsburgh, Pa., Carnegie Press, 1953.

[223] Eley, D.D., *Trans. Faraday Soc.* 1939, **35**, 1281–1293.

[224] Eley, D.D., *Trans. Faraday Soc.* 1939, **35**, 1421–1432.

[225] Deno, N.C. and Berkheimer, H.E., *J. Chem. Engng. Data* 1960, **5**, 1–5.

[226] Deno, N.C. and Berkheimer, H.E., *J. Org. Chem.* 1963, **28**, 2143–2144.

[227] London, E., *Trans. Faraday Soc.* 1937, **33**, 8–26.

[228] Collander, R., *Acta. Chem. Scand.* 1949, **3**, 717–747.

[229] Collander, R., *Acta Chem. Scand.* 1950, **4**, 1085–1098.

[230] McGowan, J.C., Ahmad, P. and Mellors, A., *Canad. J. Pharm. Sci.* 1979, **14**, 72–74.

[231] Flynn, G.L., *J. Pharm. Sci.* 1971, **60**, 345–353.

[232] Dunn, W.J. and Wold, S., *Acta Chem. Scand. B,* 1978, **32**, 536–542.

[233] Kablukov, I.A. and Milischeva, V.T., *J. Am. Chem. Soc.* 1925, **47**, 1553–1561.

[234] Takenaka, N. and Arakawa, K., *Bull. Chem. Soc. Japan* 1974, **67**, 566–570.

[235] Dryssen, D. and Hay, L.D., *Acta Chem. Scand.* 1960, **14**, 1091–1099.

[236] Collander, R., *Acta Chem. Scand.* 1951, **5**, 774–780.

[237] Leo, A., Hansch, C. and Elkins, D., *Chem. Rev.* 1971, **71**, 571–616.

[238] Currie, D.J., Lough, C.E., Silver, R.F. and Holmes, H.L., *Canad. J. Chem.* 1966, **44**, 1035–1043.

[239] Dolezalek, F., *Z. Physik. Chem.* 1908, **64**, 727–747.

[240] Zawidski, J.V., *Z. Physik. Chem.* 1900, **35**, 129–203.
[241] Dolezalek, F. and Schulze, A., *Z. Physik. Chem.* 1913, **83**, 45–78.
[242] Kohnstamm, P. and Dalfsen, B.M. van, *Proc. Acad. Wet.* 1901, **29**, 156.
[243] Ibbotson, D.A. and Moore, L.F., *Chem. Commun.* 1965, No. 15, 339–340.
[244] Kunst, M., Duijn, D. van and Bordewijk, P., *Ber. Bunsen. Ges.* 1976, **80**, 839–846.
[245] Salamon, T., Liszi, J. and Ratkovics, F., *Acta Chim. Acad. Sci. Hungar.* 1975, **87**, 137–159.
[246] Satterfield, C.N., Powell, J.H., Oster, E.A. and Noyes, J.P., *Ind. Eng. Chem.* 1955, **47**, 1458–1462.
[247] Ligny, C.L. de, Denessen, H.J.M. and Alfenaar, M., *Rec. Trav. Chim.* 1971, **90**, 1265–1284.
[248] Box, D., Ligny, C.L. de, Alfenaar, M., *Rec. Trav. Chim.* 1972, **91**, 452–476.
[249] Bonner, W.D., *J. Phys. Chem.* 1910, **14**, 738–789.
[250] Voro'beva, A.I. and Karapet'yants, M. Kh., *Russ. J. Phys. Chem.* 1966, **40**, 1619–1622.
[251] Hermann, R.B., *J. Phys. Chem.* 1972, **76**, 2754–2759.
[252] Amidon, G.L., Yalkowsky, S.H., Amik, S.T. and Valvani, S.C., *J. Phys. Chem.* 1975, **79**, 2339–2346.
[253] Harris, M.J., Higuchi, T. and Rytting, J.H., *J. Phys. Chem.* 1973, **77**, 2694–2703.
[254] Leo, A., Hansch, C. and Jow, P.Y.C., *J. Med. Chem.* 1976, **19**, 611–615.
[255] Kemula, W. and Buchowski, H., *Roczinki Chemii* 1937, **29**, 718–729.
[256] Schulz, G.V., *Z. Physik. Chem.* 1937, **179A**, 321–355.
[257] Consden, R., Gordon, A.H. and Martin, A.J.P., *Biochem. J.* 1944, **38**, 224–232.
[258] Procházka, Z., *Some General Problems of Paper Chromatography.* Symposium Liblice, 23rd June, 1961 (I.M. Hais and K. Macek, eds.). Prague, 1962, pp. 113–116.
[259] Bate-Smith, E.C. and Westfall, R.G., *Biochim. Biophys. Acta* 1950, **4**, 427–440.
[260] Boyce, C.B.C. and Milborrow, B.V., *Nature, Lond.* 1965, **208**, 537–539.
[261] Turner, N.J. and Battershill, R.D., *Contributions from Boyce Thompson Institute* 1969, **24**, 139–147.
[262] Soczewinski, E. and Wachtmeister, C.A., *J. Chromatography* 1962, **7**, 311–320.
[263] Soczewinski, E., *J. Chromatography* 1963, **11**, 275–277.
[264] Purnell, J.H. and Andrade, J.M.V. de., *J. Am. Chem. Soc.* 1975, **97**, 3585–3593.

[265]   Laub, R.J. and Purnell, J.H., *J. Am. Chem. Soc.* 1976, **98**, 30–35, 35–39.

[266]   Harbison, M.W.P., Laub, R.J., Martire, D.E., Purnell, J.H. and Williams, P.S., *J. Phys. Chem.* 1979, **83**, 1262–1268.

[267]   Meyer, E.F. and Meyer, J.A., *J. Phys. Chem.* 1981, **85**, 94–97.

[268]   Littlewood, A.B., *Anal. Chem.* 1964, **36**, 1441–1451.

[269]   Littlewood, A.B. and Willmott, F.W., *Anal. Chem.* 1966, **38**, 1031–1041.

[270]   Martire, D.E. and Riedl, P., *J. Phys. Chem.* 1968, **72**, 3478–3488.

[271]   Tammann, G., *Uber die Beziehung zwischen inneren Kräften und Eigenschaften der Lösungen.* L. Voss, Hamburg, 1907.

[272]   Tammann, G., *Z. Anorg. Chem.* 1928, **174**, 231–243.

[273]   Tammann, G., *Z. Physik. Chem.* 1893, **11**, 676–692.

[274]   Euler, H., *Z. Physik. Chem.* 1899, **31**, 360–369.

[275]   Geffeken, G., *Z. Physik. Chem.* 1904, **49**, 257–302.

[276]   Euler, H., *Z. Physik. Chem.* 1904, **49**, 303–316.

[277]   Tammann, G., *Z. Anorg. Chem.* 1919, **107**, 1–239.

[278]   Setschenow, J., *Z. Physik. Chem.* 1889, **4**, 117–125.

[279]   Setschenow, J., *Ann. Chim. Phys.* [6] 1891, **25**, 226–270.

[280]   Deno, N.C. and Spink, C.H., *J. Phys. Chem.* 1963, **67**, 1347–1349.

[281]   Long, F.A. and Bergen, R.L., *J. Phys. Chem.* 1956, **60**, 1131–1135.

[282]   McDevit, W.F. and Long, F.A., *J. Am. Chem. Soc.* 1952, **74**, 1773–1777.

[283]   Long, F.A. and McDevit, W.F., *Chem. Rev.* 1952, **51**, 119–169.

[284]   Lunden, B., *Z. Physik. Chem.* 1943, **192**, 345–378.

[285]   Tait, P.G., *Proc. Roy. Soc. Edinburgh* 1884, **12**, 45–46.

[286]   Tait, P.G., *Proc. Roy. Soc. Edinburgh* 1884, **12**, 223–224.

[287]   Tait, P.G., *Proc. Roy. Soc. Edinburgh* 1884, **12**, 757–758.

[288]   Tait, P.G., *Proc. Roy. Soc. Edinburgh* 1893, **20**, 63–68.

[289]   Tait, P.G., *Proc. Roy. Soc. Edinburgh* 1893, **20**, 141–144.

[290]   Tait, P.G., *The Voyage of H.M.S. Challenger. Physics and Chemistry*, Vol. 2, Part 4. 1888, HMSO, pp. 1–73.

[291]   Hayward, A.T.J., *Brit. J. Appl. Physics* 1967, **18**, 965–977.

[292]   Tammann, G., *Z. Physik. Chem.* 1895, **17**, 620–636.

[293]   Neece, C.A. and Squire, D.R., *J. Phys. Chem.* 1968, **72**, 128–136.

[294]   Gibson, R.E., *J. Am. Chem. Soc.* 1934, **56**, 4–14.

[295]   Gibson, R.E., *J. Am. Chem. Soc.* 1934, **56**, 865–870.

[296]   Blandamer, M.J., Burgess, J. and McGowan, J.C., *J. Chem. Soc. Dalton* 1980, 616–619.

[297]   Bischoff, F. and Pilhorn, H.R., *J. Biol. Chem.* 1948, **174**, 663–682.

[298]   Krevelen, D.W. van and Hoftijzer, P.J., *21 Congr. Int. Chim. Ind.* Brussels, 1948: *Chimie et Industrie* 1950, **63**, 168–173.

[299]   Krevelen, D.W. van, *Zeit. Elektrochem.* 1953, **57**, 502–512.

[300]   Saylor, J.H., Whitten, A.L., Clairborne, I. and Gross, P.M., *J. Am. Chem. Soc.* 1952, **74**, 1778–1781.

[301] Brønsted, J.N., Delbanco, A. and Volquartz, K., *Z. Physik. Chem.* 1932, **162**, 128–146.

[302] Rothmund, V., *Z. Physik. Chem.* 1910, **69**, 523–546.

[303] McGowan, J.C., *Nature, Lond.* 1974, **252**, 296–297.

[304] Burgess, J., Morton, N. and McGowan, J.C., *J. Chem. Soc. Dalton* 1977, 1775–1777.

[305] Flatt, R. and Jordan, A., *Helv. Chim. Acta* 1933, **16**, 37–53.

[306] De Ligny, C.L., Box, D., Alfenaar, M. and Elferink, M.G.L., *Rec. Trav. Chim.* 1969, **88**, 1183–1200.

[307] Thin, R.G. and Cumming, A.C., *J. Chem. Soc.* 1915, **107**, 361–366.

[308] Willard, H.H. and Smith, G.F., *J. Am. Chem. Soc.* 1923, **45**, 286–297.

[309] Herz, W. and Anders, G., *Z. anorg. Chem.* 1907, **55**, 271–278.

[310] McGowan, J.C. and Mellors, A., *J. Appl. Biochemistry* 1979, **1**, 423–429.

[311] Cohn, E.J., McMeekin, T.L., Edsall, J.T. and Weare, J.H., *J. Am. Chem. Soc.* 1934, **56**, 2270–2282.

[312] Dunn, M.S. and Ross, F.J., *J. Biol. Chem.* 1938, **125**, 309–333.

[313] Amis, E.S. and Hinton, J.F., *Solvent Effects in Chemical Phenomena*, Vol. I. Academic Press, New York, 1973.

[314] Christian, S.D., Taha, A.S. and Gash, B.W., *Quart. Rev. Chem. Soc.* 1970, **24**, 20–36.

[315] Uitert, C.E. van, Spicer, L.D. and Uitert, J. van, *J. Phys. Chem.* 1977, **81**, 40–47.

[316] Hollenberg, J.L. and Ifft, J.B., *J. Phys. Chem.* 1982, **86**, 1938–1941.

[317] Yasunga, T., Usui, I., Iwata, K. and Miura, M., *Bull. Chem. Soc. Japan* 1964, **37**, 1658–1660.

[318] Millero, F.J., Ward, G.K., Lepple, F.K. and Hoff, E.W., *J. Phys. Chem.* 1974, **78**, 1636–1643.

[319] Millero, F.M., La Surdo, A. and Shin, C., *J. Phys. Chem.* 1978, **82**, 784–792.

[320] Shahidi, F. and Farrell, P.G., *J. Chem. Soc. Faraday Trans I* 1981, **77**, 963–968.

[321] Burgess, J., *Metal Ions in Solution.* Ellis Horwood, Chichester, 1978.

[322] Oss, C.J. van, Absolom, D.R. and Neumann, A.W., *Colloid and Polymer Science* 1980, **258**, 424–427.

[323] Colacicco, G., *Ann. N.Y. Acad. Sci.* 1972, **195**, 224–261.

[324] Nozaki, Y. and Tanford, C., *J. Biol. Chem.* 1971, **246**, 2211–2217.

[325] Abraham, M.H., *J. Am. Chem. Soc.* 1979, **101**, 5477–5484.

[326] Abraham, M.H., *J. Am. Chem. Soc.* 1980, **102**, 5910–5912.

[327] Wertz, D.H., *J. Am. Chem. Soc.* 1980, **102**, 5316–5322.

[328] Cramer, R.D., *J. Am. Chem. Soc.* 1977, **99**, 5408–5412.

[329] Cramer, R.D., *J. Am. Chem. Soc.* 1980, **102**, 1837–1849.

[330] Hildebrand, J.H., *Proc. Natl. Acad. Sci. U.S.A.* 1979, **76**, 194.

[331] Hildebrand, J.H., *J. Phys. Chem.* 1968, **72**, 1841–1842.

[332] Dehmlow, E.V., *Angew. Chem. Internat. Ed.* 1974, **13**, 170–179.

[333] Davies, J.T., *J. Phys. Chem.* 1950, **54**, 185–204.

[334] Eisenman, G., *Anal. Chem.* 1968, **40**, 310–320.

[335] Eisenman, G., *Ion-Selective Electrodes.* Proceedings of a symposium, N.B.S. Special Publication No. 314 (R.A. Derst, ed.). National Bureau of Standards, Gaitherburg, Maryland, 1969, pp. 1–56.

[336] Goldman, S. and Duer, W.C., *Canad. J. Chem.* 1974, **52**, 3918–3931.

[337] Iwamoto, E., Ito, K. and Yamamoto, Y., *J. Phys. Chem.* 1981, **85**, 894–901.

[338] Walden, P., *Z. Physik. Chem.* 1906, **55**, 683–720.

[339] Danil de Namor, A.F. and Hill, T., *J. Chem. Soc., Faraday Trans. I.* 1983, **79**, 2713–2722.

[340] Abraham, M.H. and Danil de Namor, A.F., *J. Chem. Soc., Faraday Trans. I.* 1976, **72**, 955–962.

[341] Abraham, M.H. and Danil de Namor, A.F., *J. Chem. Soc., Faraday Trans. I.* 1978, **74**, 2101–2110.

[342] Tomlinson, E., Jefferies, T.M. and Riley, C.M., *J. Chromatography* 1978, **159**, 315–358.

[343] Schill, G., *Ion Exchange and Solvent Extraction*, Vol. 6. Marcel Dekker, New York, 1974, pp. 1–57.

[344] Purcell, W.P., Beasley, J.G., Quintana, R.P. and Singer, J.A., *J. Med. Chem.* 1966, **9**, 297–303.

[345] Quintana, R.P., *J. Pharm. Sci.* 1965, **54**, 462–463.

[346] Gavaudan, P., Dodé, M. and Poussel, H., *Mém. Services chim. état (Paris)* 1944, **31**, 384–423.

[347] Seeman, P., *Pharmacol. Rev.* 1972, **24**, 583–655.

[348] Levan, A., *Hereditas* 1938, **24**, 471–486.

[349] Levan, A. and Östergren, G., *Hereditas* 1943, **29**, 381–443.

[350] Östergren, G. and Levan, A., *Heriditas* 1943, **29**, 496–498.

[351] Östergren, G., *Hereditas* 1944, **30**, 429–467.

[352] Overton, E., *Studien über die Narkose.* Jena, 1901, p. 77.

[353] Bateman, E., *The Effect of Concentration on the Toxicity of Chemicals to Living Organisms.* United States Department of Agriculture Technical Bulletin No. 346, Washington, D.C., 1939.

[354] Miller, K.W., Paton, W.D.M., Smith, E.G. and Smith, R.A., *Anesthesiology* 1972, **36**, 339–351.

[355] Gavaudan, P., Poussel, H. and Dodé, M., *C.R. de la Soc. de Biol.* 1944, **138**, 267–268.

[356] Bauch, R., *Wochschr. Brau.* 1941, **59**, 1–7, 9–11.

[357] Bauch, R., *Naturwissen.* 1942, **30**, 420–421.

[358] Fühner, H., *Arch exp. Pathol. Pharm.* 1905, **52**, 69–82.

[359] Corman, I., *J. Nat. Cancer Inst.* 1950, **10**, 1128–1138.

[360] Nettleship, A., Henshaw, P.S. and Meyer, H.L., *J. Nat. Cancer Inst.* 1943, **4**, 309–319.

[361] Henshaw, P.S. and Meyer, H.L., *J. Nat. Cancer Inst.* 1944, **4**, 523–525.

[362] Henshaw, P.S. and Meyer, H.L., *J. Nat. Cancer Inst.* 1945, **5**, 415–417.

[363] Orr, J.W., *Brit. J. Cancer* 1947, **1**, 311–322.
[364] Cowen, P.N., *Brit. J. Cancer* 1947, **1**, 401–405.
[365] Jaffe, W.G., *Cancer Research* 1947, **7**, 107–112.
[366] Selbie, F.R., Thackray, A.C., *Brit. J. Cancer* 1948, **2**, 380–385.
[367] Pepper, J.H., *J. Econ. Entom.* 1937, **30**, 380.
[368] Yasuda-Yasaki, Y., Namiki-Kanie, S. and Hachisuka, Y., *J. Bact.* 1978, **136**, 484–490.
[369] McLennan, H. and Elliott, K.A.C., *J. Pharmacol. Exptl. Therap.* 1951, **103**, 35–43.
[370] Doebbler, G.F., Mohlke, M.F., McMullen, L.M. and Schreiner, H.R., *Fed. Proc.* 1967, **26**, 650.
[371] Schreiner, H.R., *Fed. Proc.* 1968, **27**, 872–878.
[372] Mellors, A. and McGowan, J.C., *Biochem. Pharmacol.* 1985, **34**, 2413–2416.
[373] McGowan, J.C. and Mellors, A., *Bull. Environ. Contam. Toxicol.* 1986, **36**, no. 6.
[374] Buccafusco, R.J., Ellis, S.J. and Leblanc, G.A., *Bull. Environ. Contam. Toxicol.* 1981, **26**, 446–452.
[375] Gershenfeld, L. and Witlin, B., *Amer. J. Pharm.* 1941, **113**, 215–236.
[376] Schaffer, J.M. and Tilley, F.W., *J. Bact.* 1927, **14**, 259–273.
[377] Tilley, F.W. and Schaffer, J.M., *J. Bact.* 1928, **16**, 279–285.
[378] Read, R.R. and Miller, E., *J. Am. Chem. Soc.* 1932, **54**, 1195–1199.
[379] Klarmann, E., Shternov, V.A. and von Wowern, J., *J. Bact.* 1929, **17**, 423–442.
[380] Klarmann, E., Gatyas, L.W. and Shternov, V.A., *J. Am. Chem. Soc.* 1932, **54**, 298–305.
[381] Klarmann, E. and Shternov, V.A., *Industr. Engng. Chem. (Analyl. Ed.)* 1936, **8**, 369–372.
[382] Klarmann, E., Gatyas, L.W. and Shternov, V.A., *J. Am. Chem. Soc.* 1931, **53**, 3397–3407.
[383] Klarmann, E., Gates, L.W. and Shternov. V.A., *J. Am. Chem. Soc.* 1932, **54**, 1204–1211.
[384] Klarmann, E., Shternov, V.A. and Gates, L.W., *J. Am. Chem. Soc.* 1933, **55**, 2576–2589.
[385] Klarmann, E., Gates, L.W., Shternov, V.A. and Cox, P.H., *J. Am. Chem. Soc.* 1933, **55**, 4657–4662.
[386] Frobisher, M., *J. Bact.* 1927, **13**, 163–182.
[387] Cooper, E.A., *Biochem. J.* 1913, **7**, 175–185, 186–196.
[388] Woodward, G.J., Ore, M., Kingery, L.B. and Williams, R.J., *J. Lab. Clin. Med.* 1934, **19**, 1216–1223.
[389] Hampil, B., *J. Infect. Dis.* 1928, **43**, 25–40.
[390] Tattersfield, F., *J. Agr. Sci.* 1927, **17**, 181–207.
[391] Baechler, R.H., *Proc. Amer. Wood Pres. Ass.* 1939, **35**, 364–372.
[392] Baechler, R.H., *Proc. Amer. Wood Pres. Ass.* 1947, **43**, 94–111.

[393] Evans, B.K., James, K.C. and Luscombe, D.K., *J. Pharm. Sci.* 1978, **67**, 277–278.

[394] Mills, J.E., *Fundamental Study of Toxicity*. Rep. No. PB 26947 of Department of Commerce, Washington 25, D.C., 1930.

[395] Cameron, G.R., Paterson, J.L.H., de Saram, G.S.W. and Thomas, J.C., *J. Path. Bact.* 1938, **46**, 95–107.

[396] Kocsis, J.J., Harkaway, S. and Snyder, R., *Ann. New York Acad. Sci.* 1975, **243**, 104–109.

[397] Sharom, F. and Mellors, A., *Biochem. Pharmacol.* 1980, **29**, 3311–3317.

[398] Huszar, L.A., Greenberg, J.H. and Mellors, A., *Mol. Pharmacol.* 1977, **13**, 1086–1091.

[399] Greenberg, J.H., Saunders, M.E. and Mellors, A., *Science* 1977, **197**, 475–476.

[400] Roth, S. and Seeman, P., *Nature New Biol.* 1971, **231**, 284–285.

[401] Roth, S. and Seeman, P., *Biochim. Biophys. Acta.* 1972, **255**, 207–219.

[402] Hyde, R.M., *J. Med. Chem.* 1975, **18**, 231–233.

[403] Hyde, R.M., *Chem. and Ind., Lond.* 1977, 859–862.

[404] Batelli, F. and Stern, L., *Biochem. Zeit.* 1913, **52**, 226–252.

[405] Hatefi, Y., *Methods Enzymol.* 1978, **53**, 27–35.

[406] Ohnishi, T., Salerno, J.C., Winter, D.B., Lim, J., Yu, C.A., Yu, L., and King, T.E., *J. Biol. Chem.* 1976, **251**, 2094–2104.

[407] Ohnishi, T., Lim., J., Winter, D.B. and King, T.E., *J. Biol. Chem.* 1976, **251**, 2105–2109.

[408] Hatefi, Y. and Hanstein, W.G., *Arch. Biochem. Biophys.* 1970, **138**, 73–86.

[409] Chazotte, B. and Vanderkooi, G., *Biochim. Biophys. Acta* 1981, **636**, 153–161.

[410] Lemon, J.S., *J. Phys. Chem.* 1920, **24**, 570–584.

[411] Laird, J.S., *J. Phys. Chem.* 1920, **24**, 664–672.

[412] Paul, T. and Krönig, B., *Z. Physik. Chem.* 1896, **21**, 414–450.

[413] Larsen, H., *The Bacteria*, Vol. 4, Chap. 8 (I. Gunsalus and R. Stanier, eds.). Academic Press, New York, 1962, pp. 297.

[414] Siegel, S.M. and Roberts, K., *Proc. Acad. Nat. Sci., U.S.A.* 1966, **56**, 1505–1508.

[415] Seidall, A., *Solubility of Inorganic, Metal-organic and Organic Compounds*, 3rd edn. Van Nostrand, New York, 1940.

[416] Bancroft, W.D. and Rutzler, J.E., *J. Phys. Chem.* 1931, **35**, 1185–1211.

[417] Ahmad, P., Fyfe, C.A. and Mellors, A., *Biochem. Pharmacol.* 1975, **24**, 1103–1109.

[418] Ahmad, P., Fyfe, C.A. and Mellors, A., *Canad. J. Biochem.* 1975, **53**, 1047–1053.

[419] Ahmad, P. and Mellors, A., *J. Steroid Biochem.* 1976, **7**, 19–28.

[420] Cooper, E.A. and Woodhouse, D.L., *Biochem. J.* 1923, **17**, 600–612.

[421] Cooper, E.A. and Forstner, G.E., *Biochem. J.* 1924, **18**, 941–947.

[422] Snegireff, S.L., Cox, J.R. and Eastwood, D.W., *Toxicity of Anaesthetics* (B.R. Fink, ed.). Williams and Wilkins, Baltimore, 1968, pp. 279–293.

[423] Nisbet, H.B., *Anaesthetics*. Royal Inst. Chem. Monographs and Reports, 1949, p. 8.

[424] McGowan, J.C., *Arch. Ind. Health* 1955, **11**, 315–323.

[425] Juszkiewicz, A., *Arch. Acoust.* 1981, **6**, 307–319.

[426] Munton, S.L., results quoted by G.G. Birch, reference [433].

[427] Yasunga, T., Hirata, Y., Kawano, Y. and Miura, M., *Bull. Chem. Soc. Japan* 1964, **37**, 867–871.

[428] Antosiewicz, J., Juszkiewicz, A. and Shugar, D., *J. Phys. Chem.* 1982, **86**, 4831–4834.

[429] Juszkiewicz, A. and Potaczek, J., *Arch. Acoust.* 1981, **6**, 401–408.

[430] Siek, T.J., Albin, I.A., Sather, L.A. and Lindsay, R.C., *J. Dairy Sci.* 1971, **54**, 1–4.

[431] Greenberg, M.J., *J. Agric. Food Chem.* 1980, **28**, 562–566.

[432] Hough, L. and Khan, R., *Trends Biochem. Sci.* 1978, 61–63.

[433] Birch, G.G., *Chem. and Ind.* 1983, 13–15.

[434] Goldman, S., *Canad. J. Chem.* 1974, **52**, 1668–1680.

[435] Merriman, R.W., *J. Chem. Soc.* 1913, **103**, 1774–1789.

[436] Donahue, D.I. and Bartlett, F.E., *J. Phys. Chem.* 1952, **56**, 480–484.

[437] Butler, J.A.V., Thomson, D.W. and Maclennan, W.H., *J. Chem. Soc.* 1933, 674–686.

[438] Pringle, M.J., Brown, K.B. and Miller, K.W., *Mol. Pharmacol.* 1981, **19**, 49–55.

[439] Gibbs, R.D., *Am. J. Bot.* 1934, **21**, 645–650.

[440] Hansch, C., Muir, J.R.M., Fujita, T., Maloney, P.P., Geiger, F. and Streich, M., *J. Am. Chem. Soc.* 1963, **85**, 2817–2824.

[441] Hansch, C. and Steward, A.R., *J. Med. Chem.* 1964, **7**, 691–694.

[442] Hansch, C., Deutsch, E.W. and Smith, R.N., *J. Am. Chem. Soc.* 1965, **87**, 2738–2742.

[443] Briggs, G.G., *J. Agric. Food Chem.* 1981, **29**, 1050–1059.

[444] Seifriz, W., *Protoplasm*. McGraw-Hill, New York and London, 1936, pp. 220–228 and 497.

[445] Bernard, C., *Lecons sur les Effects des Substances Toxique et Médicamenteuses*. J.B. Baillière et fils, Paris, 1875.

[446] Bernard, C., *La Science Expérimentale*. Paris, 1906.

[447] Bancroft, W.D. and Richter, G.H., *J. Phys. Chem.* 1931, **35**, 215–268.

[448] Harvey, E.N., *Biol. Bull.* 1915, **29**, 308–311.

[449] Johnson, F.H., Brown, D.E.S. and Marsland, D.A., *J. Cell Comp. Physiol.* 1942, **20**, 269–276.

[450] Johnson, F.H. and Flagler, E.A., *Science* 1950, **112**, 91–92.

[451] Johnson, S.M. and Miller, K.W., *Nature* 1970, **228**, 75–76.

[452]   Eyring, H., *Science* 1966, **154**, 1609–1613.

[453]   Ueda, I. and Kamaya, H., *Anesthesiol.* 1973, **38**, 425–434.

[454]   White, D.C., *Molecular Mechanisms in General Anaesthesia* (M.J. Halsey, R.A. Millar and J.A. Sutton, eds.). Churchill-Livingstone Ltd, Edinburgh, 1974, pp. 209–225.

[455]   Nicol, L.W., Jackson, W.H. and Winzor, D.J., *Biochemistry* 1972, **11**, 585–591.

[456]   White, D.C., Wardley-Smith, B. and Adey, G., *Life Sci.* 1973, **12**, 453–460.

[457]   Dixon, M. and Webb, E.C. *The Enzymes* , 2nd edn. Longmans, London, 1964, p. 467.

[458]   Settle, W., *A Guide to Molecular Pharmacology and Toxicology*, Part II (R.M. Featherstone, ed.). M. Dekker, New York, 1973, p.477.

[459]   Yielding, I.L. and Tomkins, G.M., *Proc. Natl. Acad. Sci. U.S.A.* 1960, **46**, 1483–1488.

[460]   Shemisa, C.A. and Fahein, L.A., *Mol. Pharm.* 1971, **7**, 8–25.

[461]   Hulands, G.H., Beard, D.J. and Brammall, A., *Molecular Mechanisms of Anesthesia* (B.R. Fink, ed.). *Progress in Anesthesiology*, Vol. 1. Raven Press, New York, 1975, pp. 501–507.

[462]   Brammall, A., Beard, D.J. and Hulands, G.H., *Brit. J. Anaesth.* 1973, **45**, 923–924.

[463]   Tappel, A.L. and Dillard, C.J., *J. Biol. Chem.* 1967, **242**, 2463–2469.

[464]   Mattson, F.H., Volpenhein, R.A. and Benjamin, L., *J. Biol. Chem.* 1970, **245**, 5335–5340.

[465]   Liu, W.-H., Beppu, T. and Arima, K., *Agr. Biol. Chem.* 1973, **37**, 2487–2492.

[466]   Mates, A., *Lipids* 1973, **8**, 549–552.

[467]   Hansch, C. and Dunn, W.J., *J. Pharm. Sci.* 1972, **61**, 1–19.

[468]   Smith, R.N., Hansch, C. and Poindexter, T.P., *Physiol. Chem. and Phys.* 1974, **6**, 323–331.

[469]   Smith, R.N., Poindexter, T.P. and Hansch, C., *Physiol. Chem. and Physics* 1975, **7**, 423–436.

[470]   Yoshimoto, M. and Hansch, C., *J. Med. Chem.* 1976, **19**, 71–98.

[471]   Tang, J., *J. Biol. Chem.* 1965, **240**, 3810–3815.

[472]   Neumann, H. and Shinitzky, M., *Biochemistry* 1971, **10**, 4335–4342.

[473]   Hegyvary, C., *Biochim. Biophys. Acta* 1973, **311**, 272–291.

[474]   Risley, E.A., Buffington, A.C. and Arnow, L.E., *J. Am. Chem. Soc.* 1944, **66**, 398–401.

[475]   Mitjavila, S., Lacombe, C. and Carrera, G., *Biochem. Pharmacol.* 1976, **25**, 625–630.

[476]   Schwert, G.W. and Eisenberg, M.A., *J. Biol. Chem.* 1949, **179**, 665–672.

[477]   Inagami, T. and Sturtevant, J.M., *Biochim. Biophys. Acta* 1960, **38**, 64–79.

[478] Kallen-Trummer, V., Hofmann, W. and Rottenberg, M., *Biochemistry* 1970, **9**, 3580–3584.

[479] Northrop, J.H., *Crystalline Enzymes*. Columbia University Press, New York, 1939, p. 92.

[480] Shilfrin, S. and Hunn, G., *Arch. Biochem. and Biophys.* 1969, **130**, 530–535.

[481] Groen, G. van der, Wouters-Leysen, J., Yola, M. and de Bruyne, C.K., *Eur. J. Biochem.* 1973, **38**, 122–129.

[482] Laidler, K.J. and Ethier, M.C., *Arch. Biochim. Biophys.* 1953, **44**, 338–345.

[483] George, H., McMahan, J., Bowler, K. and Elliott, M., *Biochim. Biophys. Acta* 1969, **191**, 466–468.

[484] Sather, S.O. and Thimann, K.V., *Plant Physiol.* 1980, **66**, 395–399.

[485] Reynolds, T., *Ann. Bot.* 1977, **41**, 637–648.

[486] Rang, H.P., *Brit. J. Pharmacol.* 1960, **15**, 185–200.

[487] Mongar, J.L. and Schild, H.O., *J. Physiol. (London)* 1957, **135**, 301–319.

[488] Miles, J.L., Robinson, D.A. and Canady, W.J., *J. Biol. Chem.* 1963, **238**, 2932–2937.

[489] Hymes, A.J., Robinson, D.A. and Canady, W.J., *J. Biol. Chem.* 1965, **240**, 134–138.

[490] Wallace, R.A., Kurtz, A.N. and Niemann, C., *Biochemistry* 1963, **2**, 824–836.

[491] Berezin, I.V., Levashov, A.V. and Martinek, K., *FEBS Letters* 1970, **7**, 20–22.

[492] Hansch, C. and Coats, E., *J. Pharm. Sci.* 1970, **59**, 731–743.

[493] Backes, W.L. and Canady, W.J., *Pharmac. Ther.* 1981, **12**, 133–158.

[494] Royer, G. and Canady, W.J., *Arch Biochem. Biophys.* 1968, **124**, 530–534.

[495] Canady, W.J., Westfall, S., Wirtz, G.H. and Robinson, D.A., *Immunochemistry* 1976, **13**, 229–233.

[496] Royer, G., Wildnauer, R., Cuppett, C.C. and Canady, W.J., *J. Biol. Chem.* 1971, **246**, 1129–1134.

[497] Torchilin, V.P., Malismenko, V.P., Sinirnov, A.V., Berezin, I.V., Klibanov, A.M. and Martinek, K., *Biochim. Biophys. Acta* 1978, **567**, 1–11.

[498] Torchilin, V.P. and Martinek, K., *Enzyme and Microbiol. Technology* 1979, **1**, 74–82.

[499] Roth, S.H., *Ann. Rev. Pharmac. and Toxicol.* 1979, **19**, 159–178.

[500] Allison, A.C. and Nunn, J.F., *The Lancet* 1968, **2**, 1326–1329.

[501] Allison, A.C., Hulands, G.F. and Nunn, J.F., *J. Cell. Sci.* 1970, **7**, 483–499.

[502] Sauberman, A.J. and Gallacher, M.L., *Anaesthesiology* 1975, **38**, 25–29.

[503] Hinkley, R.E. and Green, L.S., *J. Neurobiol.* 1971, **2**, 97–105.

[504]   Jost, P.C., Griffith, O.H., Capaldi, R.A. and Vanerkooi, G., *Proc. Nat. Acad. Sci., U.S.A.* 1973, **70**, 480–484.

[505]   Warren, G.B., Toon, P.A., Birdsall, N.J.M., Lee, A.G. and Metcalfe, J.C., *Biochemistry* 1974, **13**, 5501–5507.

[506]   Lee, A.G., *Nature, Lond.* 1976, **262**, 545–548.

[507]   Franks, N.P. and Lieb, W.R., *Nature, Lond.* 1978, **274**, 339–342.

[508]   McGowan, J.C. and Mellors, A., Manuscript submitted.

[509]   Garel, J.P., Filliol, D. and Mandel, P., *J. Chromatography* 1973, **78**, 381–390.

[510]   Steele, R. and Pacsu, E., *Textile Res. J.* 1949, **19**, 784–790.

[511]   Hoskins, M. and Guillet, J.E., *J. Macromol. Sci. A.* 1968, **2**, 1441–1455.

[512]   Smidsnød, O. and Guillet, J.E., *Macromolecules* 1969, **2**, 272–277.

[513]   Chiklis, C.K. and Grasshoff, J.M., *J. Polym. Sci. A.* 1970, **7**, 1617–1626.

[514]   Taylor, L.D. and Cerankowski, L.D., *J. Polym. Sci. A1* 1975, **13**, 2551–2570.

[515]   Kurtz, J., Berger, L.A. and Katchalski, E., *Nature, Lond.* 1956, **178**, 1066–1067.

[516]   Davis, N.G. and Model, P., *Cell* 1985, **41**, 607–614.

[517]   Heijne, G. von., *Eur. J. Biochem.* 1981, **116**, 419–422.

[518]   Davis, N.G., Boeke, J.D. and Model, P., *J. Mol. Biol.* 1985, **181**, 111–121.

[519]   Gething, M.J. and Sambrook, J., *Nature* 1982, **300**, 598–600.

[520]   Gething, M.J., Bye, J.M., Skehal, J.J. and Waterfield, M., *Nature* 1980, **287**, 301–306.

[521]   Blobel, G., *Proc. Natl. Acad. Sci., U.S.A.* 1980, **77**, 1496–1500.

[522]   Stull. D.R., *Indust. and Eng. Chem.* 1967, **39**, 517–550.

[523]   Roark, R.C. and Cotton, R.T., *Tests of Various Aliphatic Compounds as Fumigants*. Technical Bulletin No. 162, United States Department of Agriculture, Washington, D.C., 1929.

[524]   Neifert, I.E., Cook, F.C., Roark, R.C., Tonkin, W.H., Back, E.A. and Cotton, R.T., *Fumigation against Grain Weevils with Various Volatile Organic Compounds*. Bulletin No. 1313, United States Department of Agriculture, Washington, D.C., 1925.

[525]   Heitmuller, P.T., Hollister, T.A. and Parrish, P.R., *Bull. Environ. Contam. Toxicol.* 1981, **27**, 596–604.

[526]   McGowan, J.C., *Rec. Trav. Chim. Pasy-Bas* 1965, **84**, 99–108.

[527]   Smith, B.E., Gaub, M.L. and Maya, F., *Anesth. Analg.* 1965, **44**, 726–732.

[528]   Smith, B.E., Gaub, M.L. and Lehrer, S.B., *Toxicity of Anesthetics* (B.R. Fink, ed.). Williams and Wilkins, Baltimore, 1968, pp. 269–278.

[529]   Smith, B.E., Gaub, M.L. and Maya, F., *Anesthesiology* 1965, **26**, 260–261.

[530]   Anderson, N.B., *Anesthesiology* 1968, **29**, 113–122.

[531] Rector, G.H.M. and Eastwood, D.W., *Anesthesiology* 1964, **25**, 109 only.

[532] Basford, A.B. and Fink, B.R., *Anesthesiology* 1968, **29**, 1167–1173.

[533] Knill-Jones, R.P., Moir, D.D., Rodrigques, L.V. and Spence, A.A., *Lancet* 1972, **i**, 1326.

[534] Plichenfelder, J.D., *Anesthesiology* 1980, **53**, 1–2.

[535] Spence, A.A., Cohen, E.N., Brown, B.W., Knill-Jones, R.P. and Himmelberger, J., *J. Am. Med. Ass.* 1977, **238**, 955–959.

[536] Sice, J., *Toxicol. Appl. Pharmacol.* 1966, **9**, 70–74.

[537] Duuren, B.L. van, Witz, G. and Goldschmidt, B.M., *Carcinogenesis. A Comprehensive Survey* (T.J. Slaga, A. Sivak and R.K. Boutwell, eds.). Raven Press, New York, 1978, pp. 491–507.

[538] House of Commons Official Report. *Parliamentary Debates (Hansard)*. 19th November, 1981. HMSO, London, Vol. 13, No. 12, p. 75.

[539] House of Commons Official Report. *Parliamentary Debates (Hansard)*. Debate (Second Reading) on local Government (Miscellaneous Provisions) Bill, 25th November, 1981. HMSO, London, Vol. 13, No. 16, pp. 903–972.

[540] House of Commons Official Report. *Parliamentary Debates (Hansard)*. 9th November, 1983. HMSO, London, pp. 381–396.

[541] King, M.D., Day, R.E., Oliver, J.S., Lush, M. and Watson, J.M., *Brit. Med. J.* 1981, **283**, 663–665.

[542] Childs, P.E., *Chem. and Ind.* 1982, 21st August, 559.

[543] Annual Meeting 1980, *American Conference of Governmental Industrial Hygienists*, Cincinnati, Ohio.

[544] Sato, A. and Nakajima, T., *Arch. Environ. Health.* 1979, **34**, 69–75.

[545] Grove, J.F. and McGowan, J.C., *Chem. and Ind.* 1949, 647–652.

[546] Hassall, K.E., *Ann. Appl. Biol.* 1953, **40**, 688–704.

[547] Hammett, L.P., *J. Am. Chem. Soc.* 1937, **59**, 96–103.

[548] Hammett, L.B., *Physical Organic Chemistry*. McGraw-Hill Book Co., New York, 1940, Chap. 7.

[549] Hansch, C., *Drug Design*, Vol. 1 (E.J. Ariens, ed.). Academic Press, New York, 1971, Chap. 2, pp. 271–404.

[550] McGowan, J.C., *J. Soc. Chem. Ind.* 1949, **68**, 253–258.

[551] McGowan, J.C., *Chem. and Ind.* 1936, **55**, 607–608.

[552] McGowan, J.C., Brian, P.W. and Hemming, H.G., *Ann. Appl. Biol.* 1948, **35**, 25–36.

[553] Brian, P.W., Grove, J.F. and McGowan, J.C., *Nature, Lond.* 1946, **158**, 876.

[554] Bosquet, E.W., Kirby, J.E. and Searle, N.E., U.S. Patent 1943, No. 2335384.

[555] Geiger, W.B. and Conn, J.E., *J. Am. Chem. Soc.* 1945, **67**, 112–116.

[556] Rindernecht, H., Ward, J.L., Bergel, F. and Morrison, A.L., *Biochem. J.* 1947, **41**, 463–469.

[557] Geiger, W.B., *Archiv. Biochem.* 1948, **16**, 423–425.

[558]   Zienty, F.B., Vineyard, B.D. and Schleppink, J., *J. Org. Chem.* 1962, **27**, 3140–3146.

[559]   Clark, N.G., Hams, A.F. and Legetter, B.E., *Nature, Lond.* 1963, **200**, 171.

[560]   Cromwell, N.H., Greger, P.L. and Cook, K.E., *J. Am. Chem. Soc.* 1956, **78**, 4412–4419.

[561]   Cramer, B.J., Schroeder, W., Moran, W.J., Nield, C.H., Edwards, M.A., Jarowski, C.I. and Puetzer, B., *J. Am. Pharm. Assoc. Sci. Ed.* 1948, **37**, 439–449.

[562]   Morgan, L.W., Cronk, D.H. and Knott, R.P., *J. Pharm. Sci.* 1969, **58**, 942–945.

[563]   Dixon, M. and Needham, D.M., *Nature, Lond.* 1946, **158**, 432–438.

[564]   Bryde, R.J.W., *Fungicides – An Advanced Treatise.* Vol. II, *Chemistry and Physiology* (D.C. Torgeson, ed.). Academic Press, New York and London, 1969, Chapt. 12.

[565]   Busvine, J.R., *Nature, Lond.* 1942, **150**, 208–209.

[566]   Haldane, J.B.S., *Science Advances.* Allen and Unwin, London, 1947, pp. 86–87.

[567]   Leggenhager, K., *Z. ges. exptl. Med.* 1950, **116**, 353–377.

[568]   Linas, A.J. and Limousin, S., *Bull. Mém. Soc. Thérap.* 1868, **2**, 32.

[569]   Douglas, C.G., Haldane, J.S. and Haldane, J.B.S., *J. Physiol.* 1912, **44**, 275–304.

[570]   Sendroy, J., Liu, A.H. and van Slyke, D.D., *Amer. J. Physiol.* 1929, **90**, 511–512.

[571]   Woolley, D.W., *Physiological Reviews* 1947, **27**, 308–333.

[572]   Woolley, D.W. and Roblin, R.O., *Chem. Rev.* 1946, **38**, 255–377.

[573]   Woolley, D.W., *Ann. N.Y. Acad. Sci.* 1950, **52**, 1197–1378.

[574]   Woolley, D.W., *A Study of Antimetabolites.* New York, 1952.

[575]   Gibson, R.E. and Loeffler, O.H., *J. Am. Chem. Soc.* 1939, **61**, 2515–2522.

[576]   Goursot, P., Girdhar, H.L. and Westrum, E.F., *J. Phys. Chem.* 1970, **74**, 2538–2541.

[577]   Marti, F.B., *Bull. Soc. Chim. Belg.* 1930, **39**, 590–626.

[578]   Vernon, H.M., *J. Physiology* 1913, **47**, 15–29.

Formula index

After the formula in this index, is given the name of the compound used by chemists today. Then in brackets may be given a name commonly used by biologists and others.

A	Argon, 28, 77, 78
BaCl$_2$	Barium chloride, 42, 108
Br$_2$	Bromine, 68
CBr$_4$	Methane, tetrabromo- (Carbon tetrabromide), 31
CCl$_3$F	Methane, trichlorofluoro-, 175
CCl$_4$	Methane, tetrachloro- (Carbon tetrachloride), 19, 20, 24, 29, 30, 31, 32, 67, 75, 76, 87, 92, 93, 101, 123, 131, 142, 174, 177, 182, 183, 214
CHBr$_3$	Methane, tribromo-, 19, 31, 68, 75
CHCl$_2$F	Methane, dichlorofluoro-, 174
CHCl$_3$	Methane, trichloro- (Chloroform), 19, 22, 23, 43, 64, 67, 75, 81, 91, 117, 118, 122, 133, 146, 174, 182, 183, 196, 214
CHI$_3$	Methane, triiodo- (Iodofrom), 31, 32
CHN	Hydrogen cyanide (Hydrocyanic acid), 182, 183
CH$_2$Br$_2$	Methane, dibromo- (Methylene dibromide), 19, 64, 87
CH$_2$Cl$_2$	Methane, dichloro- (Methylene dichloride), 19, 20, 124, 142, 146, 174, 214
CH$_2$O	Methanal (Formaldehyde), 88
CH$_3$Br	Methane, bromo- (Methyl bromide), 214
CH$_3$Cl	Methane, chloro- (Methyl chloride), 178, 179, 182
CH$_3$I	Methane, iodo- (Methyl iodide), 19
CH$_3$NO	Formic acid amide (Formamide), 88
CH$_3$NO$_2$	Methane, nitro-, 176, 414
CH$_4$	Methane, 35, 97
CH$_4$N$_2$O	Carbamide (Urea), 38
CH$_4$N$_2$S	Urea, 2-thio-, 37, 38
CH$_4$O	Methanol (Methyl alcohol), 38, 39, 67, 77, 78, 88, 92, 96, 100, 101, 103, 104, 108–110, 112–114, 122, 136, 150, 156–159, 175, 177, 184, 196, 197, 212–214
CI$_4$	methane, tetraiodo- (Carbon tetraiodide), 31, 32
CNNa	Sodium cyanide, 114
CNNaS	Sodium thiocyanate, 137
CO	Carbon monoxide, 185
CO$_2$	Carbon dioxide 68, 104, 214
CS$_2$	Carbon disulphide, 68, 69, 75, 76, 81, 176, 178, 182, 191–193, 214
C$_2$BrI$_3$	Ethene, bromo-triiodo, 32
C$_2$Br$_2$I$_2$	Ethene, 1,1-dibromo-2,2-diiodo-, 32
C$_2$Br$_4$	Ethene, tetrabromo- (tetrabromoethylene), 32

$C_2Cl_2F_4$ Ethane,1,2-dichloro-1,1,2,2,-tetrafluoro-, 174
$C_2Cl_3KO_2$ Ethanoic acid, trichloro- potassium salt (Potassium trichloracetate), 162
C_2Cl_4 Ethene, tetrachloro- (Tetrachloroethylene), 32, 124, 174, 182, 183
$C_2HBrClF_3$ Ethane, 2-bromo-2-chloro-1,1,1-trifluoro- ("Halothane"), 162
C_2HCl_3 Ethene, trichloro- (Trichlorethylene), 174, 182, 183, 214
C_2HCl_5 Ethane, pentachloro-, 20
C_2H_2 Ethyne (Acetylene), 35
C_2H_2Br Ethane, 1,1,2,2-tetrabromo-, 87
$C_2H_2Cl_2$ Ethene, 1,1-dichloro-, 124
$C_2H_2Cl_2$ Ethene, 1,2-dichloro-, 67, 75, 124, 182
$C_2H_2Cl_4$ Ethane, 1,1,1,2-tetrachloro-, 124
$C_2H_2Cl_4$ Ethane, 1,1,2,2-tetrachloro-, 9, 124
$C_2H_2I_2$ Ethene, 1,2-diiodo-, 32
$C_2H_3Cl_3$ Ethane, 1,1,1-trichloro-, 20, 87, 142
$C_2H_3Cl_3O$ 1,1-Ethanediol, 2,2,2-trichloro- (Chloral hydrate), 18
C_2H_3N Acetic acid nitrile (Acetonitrile), 38
$C_2H_3NaO_2$ Sodium acetate, 137
C_2H_4 Ethene (Ethylene), 31, 35, 214
$C_2H_4Br_2$ Ethane, 1,2-dibromo- (Ethylene dibromide), 65, 68, 75, 76, 178, 214
C_2H_4ClNO Chloracetic acid amide (Acetamide, 2-chloro-), 89
$C_2H_4Cl_2$ Ethane, 1,1-dichloro- (Ethylidene chloride), 19, 67, 75, 117
$C_2H_4Cl_2$ Ethane, 1,2-dichloro- (Ethylene chloride), 19, 67, 75, 76, 116, 123, 142, 174, 214
C_2H_4O Oxirane (Ethylene oxide), 183
$C_2H_4O_2$ Ethanoic acid (Acetic acid), 69, 164, 214
C_2H_5Br Ethane, bromo- (Ethyl bromide), 19, 56, 182
C_2H_5Cl Ethane, chloro- (Ethyl chloride), 19, 182, 214
C_2H_5I Ethane, iodo- (Ethyl iodide), 19, 71
C_2H_5NO Ethanamide (Acetamide), 37, 38, 88
C_2H_5NO Formamide, N-methyl-, 96, 97
$C_2H_5NO_2$ Ethane, nitro-, 176
$C_2H_5NO_2$ Aminoethanoic acid (Glycine), 49, 50, 110, 164
$C_2H_5NO_2$ Carbamic acid methyl ester (Methyl urethane), 197, 212
C_2H_6 Ethane, 35
C_2H_6O Ethanol (Ethyl alcohol), 18, 38, 67, 78, 88, 92, 93, 96–101, 103, 104, 108–114, 122, 136, 148, 150, 156–159, 164, 175, 184, 196, 197, 212–214
C_2H_6O Methane, methoxy- (Dimethyl ether), 214
$C_2H_6O_2$ Ethane 1,2-diol (Glycol), 38, 39, 139, 140, 164, 214
C_2H_6S Ethane thiol (Ethyl mercaptan), 38
C_2H_6SO Methane sulphinylbis- (Dimethylsulphoxide), 102, 157, 158, 214
C_2H_7N Ethanamine (Ethylamine), 23
C_2H_7N Methanamine, N-methyl- (Dimethylamine), 23
C_2I_4 Ethene tetraiodo- (Tetraiodoethylene), 32
$C_2Na_2O_4$ Ethanedioic acid, sodium salt (Sodium oxalate), 42
C_3F_8 Propane, octafluoro-, 121
$C_3H_4Cl_2$ Propene, 1,3-dichloro-, 124
$C_3H_5Cl_3$ Propane, 1,2,3-trichloro-, 20
$C_3H_6ClNO_2$ Propane, 1-chloro-1-nitro-, 176
$C_3H_6Cl_2$ Propane, 1,2-dichloro-, 214
C_3H_6O 2-Propen-1-ol (Allyl alcohol), 38, 136
C_3H_6O 2-Propanone (Acetone), 38, 39, 67, 78, 81, 88, 91, 102, 157, 158, 164, 175, 214
C_3H_6O Propanal (Propionaldehyde), 88
$C_3H_6O_2$ Ethanoic acid methyl ester (Methyl acetate), 38, 71, 88, 94, 175, 182, 183
$C_3H_6O_2$ Methanoic acid ethyl eser (Ethyl formate), 95
$C_3H_6O_3$ Carbonic acid dimethyl ester (Dimethyl carbonate), 42, 43
C_3H_7Br Propane, 1-bromo- (n-Propyl bromide), 19
C_3H_7Br Propane, 2-bromo- (Isopropyl bromide), 19
C_3H_7Cl Propane, 1-chloro- (n-Propyl chloride), 19
C_3H_7Cl Propane, 2-chloro- (Isopropyl chloride), 17
C_3H_7I Propane, 1-iodo- (n-Propyl iodide), 19, 87
C_3H_7NO Propanoic acid amide (Propionamide), 89

C$_3$H$_7$NO$_2$ 2-Amino-propanoic acid (Alanine), 49, 50, 109, 111, 112, 123
C$_3$H$_7$NO$_2$ Carbamic acid, ethyl ester (Urethane), 123, 164, 197, 212, 215
C$_3$H$_7$NO$_2$ Propane, 2-nitro, 176
C$_3$H$_7$NO$_2$S Propionic acid, 2-amino-3-mercapto- (Cysteine), 181
C$_3$H$_7$NO$_3$ 2-Amino-3-hydroxy-propanoic acid (Serine), 164
C$_3$H$_8$ Propane, 64
C$_3$H$_8$O 1-Propanol (n-Propyl alcohol), 38, 88, 103, 104, 117, 122, 136, 148, 150, 156–159, 184, 196, 197, 212, 213, 215
C$_3$H$_8$O 2-Propanol (Isopropyl alcohol), 38, 67, 104, 157, 158, 175
C$_3$H$_8$O$_2$ Ethanol, 2-methoxy-, 164, 176
C$_3$H$_8$O$_2$ Methane, dimethoxy-, 176
C$_3$H$_8$O$_3$ 1,2,3-Propanetriol (Glycerol), 38, 39, 95, 139, 140, 157, 158, 215
C$_3$H$_9$N Methanamine, N,N-dimethyl-, (Trimethylamine), 23
C$_3$H$_{10}$BrN N,N-Dimethylmethanium bromide (Trimethylammonium bromide), 162
C$_4$H$_4$S Thiophene, 215
C$_4$H$_5$NS Isothiocyanic acid propenyl ester, (Allyl isothio-cyanate), 173
C$_4$H$_5$NO$_2$S Thiocyanoacetic acid methyl ester, 179
C$_4$H$_6$O 2-Butenal (Crotonaldehyde), 180
C$_4$H$_6$O$_2$S Ethene, 1,1'-sulphonylbis- (Diethenyl sulphone), 180
C$_4$H$_6$O$_4$ Butanedioic acid (Succinic acid), 134, 135, 153
C$_4$H$_7$Cl$_3$O 2-Propanol, 2-methyl-1,1,1-trichloro- (Chloreton), 18
C$_4$H$_7$N Butanoic acid nitrile (Butyronitrile), 89
C$_4$H$_7$NO$_4$ Butanedioic acid 2-amino- (Aspartic acid), 164
C$_4$H$_8$O 2-Butanone (Methylethyl ketone), 94, 175, 215
C$_4$H$_8$O 1,4-Epoxybutane (Tetrahydrofuran), 158
C$_4$H$_8$O$_2$ Ethanoic acid ethyl ester (Ethyl acetate), 18, 38, 39, 71, 88, 94, 104, 117, 128, 142, 172, 175, 182, 183, 197, 212, 215
C$_4$H$_8$O$_2$ Methanoic acid propyl ester (n-propyl formate), 38
C$_4$H$_8$O$_2$ Propanoic acid methyl ester (Methyl propionate), 38
C$_4$H$_8$O$_2$ 1,4-Dioxane, 156–158, 176
C$_4$H$_9$Br Propane, 1-bromo-2-methyl- (Isobutyl bromide), 87
C$_4$H$_9$Cl Butane, 1-chloro- (n-Butyl chloride), 142
C$_4$H$_9$Cl Propane, 1-chloro-2-methyl- (Isobutyl chloride), 87
C$_4$H$_9$Cl Propane, 2-chloro-2-methyl- (t-Butyl chloride), 179
C$_4$H$_9$NO Butanoic acid amide (n-Butyramide), 89
C$_4$H$_9$NO$_2$ Carbamic acid propyl ester (Propyl urethane), 197, 212
C$_4$H$_9$NO$_2$ Butanoic acid, 2-amino- (α-Aminobutyric acid), 49, 50, 109, 111, 163
C$_4$H$_9$NO$_3$ Butanoic acid, 2-amino-3-hydroxy- (Threonine), 164
C$_4$H$_{10}$ Butane, 96, 215
C$_4$H$_{10}$O 1-Butanol (Butyl alcohol), 18, 71, 88, 94, 103, 104, 122, 132, 133, 136, 142, 148, 150, 154, 158, 159, 164, 175, 184, 194–197, 212, 213, 215
C$_4$H$_{10}$O 1-Propanol, 2-methyl- (Isobutyl alcohol), 18, 38, 88, 136, 158, 196
C$_4$H$_{10}$O 2-Butanol (sec-Butyl alcohol), 88, 104
C$_4$H$_{10}$O 2-Propanol, 2-methyl- (t-Butyl alcohol), 88, 104, 156, 157
C$_4$H$_{10}$O Ethane, 1,1'-oxybis- (Ether), 18, 23, 67, 71, 76, 81, 88–91, 95, 96, 98, 104, 111, 112, 122, 123, 128, 142, 162, 163, 195, 196, 215
C$_4$H$_{10}$O$_3$ Ethanol, 2,2'-oxybis- (Diethylene glycol), 102
C$_4$H$_{10}$O$_4$ Butane, 1,2,3,4-tetrahydroxy- (Erythritol), 38, 139, 140
C$_4$H$_{11}$N Ethanamine, N-ethyl- (Diethylamine), 23
C$_4$H$_{12}$BrN N,N,N-Trimethylmethanamium bromide (Tetramethyl-ammonium bromide), 108
C$_4$H$_{12}$ClN N,N,N-Trimethylmethanamium chloride (Tetramethyl-ammonium chloride), 42
C$_4$H$_{12}$ClNO$_4$ N,N,N-Trimethylmethanamium perchlorate (Tetra-methylammonium perchlorate), 109, 114
C$_4$H$_{12}$Ge Germane, tetramethyl-, 97
C$_4$H$_{12}$Si Silane, tetramethyl-, 97
C$_4$H$_{12}$Sn Stannane, tetramethyl-, 97
C$_7$H$_7$NO$_2$S Thiocyanoacetic acid, ethyl ester, 179
C$_5$H$_8$N$_2$O$_3$ α-Aminosuccinamic acid (Asparagine), 167
C$_5$H$_8$O$_2$ Ethanoic acid propenyl ester (Allyl acetate), 38
C$_5$H$_9$NO$_2$ 2-Pyrrolidine carboxylic acid (Proline), 164

$C_5H_9NO_4$ 2-Aminopentanedioic acid (Glutamic acid), 164
C_5H_{10} 1-Pentene, 103
C_5H_{10} Cyclopentane, 20
$C_5H_{10}N_2O_3$ 2-Aminoglutaramic acid (Glutamine), 167
$C_5H_{10}O$ 2-Pentanone, 95, 175, 215
$C_5H_{10}O$ 3-Pentanone, 95
$C_5H_{10}O$ 2-Butanone, 3-methyl-, 94
$C_5H_{10}O_2$ Butanoic acid, methyl ester (Methyl n-Butyrate), 215
$C_5H_{10}O_2$ Ethanoic acid, 1-propyl ester (n-Propyl acetate), 18, 38, 94, 128, 175, 197, 212, 215
$C_5H_{10}O_2$ Ethanoic acid, 2-propyl ester (Isopropyl acetate), 18
$C_5H_{10}O_2$ Propanoic acid, ethyl ester (Ethyl Propionate), 215
$C_5H_{10}O_3$ Ethanol, 2-methoxy-, acetate, 76
$C_5H_{10}O_3$ Carbonic acid, diethyl ester, 172
$C_5H_{10}O_4$ Propane, 1,2,3-triol monoethanoate (Glycerol monoacetate), 140
$C_5H_{10}O_5$ Arabinose, 138, 139
$C_5H_{10}O_5$ Ribose, 138
$C_5H_{10}O_5$ Xylose, 38, 138, 139
$C_5H_{11}Cl$ Pentane, 1-chloro- (n-Amyl chloride), 215
$C_5H_{11}Cl$ Butane, 2-methyl-2-chloro-, 179
$C_5H_{11}N$ Pentamethyleneimine (Piperidine), 23
$C_5H_{11}NO_2$ Butanoic acid, 2-amino-3-methyl- (Valine), 164
$C_5H_{11}NO_2$ Carbamic acid, butyl ester (n-Butyl urethane), 197, 212
$C_5H_{11}NO_2S$ Butanoic acid, 2-amino-4(methylthio)- (Methionine), 164
C_5H_{12} Pentane, 64, 84, 103, 160, 175, 215
C_5H_{12} Butane, 2-methyl- (Isopentane), 103, 215
C_5H_{12} Propane, 2,2-dimethyl- (Neopentane), 61, 62, 97
$C_5H_{12}N_2O_2$ Pentanoic acid, 2,5-diamino- (Ornithine), 164
$C_5H_{12}O$ 1-Pentanol (n-Amyl alcohol), 92, 117, 129, 133, 136, 142, 148, 150, 154, 158, 159, 196, 197, 212, 213, 215
$C_5H_{12}O$ 1-Butanol, 2-methyl-, 136
$C_5H_{12}O$ 1-Butanol, 3-methyl-, 18, 38
$C_5H_{12}O$ 2-Butanol, 2-methyl-, 18, 38
$C_5H_{12}O_3$ 2,3-Propanediol, 1-ethoxy-, 140
$C_5H_{12}O_4$ 1,3-Propanediol, 2,2-bishydroxymethyl- (Pentaerythritol), 140
$C_5H_{13}N$ Pentamine (n-Amylamine), 23
C_6F_6 Benzene, hexafluoro-, 67, 78
$C_6H_2Cl_4$ Benzene, 1,2,3,5-tetrachloro-, 21
$C_6H_3Cl_3$ Benzene, 1,2,3-trichloro-, 20
$C_6H_4ClNO_2$ Benzene, 1-chloro-2-nitro-, 101
$C_6H_4ClNO_2$ Benzene, 1-chloro-4-nitro-, 101
$C_6H_4Cl_2$ Benzene, 1,2-dichloro-, 124, 142, 174, 177, 215
$C_6H_4Cl_2$ Benzene, 1,3-dichloro-, 124
$C_6H_4Cl_2$ Benzene, 1,4-dichloro-, 215
$C_6H_4O_2$ 2,5-Cyclohexadiene-1,4-dione (p-Benzoquinone), 184
C_6H_5Br Benzene, bromo-, 67, 78, 81, 215
C_6H_5Cl Benzene, chloro-, 20, 64, 67, 78, 81, 122, 131, 146, 160, 174, 189, 190, 215
C_6H_5ClO Benzene, 1-hydroxy-4-chloro-, 133
C_6H_5F Benzene, fluoro-, 78
C_6H_5FO Benzene, 1-hydroxy-4-fluoro-, 133
C_6H_5I Benzene, iodo-, 68, 76, 78, 215
$C_6H_5NO_2$ Benzene, nitro-, 43, 68, 72, 78, 81, 107, 114–116, 142, 160, 176, 216
$C_6H_5NO_3$ Benzene, 1-hydroxy-4-nitro- (4-nitrophenol), 184
C_6H_6 Benzene, 18, 20, 24, 35, 67, 69, 72, 75, 76, 78, 81, 86, 87, 100, 105, 107, 108, 114, 122, 131, 142, 146, 160, 161, 172, 177, 182, 183, 216
$C_6H_6N_2O$ Benzenamine, 4-nitroso-, (p-Nitrosoaniline), 184
C_6H_6O Benzene, hydroxy- (Phenol), 38, 72, 89, 133, 175, 184, 216
$C_6H_6O_2$ Benzene, 1,2-dihydroxy- (Catechol), 38, 128
$C_6H_6O_2$ Benzene, 1,3-dihydroxy- (Resorcinol), 38, 129
$C_6H_6O_2$ Benzene, 1,4-dihydroxy- (Hydroquinone), 38, 129
$C_6H_6O_3$ Benzene, 1,2,3-trihydroxy- (Pyrogallol), 39
$C_6H_6O_3$ Benzene, 1,3,5-trihydroxy- (Phloroglucinol), 39

C_6H_7N	Benzamine (Aniline), 68, 176, 216
$C_6H_8O_2$	2,4-Hexadienoic acid (Sorbic acid), 180–182
$C_6H_8O_2$	*trans*-Butenedioic acid methyl ester (Dimethyl fumarate), 180
$C_6H_9N_3O_2$	Propanoic acid, 2-amino-3-(4-imidazol)- (Histidine), 164
C_6H_{10}	Cyclohexene, 160, 174
$C_6H_{10}O$	Cyclohexanone, 175
$C_6H_{10}O_3$	Butanoic acid, 3-oxo-, ethyl ester (Ethyl acetoacetate), 38
$C_6H_{10}O_4$	1,2-Ethanediol diethanoate (Glycol diacetate), 140
$C_6H_{10}O_5$	Cyclohexane 1,2,3,4,5-pentahydroxy (Quercitol), 38
C_6H_{12}	Cyclopentane, methyl-, 20
C_6H_{12}	Cyclohexane, 20, 59–62, 64, 67, 78, 81, 142, 160, 174, 216
$C_6H_{12}O$	Cyclohexanol, 67, 78, 94, 175, 216
$C_6H_{12}O$	3-Pentanone 2-methyl-, 95
$C_6H_{12}O$	2-Hexanone, 95, 175
$C_6H_{12}O$	3-Hexanone, 95
$C_6H_{12}O$	2-Pentanone 3-methyl-, 95
$C_6H_{12}O$	2-Pentanone, 4-methyl-, 95, 175
$C_6H_{12}O_2$	Ethanoic acid butyl ester (n-Butyl acetate), 94, 128, 175, 197, 212
$C_6H_{12}O_2$	Butanoic acid ethyl ester (Ethyl butyrate), 94
$C_6H_{12}O_2$	Ethanoic acid 2-methyl-1-propyl ester, 18, 175
$C_6H_{12}O_2S$	Sulphone, butyl-ethenyl-, 180, 181
$C_6H_{12}O_3$	1,3,5-Trioxane,2,4,6-trimethyl- (Paraldehyde), 18, 216
$C_6H_{12}O_5$	Rhamnose, 138, 139
$C_6H_{12}O_6$	Glucose, 38, 50, 51, 138, 139
$C_6H_{12}O_6$	Galactose, 139
$C_6H_{12}O_6$	Mannose, 139
$C_6H_{12}O_6$	Fructose, 38, 50, 51, 139
$C_6H_{13}NO_2$	Pentanoic acid, 2-amino-4-methyl (Leucine), 111, 112, 163, 164
$C_6H_{13}NO_2$	Pentanoic acid, 2-amino-3-methyl (Isoleucine), 110, 164
$C_6H_{13}NO_2$	Carbamic acid, pentyl ester (*n*-Amyl urethane), 197, 212
C_6H_{14}	Hexane, 20, 56, 60, 67, 75, 81, 84, 86, 96, 100, 103, 146, 153, 172, 174, 191, 192, 216
C_6H_{14}	Pentane, 2-methyl-, 103
C_6H_{14}	Pentane, 3-methyl-, 20, 104
C_6H_{14}	Butane, 2,2-dimethyl-, 104
C_6H_{14}	Butane, 2,3-dimethyl-, 104
$C_6H_{14}N_2O_2$	Hexanoic acid, 2,6-diamino- (Lysine), 164
$C_6H_{14}N_4O_2$	Pentanoic acid, 2-amino-5-guanidino- (Arginine), 164
$C_6H_{14}O$	1-Hexanol, 92, 94, 95, 128, 132, 133, 136, 142, 154, 158, 159, 172, 196, 197, 212, 213, 216
$C_6H_{14}O$	2-Hexanol, 150
$C_6H_{14}O$	1-Butanol, 1,3-dimethyl-, 175
$C_6H_{14}O$	Propane, 1,1'-oxybis- (Di-n-propyl ether), 92, 94, 128, 216
$C_6H_{14}O$	Propane, 2,2'-oxybis- (Di-siopropyl ether), 102, 176
$C_6H_{14}O_2$	Ethanol, 2-butoxy-, 164, 176
$C_6H_{14}O_6$	Hexane, 1,2,3,4,5,6-hexol- (Mannitol), 38
$C_6H_{15}ClN_2O_2$	2[(Aminocarbonyl)oxyl]-*N,N,N*-trimethylethanaminium chloride, 125, 158
$C_6H_{15}N$	Ethanamine, *N,N*-diethyl- (Triethylamine), 23
C_7F_{14}	Cyclohexane, hendecafluoro-trifluoromethyl-, 67, 75, 78
C_7F_{16}	Heptane, hexadecafluoro-, 67, 76
$C_7H_5O_2Na$	Sodium benzoate, 135, 137
C_7H_6O	Benzaldehyde (Benzenecarbonal), 94
C_7H_7Cl	Benzene, 1-chloro-2-methyl- (Toluene, 2-chloro-), 175
$C_7H_7NO_2$	Benzene, 1-methyl-2-nitro- (Toluene, nitro-), 176
$C_7H_7NO_2$	Benzoic acid, 4-amino-, 181
C_7H_8	Benzene, methyl- (Toluene), 20, 67, 76, 78, 124, 131, 146, 160, 161, 175, 182, 183, 216
C_7H_8O	Benzene, hydroxy-methyl- (Cresol), 175
C_7H_8O	Benzene, 1-hydroxy-2-methyl- (*o*-Cresol), 38, 95, 128, 216
C_7H_8O	Benzene, 1-hydroxy-3-methyl- (*m*-Cresol), 38, 95, 128, 216
C_7H_8O	Benzene, 1-hydroxy-4-methyl- (*p*-Cresol), 38, 128, 133, 213
C_7H_8O	Benzene, methoxy- (Anisole), 92

C_7H_8O Benzenemethanol (Benzyl alcohol), 94, 133, 136, 184, 216
$C_7H_8O_2$ Benzene, 1-hydroxy-2-methoxy- (o-Methoxyphenol), 129
$C_7H_8O_2$ Benzene, 1-hydroxy-4-methoxy- (p-Methoxyphenol), 129, 133
C_7H_9N Benzamine, methyl- (Toluidine), 176
$C_7H_{11}NO_2S$ Thiocyanoacetic acid, butyl ester, 179
$C_7H_{12}O$ Cyclohexanone, methyl-, 175
$C_7H_{12}O_5$ 1,2,3-Propanetriol diethanoate (Glycerol diacetate), 140
C_7H_{14} Cyclohexane, methyl-, 20, 67, 78, 174, 216
$C_7H_{14}O$ 3-Pentanone,2,4-dimethyl-, 95
$C_7H_{14}O$ 2-Heptanone, 95
$C_7H_{14}O$ 3-Heptanone, 95
$C_7H_{14}O$ Cyclohexanol, methyl-, 175
$C_7H_{14}O_2$ Ethanoic acid, pentyl ester (n-Amyl acetate), 197, 212
$C_7H_{14}O_2$ Ethanoic acid, 3-methylbutyl ester (Isoamyl acetate), 175
$C_7H_{14}O_6$ Methyl-D-glucopyranoside (methyl glucoside), 140
$C_7H_{15}Cl$ Heptane, 1-chloro- (n-Heptyl chloride), 216
C_7H_{16} Heptane, 67, 75, 76, 84, 96, 101, 103, 104, 153, 172, 174, 216
C_7H_{16} Hexane, 3-methyl-, 104
C_7H_{16} Pentane, 2,4-dimethyl-, 104
$C_7H_{16}O$ 3-Pentanol, 3-ethyl-, 92
$C_7H_{16}O$ 1-Hetanol (n-Heptyl alcohol), 18, 92, 95, 122, 133, 142, 148, 158, 159, 184, 196, 197, 212, 213, 216
$C_7H_{16}O_3$ 2-Propanol, 1,3-diethoxy-, 140
$C_8H_6ClNO_2$ Benzene, 1-ethenylnitro-4-chloro-, 180
$C_8H_7NO_2$ Benzene, ethenylnitro- (β-Nitrostyrene), 180, 181
C_8H_8O Ethanone, 1-phenyl- (Acetophenone), 95
$C_8H_8O_2$ Benzoic acid, methyl ester, 172
$C_8H_8O_3$ Benzoic acid, 4-hydroxy-, methyl ester, 133
$C_8H_8O_4$ 2,4-Pyrandione, 3-acetyl-6-methyl- (Dehydracetic acid), 180–182
C_8H_9NO Acetamide, N-phenyl- (Acetanilide), 89
C_8H_{10} Benzene, ethyl-, 20, 160, 174
C_8H_{10} Benzene, 1,3-dimehtyl- (o-Xylene), 131, 216
C_8H_{10} Benzene, 1,4-dimethyl- (p-Xylene), 20, 131, 146, 172, 216
C_8H_{10} benzene, 1,3-dimethyl- (m-Xylene), 22, 23, 64, 67, 76, 123, 131, 174, 216
$C_8H_{10}O$ Benzene, 1-hydroxy-3,4-dimethyl-, 128
$C_8H_{10}O$ Benzene, 1-hydroxy-3,5-dimethyl-, 133
$C_8H_{11}N$ Benzamine, N,N-dimethyl- (Dimethyl anilinel), 176
$C_8H_{12}N_2O_3$ 5,5-Diethyl-2,4,6-(1H,3H,5H)-pyrrimidinetrione (Veronal), 18
$C_8H_{12}O_4$ trans-Butenedioic acid ethyl ester (Ethyl fumarate), 180
$C_8H_{15}NO_3$ Butanoic acid, 2-acetamido-3-methyl- methyl ester (N-Acetylvaline methyl ester), 161
C_8H_{16} Cyclooctane, 20
$C_8H_{16}O_2$ Hexanoic acid ethyl ester, 95
$C_8H_{16}O_2$ Ethanoic acid 1-methylpentyl ester, 175
$C_8H_{17}Cl$ Octane, 1-chloro-, 114, 132, 217
C_8H_{18} Octane, 21, 67, 78, 84, 97, 99, 147, 172, 175, 217
C_8H_{18} Heptane, 3-methyl-, 67
C_8H_{18} Pentane, 2,2,4-trimethyl-, 75, 101, 217
$C_8H_{18}O$ 1-Octanol, 67, 78, 91, 97, 122, 132, 133, 142, 145, 148, 150, 154, 158, 159, 161, 196, 212, 217
$C_8H_{18}O$ 2-Octanol, 150
$C_8H_{18}O$ Butane, 1,1'-oxybis- (Di-n-butyl ether), 102, 128, 139, 217
$C_8H_{19}O_4P$ Phosphoric acid, di-n-butyl ester, 90
$C_8H_{20}BrN$ N,N,N-Triethylethanamium bromide (Tetraethylammonium bromide), 108
$C_8H_{20}ClN$ N,N,N-Triethylethanamium chloride (Tetraethylammonium chloride), 42
$C_8H_{20}ClNO_4$ N,N,N-Triethylethanamium perchlorate (Tetraethylammonium perchlorate), 114
$C_8H_{20}IN$ N,N,N-Tetraethylethanamium iodide (Tetraethylammonium iodide), 116
$C_8H_{20}SI$ Silane, tetraethyl-, 97
$C_8H_{20}Sn$ Stannane, tetraethyl-, 97
$C_8H_{24}O_4Si_4$ Octamethylcyclotetrasiloxane, 67, 75, 76
C_9H_7NO 8-Quinolinol (8-Hydroxyquinoline), 102

C_9H_8 Indene, 160
C_9H_8O 2-Propenal, 3-phenyl- (Cinnamaldehyde), 180
$C_9H_8O_2$ 2-Propenoic acid, 3-phenyl (Cinnamic acid), 180
$C_9H_9NO_2$ Benzene, 2-nitro-1-propenyl-, 181
$C_9H_9NO_3$ Benzene, 1-ethenylnitro-4-methoxy- (4-methoxy-β-nitrostyrene), 180
$C_9H_{10}O_2$ Benzoic acid, ethyl ester, 94, 122
$C_9H_{11}NO_2$ Propanoic acid, 2-amino-3-phenyl- (Phenylalanine), 164
$C_9H_{11}NO_3$ Propanoic acid, 2-amino-3-(4-hydroxyphenyl)- (Tyrosine), 164
C_9H_{12} Benzene, 1,2,4-trimethyl- (Pseudocumene), 131, 217
C_9H_{12} Benzene, 1,3,5-trimethyl- (Mesitylene), 131, 146, 170, 174, 217
C_9H_{12} Benzene, 1-ethyl-2-methyl-, 21
C_9H_{12} Benzene, 1-ethyl-4-methyl-, 21
C_9H_{12} Benzene, propyl-, 21
C_9H_{12} Benzene, 1-methylethyl- (Cumene), 21, 174
$C_9H_{14}O_6$ 1,2,3-Propanetriol triethanoate (Glycerol triacetate), 140
$C_9H_{15}NO_2S$ Thiocyanoacetic acid hexyl ester, 179
$C_9H_{16}O$ 2-Cyclohexene-1-one, 3,5,5-trimethyl-, 175
C_9H_{20} Nonane, 67, 96, 97, 99, 217
C_9H_{20} Pentane, 3,3-diethyl-, 97
$C_9H_{20}O$ 1-Nonanol, 132, 133, 148, 217
$C_{10}H_7Br$ Naphthalene, 1-bromo-, 217
$C_{10}H_7Cl$ Naphthalene, 1-chloro-, 124, 217
$C_{10}H_8$ Naphthalene, 20, 35, 121, 122, 144, 146, 160, 170, 217
$C_{10}H_8$ Bicyclo-[5,3,0]-deca-2,4,6,8,10-pentaene (Azulene), 160
$C_{10}H_8O$ 1-Naphthalenol (α-Naphthol), 102
$C_{10}H_8O$ 2-Naphthalenol (β-Naphthol), 102
$C_{10}H_8O_3$ 2-Butenoic acid, 4-oxo-4-phenyl- (Benzoylacrylic acid), 181
$C_{10}H_{10}O$ 3-Buten-2-one, 4-phenyl- (Benzalacetone), 180
$C_{10}H_{11}NO_2$ Benzene, 2-nitro-1-butenyl-, 181
$C_{10}H_{11}NO_3$ Aminoethanoic acid, N-benzoyl-, methyl ester (Methyl hippurate), 160, 161
$C_{10}H_{12}O_2$ Benzene, 1-hydroxy-2-methoxy-5-propenyl- (Eugenol), 128
$C_{10}H_{14}$ Benzene, 1,2,4,5-tetramethyl-, 21, 121, 144–146, 217
$C_{10}H_{14}$ Benzene, butyl-, 21, 87, 172
$C_{10}H_{14}$ Benzene, 2-methylpropyl-, 21
$C_{10}H_{14}$ Benzene, 1-methyl-4-(2-propyl)-, 146, 170
$C_{10}H_{14}O$ Benzene, 1-butyl-4-hydroxy-, 95
$C_{10}H_{14}O$ Benzene, 1-hydroxy-4 (dimethylethyl), 133
$C_{10}H_{14}O$ Benzene, 1-hydroxy-2-methyl-5-(1-methylethyl)-, 95
$C_{10}H_{14}O$ Benzene, 1-hydroxy-2-(1-methylethyl)-5-methyl- (Thymol), 129
$C_{10}H_{16}O$ 1,7,7-Trimethylbicyclo[2,2,1]heptan-2-one (Camphor), 121, 128
$C_{10}H_{18}$ Bicyclo[4,4,0]decane (Decalin), 21, 102
$C_{10}H_{20}O_2$ Octanoic acid, ethyl ester, 95
$C_{10}H_{21}Cl$ Decane, 1-chloro-, 132
$C_{10}H_{22}$ Decane, 21, 59, 60, 67, 78, 84, 96, 147, 172, 217
$C_{10}H_{22}O$ 1-Decanol, 67, 78, 123, 132, 133, 148, 154
$C_{10}H_{22}O$ Pentane, 1,1'-oxybis- (Di-n-pentyl ether), 102
$C_{11}H_{12}$ Naphthalene, 1-methyl-, 21
$C_{11}H_{12}$ Naphthalene, 2-methyl-, 21
$C_{11}H_{12}N_2O_2$ 2-Amino-3-indolyl-propanoic acid (Tryptophan), 157, 164
$C_{11}H_{13}NO_2$ Benzene, (2-nitro-1-pentenyl)-, 181
$C_{11}H_{13}NO_3$ Aminoethanoic acid, N-benzoyl- ethyl ester (Ethyl hippurate), 160
$C_{11}H_{15}NO$ Nitrone, N-t-butyl-α-phenyl-, 31
$C_{11}H_{15}N_4O_7$ N,N,N-trimethylethanamium salt of Benzene, 1-hydroxy-2,4,6-trinitro- (Trimethylethylammonium picrate), 117, 118
$C_{11}H_{15}N_4O_7$ 2-Hydroxy-N,N,N-trimethylethanamium salt of Benzene, 1-hydroxy-2,4,5-trinitro- (Choline picrate), 117, 118
$C_{11}H_{16}$ Benzene, 2-methylpropyl-4-methyl-, 174
$C_{11}H_{18}N_2O_3$ 5-Ethyl-5-(1-methylbutyl)-2,4,6(1H,3H,5H)-pyrimidinetrione (Pentobarbital), 162
$C_{11}H_{19}NO_2S$ Thiocyanoacetic acid, octyl ester, 179
$C_{11}H_{24}$ Undecane, 217
$C_{11}H_{24}O$ Undecanol, 145, 148

$C_{12}H_2Cl_8$ Biphenyl, 2,2′,3,4,4′,5,6,6′-octachloro-, 132

$C_{12}H_3Cl_7$ Biphenyl, 2,2′,3,4,4′,5,6′-heptachloro-, 132

$C_{12}H_4Cl_6$ Biphenyl, 2,2′4,4′,5,6′-hexachloro-, 132

$C_{12}H_5Cl_5$ Biphenyl, 2,2′,3,4,5′-pentachloro-, 132

$C_{12}H_6Cl_4$ Biphenyl, 2,2′,4,5′-tetrachloro-, 132

$C_{12}H_7Cl_3$ Biphenyl, 2,4,5-trichloro-, 132

$C_{12}H_8Cl_2$ Biphenyl, 2,2′-dichloro-, 132

$C_{12}H_9Cl$ Biphenyl, 4-chloro-, 132

$C_{12}H_{10}$ Biphenyl, 21, 121, 144–146, 217

$C_{12}H_{10}$ 1,2-Dihydroacenaphthylene (Acenaphtene), 121, 122, 144–146, 217

$C_{12}H_{12}N_2O_3$ 2,4,6(1H,3H,5H)-Pyrimidinetrione, 5-ethyl-5-phenyl- (Phenobarbital), 162

$C_{12}H_{15}NO_3$ Aminoethanoic acid N-benzoyl-, 1-propyl ester (n-Propyl hippurate), 160

$C_{12}H_{15}NO_3$ Aminoethanoic acid N-benzoyl-, 2-propyl ester (Isopropyl hippurate), 160

$C_{12}H_{15}NO_8$ Benzene, 1-hydroxy-2-nitro-, D-galactopyranoside, 157

$C_{12}H_{16}N_5O_3P_3$ Purine 6-amino-D-ribofuranoside-, triphosphate (Adenosine triphosphate), 155–157, 195–197, 213

$C_{12}H_{22}O_{11}$ β-D-Fructofuranosyl-α-D-glucopyranoside (Sucrose), 38, 50, 51, 52, 138, 139

$C_{12}H_{22}O_{11}$ β-D-Glucopyranosyl-β-D-glucopyranoside (Cellobiose), 50

$C_{12}H_{22}O_{11}$ β-D-Galactopyranosyl-β-D-glucopyranoside (Lactose), 138, 139

$C_{12}H_{22}O_{11}$ α-D-Glucopyranosyl-α-D-glucopyranoside (Maltose), 50, 51, 138, 139

$C_{12}H_{26}$ Dodecane, 21, 147, 153, 172

$C_{12}H_{26}O$ 1-Dodecanol, 123, 132, 148, 154, 172

$C_{12}H_{27}N$ 1-Dodecanamine (1-Decylamine), 115

$C_{12}H_{28}BrN$ N,N,N-Tripropylpropanamium bromide (Tetra-n-propyl-ammonium bromide), 108

$C_{12}H_{28}ClNO_4$ N,N,N-Tripropylpropanamium perchlorate (Tetra-n-propylammonium perchlorate), 114

$C_{12}H_{28}IN$ N,N,N-Tripropylpropanamium iodide (Tetra-n-propylammonium iodide), 116

$C_{13}H_{12}$ Benzene, 1,1′-methylenebis- (Diphenylmethane), 87

$C_{13}H_{13}O_4P$ Phosphoric acid, methyl diphenyl ester, 84

$C_{13}H_{17}NO_4$ Propanoic acid, 2-acetylamino-3-(4-hydroxyphenyl)-, ethyl ester (N-Acetyl-tyrosine ethyl ester), 161, 162

$C_{13}H_{20}O_8$ 2,2-Bishydroxymethyl-1,3-propanediol tetraacetate (Pentaerythritol tetraacetate), 140

$C_{13}H_{23}NO_2S$ Thiocyanoacetic acid decyl ester, 179

$C_{14}H_{10}$ Anthracene, 21, 81, 147, 160, 191–193, 217

$C_{14}H_{10}$ Phenanthrene, 21, 87, 144, 147

$C_{14}H_{12}$ Benzene, 1,1′-(1,2-ethenediyl)bis- (Diphenylethene), 87

$C_{14}H_{20}N_4O_3$ Pentanoic acid, 2-benzoylamino-5-guanidino-, methyl ester (Benzoylarginine methyl ester), 156

$C_{14}H_{30}$ Tetradecane, 21, 59, 60, 172

$C_{14}H_{30}O$ 1-Tetradecanol, 132, 148

$C_{15}H_{22}N_4O_3$ Pentanoic acid, 2-benzoylamino-5-guanidino-, ethyl ester (Benzoylarginine ethyl ester), 156

$C_{15}H_{27}NO_2S$ Thiocyanoacetic acid dodecyl ester, 179

$C_{16}H_{10}$ Pyrene, 21

$C_{16}H_{22}O_{11}$ Glucose pentaacetate, 140

$C_{16}H_{33}Cl$ Hexadecane, 1-chloro-, 103, 217

$C_{16}H_{34}$ hexadecane, 217

$C_{16}H_{34}O$ 1-Hexadecanol, 103, 154

$C_{16}H_{34}O$ Octane, 1,1′-oxybis- (Di-n-octyl ether), 103, 104, 217

$C_{16}H_{36}BrN$ N,N,N-Tributylbutanamium bromide (Tetrabutylammonium bromide), 118

$C_{16}H_{36}ClN$ N,N,N-Tributylbutanamium chloride (Tetrabutyl-ammonium chloride), 118

$C_{16}H_{36}ClNO_4$ N,N,N-Tributylbutanamium perchlorate (Tetrabutylammonium perchlorate), 188

$C_{16}H_{36}IN$ N,N,N-Tributylbutanamium iodide (Tetrabutylammonium iodide), 118

$C_{16}H_{36}N_2O_3$ N,N,N-Tributylbutanamium nitrate (Tetrabutylammonium nitrate), 118

$C_{17}H_{19}ClN_2S$ 2-Chloro-N,N-dimethyl-10H-phenathiazine-10-Propanamine (Chlorpro-

	mazine), 118
$C_{17}H_{34}O$	9-Heptadecanone (Di-n-octyl ketone), 103, 104, 217
$C_{17}H_{36}$	Heptadecane
$C_{18}H_{12}$	Benzanthracene
$C_{18}H_{20}$	2-Pentene, 2,4-diphenyl-4-methyl-
$C_{18}H_{21}NO_3$	7,8-Didehydro-4,5-epoxy-3-methoxy-17-methylmorphinan-6-ol (Codeine)
$C_{18}H_{22}O_2$	Estra-1,3,5(10)-trien-17-one, 3-hydroxy- (Estrone)
$C_{18}H_{24}O_2$	Estra-1,3,5(10)-trien-3,17-diol (Estradol)
$C_{18}H_{34}O_2$	9-Octadecenoic acid (Oleic acid)
$C_{18}H_{37}BrN_2O$	N,N-Dimethyl-1-decyl-3(carbamoyl)pyridinium bromide
$C_{18}H_{38}$	Octadecane
$C_{19}H_{36}O_2$	9-Octadecenoic acid, methyl ester (Methyl oleate)
$C_{20}H_{16}$	7,12-Dimethylbenz[a]anthracene
$C_{20}H_{21}NO_4$	1- (3,4-dimethoxyphenyl)methyl -6,7-dimethoxy-isoquinoline (Papaverine)
$C_{20}H_{30}O$	3,7-Dimethyl-9-(2,6,6-trimethyl-1-cyclohexen-1-yl) -2,4,6,8-nonatetraen-1-ol (Vitamin A)
$C_{20}H_{41}BrN_2O$	N,N-Diethyl-1-decyl-3-(carbamoyl)pyridinium bromide, 119
$C_{20}H_{44}ClNO_4$	N,N,N-Tripentylpentanamium perchlorate (Tetraamylammonium perchlorate), 114
$C_{20}H_{44}IO$	N,N,N-Tris(3-methylbutyl)-3-methylbutanamine iodide, 116
$C_{21}H_{26}O_2$	6H-Benzo [b,d] pyran-1-ol, 6,6,9-trimethyl-3-pentyl- (Cannabinol), 133
$C_{21}H_{27}NO$	3-Heptanone, 6-dimethylamino-4,4-diphenyl- (Methadone), 118
$C_{21}H_{28}O_5$	Pregna-1,4-dien-3,20-dione, 11,17,21-trihydroxy- (Prednisolone), 89
$C_{21}H_{30}O_2$	Δ^8-Tetrahydrocannabinol, 133
$C_{21}H_{30}O_2$	Δ^9-Tetrahydrocannabinol, 133
$C_{21}H_{30}O_2$	1,3-Benzenediol, 2-[3-methyl-6-(1-methylethenyl)-2-cyclohexen-1-yl]-5-pentyl- (Cannabidiol), 133
$C_{21}H_{30}O_3$	Δ^9-Tetrahydrocannabinol, 11-hydroxy-, 133
$C_{21}H_{30}O_5$	Pregna-4-ene-3,20-dione, 11,17,21-trihydroxy- (Hydrocartisone), 89
$C_{21}H_{30}O_2$	1,3-Benzenediol, 2-(3,7-dimethyul-2,6-octadienyl)-5-pentyl- (Cannabigerol), 133
$C_{21}H_{41}BrN_2O$	N,N-Pentamethylene-1-decyl-3(carbamoyl)pyridinium bromide, 119
$C_{22}H_{14}N_6Fe$	Bis)2,2'-bipyridyl)biscyanoiron(II),107
$C_{22}H_{25}NO_6$	N-(5,6,7,9-Tetrahydro-1,2,3,10-tetramethoxy-9-oxobenzo[a]heptalen-7-yl)acetamide (Cochicine), 162
$C_{22}H_{32}O_2$	6H-Dibenzo[b,d]pyran-1-ol, 3-hexyl-7,8,9,10-tetrahydro-6,6,9-trimethyl- (Synhexyl), 133
$C_{22}H_{38}N_4O_7$	N,N,N-Tributylbutanamium salt of Benzene, 1-hydrox-2,4,6-trinitro- (Tetra-n-butylammonium picrate), 118
$C_{22}H_{43}BrN_2O$	N,N-Hexamethylene-1-decyl-3(carbamoyl)pyridinium bromide, 118
$C_{22}H_{45}BrN_2O$	N,N-Dipropyl-1-decyl-3(carbamoyl)pyridinium bromide, 118
$C_{23}H_{22}N_2O_7$	N-Carbobenzoxy-L-glutamyl-L-tyrosine, 155, 156, 184
$C_{24}H_{52}ClNO_4$	N,N,N-Trihexylhexanamium perchlorate (Tetra-n-hexylammonium perchlorate), 114
$C_{26}H_{14}N_8O_4Fe$	Dicyanobis(5-nitrophenanthroline)iron(II), 107
$C_{28}H_{18}Br_4O_4$	2,4,7,9-Tetrabromo-3,8-dimethoxy-5a,10b-diphenylcoumarano-2,3,2',3'-coumaran, 65
$C_{28}H_{20}Br_2O_4$	2,9-Dibromo-3,8-dimethoxy-5a,10b-diphenylcoumarano-2,3,2'3'-coumaran, 65
$C_{28}H_{44}O$	Δ-5,7,22-Ergostatrien-3β-ol (Ergosterol), 31
$C_{28}H_{44}O$	Vitamin D, 31
$C_{28}H_{60}BrP$	Tributylhexadecylphosphonium bromide, 114
$CaCl_2$	Calcium chloride, 42, 46, 48
Cl_3P	Phosphorus trichloride, 56
$CoH_9N_6O_6$	Trinitrotriamionecobalt, 107
$CsClO_4$	Caesium perchlorate, 109
$CsCl_4Re$	Caesium tetrachlororhenate, 30
CsO_4Re	Caesium tetraoxorhenate (VII), 108
Cs_2Br_6Re	Caesium hexabromorhenate (IV), 108
Cs_2Cl_6Re	Caesium hexachlororhenate (IV), 108
H_3N	Ammonia, 176, 182, 183
H_4NCl	Ammonium chloride, 49

$H_8N_2O_4S$	Ammonium sulphate, 49	
H_2O	Water, 17, 22, 36–52, 68, 69, 71, 72, 77, 78, 85–102, 105–118, 138–142, 144–148, 164, 165, 217	
H_2S	Hydrogen sulphide, 68	
I_2	Iodine, 68, 74–76, 217	
KBr	Potassium bromide, 41, 44, 46, 108, 137	
KCl	Potassium chloride, 41, 44, 45, 108, 109, 137, 160–162	
$KClO_4$	Potassium perchlorate, 109	
KF	Potassium fluoride, 42	
KOH	Potassium hydroxide, 42	
KI	Potassium iodide, 41, 137	
KNO_3	Potassium nitrate, 41	
K_2SO_3	Potassium sulphite, 40	
K_2SO_4	Potassium sulphate, 40, 41	
K_2SeO_3	Potassium selenite, 40	
K_2SeO_4	Potassium selenate, 40	
Kr	Krypton, 28, 56, 123	
LiCl	Lithium chloride, 42, 108, 135, 137	
$LiNO_3$	Lithium nitrate, 42	
Mo_2Cl_{10}	Molybdenum pentachloride, 29, 30	
$MgCl_2$	Magnesium chloride, 46, 47	
$MgSO_4$	Magnesium sulphate, 49	
N_2	Nitrogen, 25, 68, 121	
N_2O	Nitrous oxide, 68, 121, 123	
$NaBrO_3$	Sodium bromate, 42	
NaCN	Sodium cyanide, 114	
NaCNS	Sodium thiocyanate, 134	
NaCl	Sodium chloride, 41, 108, 135, 137, 161, 162	
$NaClO_3$	Sodium chlorate, 41	
$NaClO_4$	Sodium perchlorate, 137	
NaF	Sodium fluoride, 42	
NaOH	Sodium hydroxide, 42, 108	
$NaIO_3$	Sodium iodate, 42	
$NaNO_3$	Sodium nitrate, 41, 137	
Na_2SO_4	Sodium sulphate, 41, 108, 162	
$Na_2S_2O_3$	Sodium thiosulphate, 42	
Na_2SeO_4	Sodium selenate, 42	
O_2	Oxygen, 68, 185	
RbCl	Rubidium chloride, 41, 108	
S_8	Sulphur, 72, 217	
SF_6	Sulphur hexafluoride, 123	
SO_2	Sulphur dioxide, 95, 96, 182, 183	
$SiCl_4$	Silicon tetrachloride, 67, 75, 217	
$SnCl_4$	Tin(IV) tetrachloride (Stannic chloride), 217	
$SrCl_2$	Strontium chloride, 42	
Xe	Xenon, 28, 56, 123	

Subject index

Acetylcholine esterase 123
Acetylcholine synthesis 123
Actinosphaerium nucleofilum 162
Agriotes species 127, 169–172
Alcohol dehydrogenase 161, 181
Alcohols 92–94, 148, 153–156
Allium cepa 121, 122, 127
Amino-acids 49, 50, 163–167
Anaesthetics 120, 121, 151, 152, 172
Anaesthetics, teratogenic effects of 172
Aphis rumicis 126
Aspergillus niger 180, 181
Associated liquids 85
Atomic and group factors for physical
    toxicity 124, 125
ATPase 155, 156, 195–197, 213
Avena sativum 157

Bacillus antracis 135, 137
Bacillus pyocyaneus see *Pseudomonas
    aeruginosa*
Bacillus subtilis 123, 155
Bacterium coli 127
Bed bug see *Cimex lectularis*
Biophase 17, 123–128, 139, 141, 159,
    168, 169, 182, 184, 185
Bluegill 123
Boiling points 17, 26, 171, 172
Botrytis allii 31, 32, 180, 181
Brain cortex 123

Calandra granaria 127, 169, 176, 182,
    183, 185
Calandra oryzae 183
Candida albicans 126
Candida tropicalis 126
Carbohydrates 138, 139
Carcinogenesis 172
Carminative action 125, 128, 129
Catechol oxidase 123
Cavitation 63
C_B 123, 125–128, 153, 169–174, 182
Cell division 120, 123
Cell membranes 166, 167
Characteristic temperature 17, 25, 67, 68,
    79, 144, 146, 147, 198, 214–218
Characteristic volume 17, 22, 25–30,
    43–52, 65–68, 86, 87, 139, 140,
    153–156, 160, 188, 198, 214–218
Chemical potential 17
Chemical toxicity 176–185
Chicken 172
Chlamydomonas angulosa 19–21, 143,
    144
Chlorella vulgaris 19–21, 143, 144
Chlorine substitution (in sugars) 139, 141
Choline esterase 117, 119
Chromatography 101–104
α-Chymotrypsin 123, 156, 160–162
Cimex lectularis 183
Clapeyron equation 73

Cl-esterase (human) 161
Clothes moth see *Tineola bisiella*
c-Mitosis 120–122
Cockroach 171
Cohesive energy density 65
Compressibility 24, 25, 44, 46, 50, 52,
    55, 56, 58–62, 100, 104, 189, 190
Concentration units 70–72
Critical volume 26
Cucurbita pepo 145
Cut-off 121, 143, 144, 169, 170

Density of liquids 25–27, 56, 57, 189,
    190, 196
Density of liquids, effect of pressure on
    56, 57
Density of liquids, effect of temperature
    on 57, 189
Distribution law 68-70, 168
Dormancy shortened 123

Ebethella typhi (see *Salmonella typhosa*)
Electrolytes, partial molar volumes of
    36–42
Enterocytes 156
Enzymes 131, 132, 152, 162
Enzyme activation 156, 157
Enzyme inhibition 123, 151–156, 181,
    195–197, 213
Ephestia kuehniella 183
Erythrocytes 127
Escherichia coli 166, 184
Ethylenic compounds, toxicity of 179–
    182

Flour beetle see *Tribolium castaneum*
Flour moth see *Ephestia knehniella*
Fomes annosus 121, 127, 144
Food preservation 182
Frog heart 18, 19, 39, 155
Fungus 'Madison 517' 127
Fusarium caeruleum 178, 179

Galactosidase 157
Genetic engineering 166, 167
Germination, inhibition of 155, 158
β-Glucoronidase 152
Glue sniffing 172, 173
Glutamate dehydrogenase 152
Grain weevil see *Calandra granaria*
Guinea pig 125, 155, 158, 159

Haemagglutinin protein 167
Haemaglobin 156, 184, 185
Haemolysis 127, 132, 155
Hammett equation 145, 147, 148, 179
Heat of fusion 57, 58, 74, 214–218
Heat of mixing liquids 54, 55
Heat of vapourisation 54, 64, 65, 72
Helianthus annuus 145

Henry's law 68, 163, 168
Hexokinase 181
House flies see *Musca domestica*
Humans, toxicity to 172–177
Humicola species 153
Hydration 138, 139
Hydration of salts 44-49
Hydration of sugars and related com-
    pounds 138–141
'Hydrophobicity' 86, 113, 167

Inhibition of enzymes 123, 151–156,
    181, 195–197
Injection into animals 129–131
Internal latent heat of vapourisation 64,
    65, 72
Internal pressure 54
Iodine, positive 31, 32, 179

Lachrymators 181
Lactuca sativum 158
Lepomis macrochirus 123
Lettuce 158
Leucine amino-peptidase 123
Lipase 153–155
Lipoxygenase 123
Liquid properties 62, 198–202
Loxostege stictalis 123
Luciferase 151, 152
Luminous bacteria 151, 152
Lupinos polyphyllus 145
Lisophosphatidylcholine acetyltransferase
    127, 132

Malate dehydrogenase 157, 158
Michaelis-Menten constant 159, 160
Microtubules 162
Molal concentrations 71
Molar concentrations 70–72
Molecular attraction constants 64–66
Molecular volumes 22–24, 36, 97, 100
Monilia albicans (see *Candida albicans*)
Monilia tropicalis (see *Candida tropicalis*)
Mouse 123, 127, 132–134, 155, 172,
    182
Musca domestica 171
Muscle contraction 158, 159
Mycobacterium tuberculosis 126
Myoglobin 152

Narcotics 17, 121, 123, 134, 169, 194–
    197, 212
Nerve impulses, transmission of 149, 150,
    184
Newt 151
5'-Nucleotidase 131, 132

1-Octanol/water partitions 145, 148, 149
Ox 134–136, 153
Oxidative phosphorylation 120

Paired ion chromatography 114, 117
Papain 181
Parachor 25–27
Paramecium species 158, 159
Partial molar volume 36–42, 137
Partition coefficients 17, 68, 69, 88–91,
  95, 137–140, 145, 148, 149, 163, 164
Pepsin 155, 156, 184
Phase transfer catalysis 114
Physical toxicity 17–19, 120–137, 141,
  151–153, 178, 182–185, 193–197,
  207–211
Physical toxicity, effects of salts on
  135–137
Physical toxicity (estimation) 123, 128,
  170, 171, 174
Pig 155–158
Pisum sativum 121, 145
Polymer properties 79, 80, 164–166
Properties of liquids 62, 198–202
Proteins 40, 151, 152
Proteins, fixation in membranes 166,
  167, 178, 179
Pseudomonas aeruginosa 127, 184
Pyruvate dehydrogenase 181

Rat 131, 134, 136, 172
Regular solutions 53–55
Respiration increase 120, 182
Respiration reduction 158, 159

Salmonella typhosa 126, 181
Sea urchin 122, 123
Setschenow equation 104–107, 135, 137
Sheep 134, 136, 153
Sitophilus oryzae 169
Solubilities in salt solutions 104–108
Solubilities in water 17, 86–88, 92–95
Solubilities in gases 76–79
Solubilities of salts 39, 108–110,
  113–118
Solubilities of solids 57, 58, 74–76, 81,
  82, 191–193, 203
Solubility parameter 55, 64, 65, 72
Solution process 85–88
Solvents, choice of 65–67, 83, 84, 191,
  203

Solvents other than water 95–97
Specific interactions 22, 85, 88–90, 184,
  185
Sporotrichum species 126
Staphylococcus aureus 126, 154, 181
Steroids 152
Strained molecules 30–34
Strongylocentrotus lividus 122
Succinic dehydrogenase 134–136, 153
Sugars 50–52, 138, 139
Sugars, compounds related to 139–141
Sulphydryl compounds 181
Surface tension 25, 26, 39, 43–51, 189,
  190, 196
Sweetness 139, 140

Tadpole 127, 134, 151, 155, 194–197,
  212
Tait equation 105
Teratogenic effects 172
Thiocyanoacetates 178, 179
Threshold limits of vapours for safety
  173–177
Tineola biselliella 183
Tranquillisers 152
Tribolium castaneum 183
Triosephosphate dehydrogenase 181
Triticum 121, 127
Trypsin 156, 157

Urease 181
Urethanes 152

Van der Waal's equation 24, 26, 34, 35,
  53, 54, 62–65
Vapour pressure 17, 73, 74, 169–172
Vapour toxicity 168–172
Viruses 166
Viscosity 26, 29, 30, 189
Volume change on mixing 58–62

Wireworm see *Agriotes* species
Work of compression of liquids 57

Yeast 121, 161

Author index

The page numbers, inorder, indicate where the work of the author is referred to in the text. Since the name of the author may not be given in the text, reference numbers are shown in brackets before the first page with the reference.

Abe, A. [41], 24
Abraham, M.H. [325], [326], 113,
   [340], 116, [341], 117
Absolom, D.R. [322], 113
Adey, G. [456], 152
Ahamad, P. [230], [259], [260], 89,
   [417], [418], [419], 138
Aicart, E. [163], 59, 60
Albin, I.A. [430], 139
Alfenaar, M. [247], [248], 96, 97,
   [306], 109
Allison, A.C. [500], [501], 162
American Conference of Governmental
   Industrial Hygienists [543], 173, 176
Amidon, G.L. [252], 97
Amik, S.T. [252], 97
Amis, E.S. [313], 110
Anders, G. [309], 109
Anderson, H.C. [180], 67
Anderson, N.B. [530], 172
Anderson, O.L. [157], 55
Andrade, J.M.V.de, [264], 102
Andrew, L.W. [110], 42, 43, 72

Antosiewicz, J. [428], 138, 139
Apelblat, A. [220], [221], 84
Arakawa, K. [234], 90
Arima, K. [465], 153
Arkel, A.E.van, [167], 63
Arnett, R.L. [222], 84
Arnow, L.E. [474], 156
Atherton, F.R. [77], 31
Atkinson, P.N. [48], 26

Back, E.A. [524], 169
Backes, W.L. [493], 161
Baechler, R.H. [391], [392], 126
Bakker, G. [139], [140], 54
Bancroft, W.D. [416], 137, [447], 151
Barlow, C.A. [152], 55
Bartlett, F.E. [436], 142
Basford, A.B. [532], 172
Batelli, F. [404], 134, 135, 136, 153
Bateman, E. [353], 121, 127, 144
Bate-Smith, E.C. [259], 102
Battershill, R.D. [261], 102
Battino, R. [212], [213], [214], 77

Bauch, R. [356], [357], 121
Beard, D.J. [461], [462], 152
Beasley, J.G. [344], 117, 119
Belton, J.W. [114], 45, [131], 49, 50
Benesi, H.A. [203], 74, 75, [208], 76
Benhamin, L. [464], 153, 154, 155
Ben-Naim, A. [198], 72
Benson, S.W. [65], 27
Beppu, T. [465], 153
Berezin, I.V. [491], [497], 161
Bergel, F. [556], 181
Bergen, R.L. [281], 105
Berger, A. [515], 165
Berkheimer, H.E. [225], [226], 86, 87, 95, 113
Bernard, C. [445], [446], 151, 185
Berthelot, M. [190], 68
Bhagwat, W.V. [112], 43, 49
Bigeleisen, J. [106], 41
Biltz, W. [43], [44], 9, 25
Birch, G.G. [433], 141
Birdsall, N.J.M. [505], 162
Bischoff, F. [297], 107
Bixler, H.J. [216], 77, 79
Blagoi, Yu.P. [160], 56
Blandamer, M.J. [296], 107
Blobel, G. [521], 167
Boeke, J.D. [518], 167
Bondi, A. [83], [84], 34, 35, 96
Bonner, W.D. [249], 96, 98
Bordewijk, P. [244], 92
Bosquet, E.W. [554], 180, 181
Bowden, S.T. [111], 42, 43
Bowler, K. [483], 157, 158
Box, D. [248], 96, [306], 109
Boyce, C.B.C. [260], 102
Bradbury, F.R. [8], 17, 18
Brammall, A. [461], [462], 152
Braun, R.M. [222], 84
Bretzel, J.J.von, [94], 39
Brian, P.W. [552], [553], 180, 181
Bridgeman, P.W. [158], 56
Briggs, G.G. [443], 148
Brink, F. [20], 17, 149, 150
Brønsted, J.N. [301], 107
Brown, B.W. [535], 172
Brown, D.E.S. [449], 151
Brown, K.B. [438], 145
Browne, C.A. [133], 50, 51
Bruyne, C.K.de, [481], 157
Bryde, R.J.W. [564], 182
Buccafusco, R.J. [374], 124
Buchowski, H. [255], 101
Buffington, A.C. [474], 156
Bunn, A. [132], 49
Burgess, J. [296], 96, 107, [304], 108, [321], 113
Burford, W.B. [180], 67
Buss, J.H. [65], 27
Busvine, J.R. [565], 182, 183

Butler, E.T. [111], 42, 43
Butler, J.A.V. [437], 142
Bye, J.M. [520], 167

Cady, G.H. [179], 67
Cameron, G.R. [395], 131
Canady, W.J. [488], [489], 159, 160, [493–496], 161
Capaldi, R.A. [504], 162
Carrera, G. [475], 156
Cerankowski, L.D. [514], 164, 165
Chazotte, B. [409], 134, 136
Chiklis, C.K. [513], 164, 165
Childs, P.E. [542], 173
Christian, S.D. [314], 110
Clairborne, I. [300], 107, 115
Clark, N.G. [559], 181
Cleaver, H.L. [211], 77
Coats, E. [492], 161
Cogswell, F.N. [51], 26, 188, [218], 79, 80
Cohen, E.N. [535], 172
Cohn, E.J. [93], 39, 40, [132], 49, [311], 109, 111
Colacicco, G. [323], 113
Collander, R. [228], 71, 88, [229], 89, 90, 111, [236], 138, 139
Conn, J.E. [555], 181
Consden, R. [257], 101
Cook, K.E. [560], 169, 181
Cook, M.A. [156], 55
Cooper, E.A. [387], 126, [420], [421], 127, 182, 184
Copley, G.N. [66], 27
Corman, I. [359], 123
Cotton, R.T. [523], [524], 169
Counsell, J.F. [183], 67
Couture, A.M. [103], 41, 137
Cowen, P.N. [364], 123
Cox, J.R. [422], 127
Cox, P.H. [385], 126
Cramer, B.J. [561], 181
Cramer, R.D. [328], [329], 113
Cresswell, T. [62], 27
Cromwell, N.H. [560], 181
Cronk, D.H. [562], 181
Cudby, M.E.A. [178], 65
Cumming, A.C. [307], 109
Cuppett, A.C. [307], 161
Cupples, C.C. [126], 47, 48
Currie, D.J. [238], 91

Danforth, W.F. [214], 77
Dalfsen, B.M.van, [242], 92
Daniel, J. [132], 49
Danil de Namor, A.F. [339], 115, [340], 116, [341], 117
Davies, J.T. [333], 114, 116
Davis, E.R. [76], 31
Davis, N.G. [516], 166, [518], 167

Day, R.E. [541], 173
Dehmlow, E.V. [332], 114
Delbanco, A. [301], 107
Denessen, H.J.M. [247], 96, 97
Deno, N.C. [225], [226], 86, 87, 95, [280], 105, 107, 108, 113
Desmyter, A. [165], 61, 62
Desnoyers, J.E. [105], 41
Deutsch, E.W. [442], 145
Diaz Pena, M. [164], 59, 60
Dillard, C.J. [463], 152
Dixon, M. [457], 152, [563], 181
Dodé, M. [346], 117, 120, [355], 121, 122, 127
Doebbler, G.F. [370], 123
Dolezalek, F. [239], [241], 91
Donahue, D.I. [436], 142
Douglas, C.G. [569], 185
Doxey, D. [32], 22, 122, 185
Dryssen, D. [235], 90
Duer, W.C. [336], 115
Duijn, D. [244], 92
Dunn, M.S. [312], 109, 111
Dunn, W.J. [232], 89, [467], 156
Dupré, A. [143], 54
Duuren, B.L.van, [537], 172

Eastwood, D.W. [422], [531], 172
Edsall, J.T. [93], 39, 40, [311], 109
Eduljee, H.E. [159], 56
Edwards, M.A. [476], 156
Einstein, A. [171], [172], 65
Eisenberg, M.A. [476], 156
Eisenman, G. [334], [335], 115
Elder, M. [73], 30
Eley, D.D. [223], [224], 85
Elferink, M.G.L. [306], 109
Elkins, D. [237], 91, 142, 148
Elliott, K.A.C. [369], 123
Elliott, M. [483], 157, 158
Ellis, S.J. [374], 124
Ethier, M.C. [482], 157
Euler, H. [274], [276], 104, 105
Evans, B.K. [393], 125, 128
Evans, F.D. [213], 77
Ewens, R.V.G. [70], 29
Exner, O. [60], [64], 27, 97
Eyring, H. [452], 152

Farrell, P.G. [320], 110
Fahein, L.A. [460], 152
Ferguson, J. [21], [22], [27], 17, 22, [30], [31], [32], 122, 159, 169, 176, 179, 185
Fergusson, J.E. [72], [73], 30
Filliol, D. [509], 164
Fink, B.R. [532], 172
Fischer, H. [192], 69
Fisher, B.B. [208], 76
Flagler, E.A. [450], 151

Flatt, R. [305], 109
Flory, P.J. [39], [40], [41], 24
Floyd, R.A. [76], 31
Flynn, G.L. [231], 89
Forbes, J.W. [94], 39
Forch, C. [129], 49
Forstner, G.E. [421], 126, 127
Fowler, R.D. [180], 67
Franks, N.P. [507], 163
Fraser, C.G. [19], 17, 135
Frobisher, M. [386], 122
Fühner, H. [10], 17, 18, 19, 39, [358], 122, 155
Fujita, T. [13], [14], [15], 17, [440], 145
Fyfe, C.A. [417], [418], 138

Gallacher, M.L. [502], 160
Garel, J.P. [509], 164
Gash, B.W. [314], 110
Gasparro, E.P. [197], 72
Gates (Gatyas), L.W. [380], [382], [383], [384], [385], 126
Gaub, M.L. [527], [528], [529], 172
Gavaudan, P. [346], 117, 120, [355], 121, 122, 127
Geffeken, G. [275], 104
Geiger, F. [440], 145
Geiger, W.B. [555], [557], 181
George, H. [483], 157, 158
Gerrard, W. [189], 68, [194], 71
Gershenfeld, L. [375], 126
Gething, M.J. [519], [520], 167
Gibbs, R.D. [439], 145
Gibson, R.E. [120], 44, 46, [294], [295], 106, [575], 190
Gilbert, E.C. [127], 48
Gilvarry, J.J. [150], [151], 55
Girdhar, H.L. [576], 192
Glende, E.A. [74], 31, 177
Goard, A.K. [115], 45
Goldman, S. [336], 115, [434], 142
Goldschmidt, B.M. [537], 172
Gordon, A.H. [257], 101
Goursat, P. [576], 192
Graham, S.A. [3], 17, 171
Grasshoff, J.M. [513], 164, 165
Green, J.H.S. [182], 67
Green, L.S. [503], 162
Greenberg, J.H. [50], 26, 127, [398], [399], 132, 133, 148, 169
Greenberg, M.J. [431], 139
Greger, P.L. [560], 181
Griffith, O.H. [504], 162
Groen, G. van der, [481], 157
Groot, W. de, [167], 63
Gross, P.M. [211], 77, [300], 107, 115
Grosse, A.V. [179], 67
Grove, J.F. [545], 178, 179, [553], 180

Guillet, J.E. [511], [512], 164
Gupta, M.M. [112], 43, 49

Hachisuka, Y. [368], 123, 155
Haldane, J.B.S. [566], [569], 185
Haldane, J.S. [569], 185
Hales, J.L. [183], 67
Hamilton, J.M. [180], 67
Hammaker, R.M. [196], 72
Hammett, L.P. [547], [548], 179
Hammick, D.L. [110], 42, 43, 72
Hampil, B. [389], 126
Hams, A.F. [559], 181
Hancock, C.R. [81], 34
Hansch, C. [13], [14], [15], [16], [17],
    17, 34, [82], [237], 91, [254],
    [440], [441], [442], 97, 142, 145,
    148, [467], [468], [469], [470], 156
    [492], 161, [549], 179
Hanstein, W.G. [408], 134
Harbison, M.W.P. [266], 102
Harkaway, S. [396], 131
Harned, H.S. [102], 41
Harris, M.J. [253], 97
Harrison, D. [149], 55
Harvey, E.N. [448], 151
Hassall, K.E. [546], 179
Hatefi, Y. [405], [408], 134
Hawkins, S.W. [31], [32], 22, 122, 185
Hawkins, W.D. [127], 48
Hay, L.D. [235], 90
Hayward, A.T.J. [291], 105, 106
Hazeldine, P.N. [181], 67
Heath, J.B.R. [95], 39, 40
Hegyvary, C. [473], 155, 195, 197, 213
Heijne, G. [517], 169
Heitmuller, P.T. [525], 169
Hellebust, J.A. [28], 19–21, 143
Hemmi, H. [6], 17, 127, 148, 155
Hemming, H.G. [552], 180, 181
Henry, W. [188], 68, 188
Henshaw, P.S. [360], [361], [362], 123
Hepler, L.G. [105], 41
Hermann, R.B. [251], 97
Herz, W. [117], 45, 46, 49, [192], 69,
    [309], 109
Higuchi, T. [253], 97
Hildebrand, J.H. [135], [136], [137],
    53, [185], [186], [199], 65, 72,
    [201], [203], [204], 74, [205],
    [207], 75, [208], [209], 76, [330],
    [331], 113
Hill, T. [339], 115
Himmelberger, J. [535], 172
Hinkley, R.E. [503], 162
Hinton, J.F. [313], 110
Hirata, Y. [427], 138
Hoff, E.W. [318], 110
Hofmann, W. [478], 157
Hoftijzer, P.J. [176], 65, 66, 107

Hollenberg, J.L. [316], 110
Hollister, T.A. [525], 169
Holmes, H.L. [238], 91
Holt, J.J.H. [1], 17, 172
Hoskins, [511], 164
Hough, L. [432], 141
House of Commons, [538], [539],
    [540], 173
Hoy, K.L. [175], 65, 66
Hruzkewycz, A.M. [74], 31, 177
Hulands, G.F. [501], 162
Hulands, G.H. [461], [462], 152
Hunn, G. [480], 157
Hurd, C.B. [184], 67
Huszar, L.A. [398], 127, 132, 133
Hutchinson, T.C. [28], 19–21, 143
Hyde, R.M. [402], [403], 134, 148
Hymes, A.J. [489], 160

Ibbotson, D.A. [243], 92
Ifft, J.B. [316], 110
Inagami, T. [477], 156
Ito, K. [337], 115, 116, 142
Iwamoto, E. [337], 115, 116, 142
Iwasa, J. [15], 17, 145
Iwata, K. [317], 110, 138

Jackson, W.H. [455], 152
Jaffe, W.G. [365], 123
James, K.C. [393], 125, 128
Janzen, E.G. [76], 31
Jarowski, C.I. [561], 181
Jefferies, T.M. [342], 117, 118
Jeffrey, G.I. [62], 26
Jenks, C.A. [202], 74, [205], 75
Johnson, F.H. [449], [450], 151
Johnson, S.M. [451], 151
Johnston, M.D. [197], 72
Jones, G. [116], 45, [128], 49
Jordan, A. [305], 109
Jost, P.C. [504], 162
Jow, P.Y.C. [254], 97
Jungfleisch, E. [190], 68
Juszkiewicz, A. [425], [428], [429],
    138, 139

Kablukov, I.A. [233], 90, 142
Kallen-Trummer, V. [478], 157
Kamaya, H. [453], 152
Karapet'yants, M.Kh. [250], 97, 99
Kasper, J.S. [180], 67
Katchalski, E. [515], 165
Kawano, Y. [427], 138
Kemula, W. [255], 101
Khan, R. [432], 141
King, M.D. [541], 173
King, T.E. [406], [407], 134
Kingery, L.B. [388], 126
Kirby, J.E. [554], 180, 181
Klarmann, E. [379–385], 126

Klibanov, A.M. [497], 161
Knaebel, E. [117], 45, 46, 49
Knill-Jones, R.P. [533], [535], 172
Knott, R.P. [562], 181
Kocsis, J.J. [396], 131
Kohnstamm, P. [242], 92
Krevelen, D.W. van, [176], 65, 66,
   [298], [299], 107
Krönig, B. [412], 135, 137
Kunst, M. [244], 92
Kuntz, I.D. [197], 72
Kurtz, A.N. [490], 161
Kurtz, J. [515], 165

Laar, J.J. van, [145], 54, [166], 63
Lacombe, C. [475], 156
Laidler, K. [103], 41, 137, [482], 157
Laird, J.S. [411], 135, 137
Lannung, A. [210], 77
Larsen, H. [413], 135
La Surdo, A. [319], 110
Laub, R.J. [265], [266], 102
Leblanc, G.A. [374], 124
Leblanc, M. [215], 77
Lee, A.G. [505], [506], 162
Legetter, B.E. [559], 181
Leggenhager, K. [567], 185
Lehrer, S.B. [528], 172
Leicester, J. [62], 27
Lemon, J.S. [410], 135
Leo, A. [237], [254], 91, 97, 142, 148
Lepie, M.P. [130], 49, 50
Lepple, F.K. [318], 110
Levan, A. [348], [349], [350], 120,
   121, 127
Levashov, A.V. [327], 161
Lewis, W.C.M. [187], 68, [193], 70, 163
Lieb, W.R. [507], 163
Liempt, J.A.M. van, [168], 63
Ligney, C.L. de, [247], [248], 96, 97,
   [306], 109
Lim, J. [406], [407], 134
Limousin, S. [568], 185
Linas, A.J. [568], 185
Lindenberg, A.B. [195], 72
Lindsay, R.C. [430], 139
Lister, [70], 29
Liszi, J. [245], 92, 93
Littlewood, A.B. [201], 74, [268],
   [269], 103, 171
Liu, A.H. [570], 185
Liu, W.-H. [465], 153
Loeffler, O.H. [575], 190
London, E. [227], 86
Long, F.A. [281], [282], [283], 105
Lorenz, R. [145], 54
Lough, C.E. [238], 91
Lunden, B. [284], 105
Luscombe, D.K. [393], 125, 128
Lush, M. [541], 173

McCarthy, M.C. [8], 17, 18
McCay, P.B. [76], 31
McDevit, W.F. [282], [283], 105
Macdonald, J.R. [152], [153], [154], 55
McDuffie, G.E. [94], 39
McGowan, J.C. [5], [23], [24], [26],
   17, 22, [37], [38], [42], [45], [47],
   [48], [49], [50], [51], [52], [67],
   24, 25, 26, 27, [85], 34, 39, [123],
   [124], 42, 44, [161], [162], [163],
   57, [169], 63, 64, 65, [178], [230],
   89, [296], [303], [304], [310], 92,
   97, 107, 108, 109, 113, [372], [373],
   124, 126, [424], 127, 128, 129, 131,
   132, 141, 143, 144, 147, 148, 149,
   [508], 161, 163, 165, 166, 168, 169,
   170, [526], 171, 173, 174, [545],
   [550], [551], [552], [553], 178,
   179, 180, 181, 185
Mackay, D. [28], [29], 19–21, 143
McLennan, H. [369], 123
Maclennan, W.H. [437], 142
McMahan, J. [483], 157, 158
McMeekin, T.L. [96], 39, 40, [311],
   109, 111
McMullen, L.M. [370], 123
Mellors, A. [50], 26, [230], 89, [310],
   108, 109, 113, [372], [373], 124,
   127, [397], [398], [399], 131, 132,
   133, [417], [418], [419], 138, 148,
   155, [508], 163, 166, 169
Merriman, R.W. [435], 142
Metcalfe, J.C. [505], 162
Meyer, D.M. [107], 41
Meyer, E.F. [267], 102
Meyer, H.L. [360], [361], [362], 123
Meyer, J.A. [267], 102
Meyer, K.H. [6], [12], 12, 17, 148, 151,
   155
Meyers, E.A. [81], 34
Milborrow, B.W. [260], 102
Michaels, A.S. [216], 77, 79
Miles, J.L. [488], 159, 160
Miller, E. [378], 126
Miller, K.W. [354], 121, [438], 145,
   [451], 151
Miller, W.L. [18], 17
Millero, F.J. [108], [109], 41, 42, 108,
   [318], [319], 110
Mills. J.E. [394], 131
Mitjavila, S. [475], 156
Miura, M. [317], 110, [427], 138
Model, P. [516], 166, [518], 167
Moelwyn-Hughes, E.A. [148], [149],
   55
Mohlke, M.F. [370], 123
Moir, D.D. [533], 172
Mongar, J.L. [487], 158
Moore, L.F. [243], 92
Moore, W. [2], [3], 17, 171

Moran, W.J. [561], 181
Morgan, L.W. [562], 181
Morrison, A.L. [556], 181
Morton, N. [304], 108
Moslen, M.T. [75], 31, 177
Muir, R.M. [13], 17, [440], 145
Muirhead, I. [78], 31, 32
Mullins, L.J. [25], 17
Mumford, S.A. [63], 27
Munton, S.L. [426], 138, 139
Murnagham, F.D. [147], 55
Mushally, M. [105], 41

Nakajima, T. [544], 177
Namiki-Kanie, S. [368], 123, 155
Neece, C. [293], 106
Needham, D.M. [563], 181
Neifert, I.E. [524], 169
Nernst, W. [191], 69
Nettleship, A. [360], 123
Neumann, A.W. [322], 113
Neumann, H. [472], 155, 156
Nicol, L.W. [455], 152
Nield, C.H. [561], 181
Niemann, C. [490], 161
Nisbet, H.B. [423], 127
Nisel'son, L.A. [69], 29, 30
Northrop, J.H. [479], 157
Noyes, J.P. [246], 95
Nozaki, Y. [324], 113
Nunn, J.F. [500], [501], 162

Obenhaus, V.M. [122], 44, 46
Ohnishi, T. [406], [407], 134
Oliver, J.S. [541], 173
Orr, J.W. [363], 123
Orwoll, R.A. [39], 24
Oss, C.J. van, [322], 113
Oster, E.A. [246], 95
Ostergren, G. [349], [350], [351], 121,
    122, 127
Overton, E. [11], 17, 18, [352], 121,
    127, 151
Owen, B.B. [102], 41

Pacsu, E. [510], 164
Peppenheimer, J.R. [130], 49, 50
Parrish, P.R. [525], 169
Partington, J.R. [53], 26, [141], [142],
    54
Paterson, J.L.H. [395], 131
Paton, W.D.M. [354], 121
Paul, T. [412], 135, 137
Penfold, B.R. [72], [73], 30
Pepper, J.H. [367], 123
Perman, E.P. [121], 44, 46, [125], 47,
    48, 50
Perron, G. [105], 41
Phillips, J.W.C. [63], 27
Pilhorn, H.R. [297], 107

Pimental, G.C. [222], 84
Pirie, H. [30], 22, 126, 169, 176, 179
Pitzer, K.S. [222], 84
Plichfelder, J.D. [534], 172
Poindexter, T.P. [468], [469], 156
Posternak, J.M. [20], 17, 149, 150
Potaczek, J. [429], 138
Poussel, H. [346], 117, 120, [355], 121,
    122, 127
Powell, J.H. [246], 95
Poyer, J.L. [76], 31
Prausnitz, J.M. [56], 26, [137], 53
Pringle, M.J. [438], 145
Procházka, Z.D. [258], 102
Puetzer, B. [561], 181
Purcell, W.P. [344], 117, 119
Purnell, J.H. [264], [265], [266], 102

Quayle, O.R. [61], 27, 31
Quintana, R.P. [344], [345], 117, 119

Rang, H.P. [486], 158, 159
Ratkovics, F. [245], 92, 93
Ray, W.A. [116], 45, [128], 49
Read, R.R. [378], 126
Recknagel, R.O. [74], 31, 177
Rector, G.H.M. [531], 172
Redlich, O. [99], [100], [101], 40,
    [106], [107], 41
Reed, T.M. [46], 26
Reid, R.C. [56], 26
Reynolds, E.S. [75], 31, 177
Reynolds, T. [485], 158
Richet, C. [7], 17, 18
Richter, G.H. [447], 151
Rider, P.E. [196], 72
Riedl, P. [270], 103, 104
Riess, J.G. [215], 77
Riley, C.M. [342], 117, 118
Rindernecht [556], 181
Risley, E.A. [474], 156
Roark, R.C. [523], [524], 169
Roberts, A.W.R. [4], 17, 169, 170, 171,
    182
Roberts, K. [414], 135
Robinson, B.H. [73], 30
Robinson, D.A. [488], 159, [489], 160,
    [495], 161
Robinson, W.T. [72], 30
Roblin, R.O. [572], 185
Rodrigues, L.V. [533], 172
Rogers, L.A. [156], 55
Rosenfeld, P. [99], [100], 40
Ross, F.J. [312], 109, 111
Ross, M. [185], 65
Rossini, F.D. [222], 84
Roth, S. [400], [401], 132, 133, 155
Roth, S.H. [499], 162
Rothmund, V. [302], 108
Rottenberg, M. [478], 157

Roux, A. [105], 41
Rowlinson, J.S. [182], 67
Royer, G. [494], [496], 161
Ruddle, L.H. [48], 26
Rutzler, J.E. [416], 137
Ryabinin, Yu. N. [155], 55
Rytting, J.H. [253], 97

Salamon, T. [245], 92, 93
Salerno, J.C. [406], 134
Sambrook, J. [519], 167
Sands, D.E. [71], 29
Saram, G.S.W. de, [395], 131
Sather, L.A. [430], 139
Sather, S.O. [484], 157
Sato, A. [544], 177
Satterfield, C.N. [246], 95
Sauberman, A.J. [502], 162
Saunders, M.E. [399], 132
Saylor, J.S. [211], [212], 77, [300],
    107, 115
Scatchard, G. [146], 54, [173], 65
Schaffer, J.M. [376], [377], 126
Schild, H.O. [487], 158
Schill, G. [343], 117
Schleppink, J. [558], 181
Schonhorn, H. [217], 79, 80, 191
Schreiner, H.R. [370], [371], 123
Schroeder, H. [54], [55], 26
Schroeder, W. [561], 181
Schulz, G.V. [256], 101
Schulze, A. [241], 91
Schwert, G.W. [476], 156
Scott, A.F. [122], 44, 46, [135], [136]
    [137], 53, [186], 65, [204], 74,
    [207], 75
Searle, N.E. [554], 180, 181
Seeman, P. [347], 120, [400], [401],
    132, 133, 155
Seidall, A. [415], 137
Seifriz, W. [444], 151
Selbie, F.R. [366], 123
Sendroy, J. [570], 185
Setschenow, J. [278], [279], 104
Settle, W. [458], 152
Shahidi, F. [320], 110
Sharom, F. [397], 131, 132, 155
Sharpe, L.H. [217], 79, 80, 191
Shemisa, C.A. [460], 152
Sherwood, T.K. [56], 26
Shilfrin, S. [480], 152
Shin, C. [319], 110
Shinitzky, M. [472], 155, 156
Shinoda, K. [209], 76
Shiu, W.Y. [28], [29], 19, 21, 143
Shorter, J. [79], 33
Shternov, V.A. [379–385], 126
Shugar, D. [428], 138, 139
Shukla, R.P. [112], 43, 49
Sice, J. [536], 172

Siegel, S.M. [414], 135
Siek, T.J. [430], 139
Silipo, C. [17], 17, 145, 156
Silver, R.F. [238], 91
Simkin, D.J. [83], 34, 96
Singer, J.A. [344], 117, 119
Singh, P.P. [105], 41
Sinirnov, A.V. [497], 161
Skehal, J.J. [520], 167
Slyke, D.D. van, [570], 185
Small, P.A. [174], 65, 66
Smidsnød, O. [512], 164
Smith, B.E. [527–529], 172
Smith, E.B. [199], 72
Smith, E.G. [206], 75, [354], 121
Smith, F. [181], 67
Smith, H.W. [33], [34], 22, 23, [35],
    [36], 90, 95
Smith, R.A. [354], 121
Smith, R.N. [442], 145, [468], [469],
    156
Snegireff, S.L. [422], 127
Snow, J. [9], 17, 18
Snyder, R. [396], 131
Soczewinski, E. [262], [263], 102
Sokolova, T.D. [69], 29, 30
Sorkin, V.A. [160], 56
Spence, A.A. [533], [535], 172
Spicer, L.D. [315], 110
Spink, C.H. [280], 105, 107, 108
Squire, D.R. [293], 106
Steele, R. [510], 164
Stefan, J. [144], 54
Stern, L. [404], 134–136, 153
Steward, A.R. [441], 145
Stocker, H. [118], 45–46, 49
Streich, M. [440], 145
Stull, D.R. [522], 169
Sturtevant, J.M. [477], 156
Suckling, C.W. [8], 17, 18
Sugden, S. [57], [58], [59], 9, 57–59

Taft, R.W. [80], 33
Taha, A.S. [314], 110
Tait, P.G. [285–290], 105
Takenaka, N. [234], 90
Tam, D. [28], 19–21, 143
Tammann, G. [271–273], [277], 104,
    [292], 106
Tanford, C. [324], 113
Tang, [471], 155, 156
Tappel, A.L. [463], 152
Tardajos, G. [164], 59, 60
Tattersfield, F. [4], 17, 127, 169–171,
    182, [390], 126
Taylor, L.D. [514], 164, 165
Taylor, R.P. [197], 72
Thacker, R. [182], 67
Thackray, A.C. [366], 123
Thimann, K.W. [484], 157

Thin, [307], 109
Thomas, W.G. [121], 44, 46
Thomson, D.W. [437], 142
Tilley, F.W. [376], [377], 126
Timmermanns, J. [68], 29, [177], 67, 68, 190, 192
Todd, A.R. [77], 31
Tomkins, G.M. [459], 152
Tomlinson, E. [342], 117, 118
Tonkin, W.H. [524], 169
Toon, P.A. [505], 162
Torchilin, V.P. [497], [498], 161
Traube, J. [86–92], 36–39, [97], 40, 41
Trouton, F.T. [200], 73
Turner, N.J. [261], 102

Ueda, I. [453], 152
Uitert, C.E. van, [315], 110
Uitert, J. van, [315], 110
Urry, W.D. [125], 47, 48, 50
Usni, I. [317], 110, 138

Valvani, S.C. [252], 97
Vanderkooi, G. [409], 134, 136, [504], 162
Vernon, H.M. [578], 194–197, 212
Vineyard, B.D. [558], 181
Vogel, A.I. [62], 27
Volpenheim, R.A. [464], 153–155
Volquartz, K. [301], 107
Voro'beva, A.I. [250], 97, 99
Vrij, A. [39], 24

Waals, J.D. vander, [138], 53
Wachmeister, C.A. [262], 102
Walden, P. [338], 115, 116
Walkley, J. [199], 72, [206], 75
Wallace, R.A. [490], 161
Ward, G.K. [318], 110
Ward, J.L. [556], 181
Wardley-Smith, B. [456], 152
Warren, [505], 162
Washburn, E.W. [113], 44, 46, 49
Waterfield, M. [520], 167
Watson, J.M. [541], 173
Watson, K.M. [170], 64
Weale, K.E. [159], 56
Weare, J.H. [311], 109, 111
Weast, R.C. [134], 50
Webb, E.C. [457], 152

Weber, D.E. [180], 67
Weeks, J.C. [162], 57
Wertz, D.H. [327], 113
Westfall, R.G. [259], 102
Westfall, S. [495], 161
Westrum, E.F. [576], 192
Whalley, E. [95], 39
Whatmough, W.H. [119], 45
White, D.C. [454], [456], 152
Whitten, A.I. [300], 107, 115
Wilcock, R.J. [214], 77
Wildnauer, R. [496], 161
Wilhelm, E. [214], 77
Willard, H.H. [308], 109
Williams, R.J. [388], 126
Willmott, F.W. [269], 103
Wilson, R.W. [122], 44, 46
Winter, D.B. [406], [407], 134
Winzor, D.J. [455], 152
Wirtz, G.H. [495], 161
Witlin, B. [375], 126
Witz, G. [537], 172
Wold, S. [232], 89
Woodhouse, D.L. [420], 126
Woodward, G.J. [388], 126
Woolley, D.W. [571–574], 185
Wooley, E.M. [105], 41
Wouters-Leysen, J. [481], 157
Wowern, J. von, [379], 126
Wunnenberg, E. [37], 25
Wyman, J. [130], 49, 50

Yalkowsky, S.H. [252], 97
Yamamoto, Y. [337], 115, 116, 142
Yasuda-Yasaki, Y. [368], 123, 155
Yasunga, T. [317], [427], 110, 138
Yeager, E. [104], 41
Yeger, B.J. [81], 34
Yielding, I.L. [459], 152
Yola, M. [481], 157
Yoshimoto, M. [470], 156
Yu, C.A. [406], 134
Yu, L. [406], 134

Zalkin, A. [71], 29
Zana, R. [104], 41
Zawidski, J.V. [240], 91
Zerbon, F.W. [133], 50, 51
Zienty, F.B. [558], 181